Oxford American Handbook of
Clinical
Examination
and
Practical Skills

About the Oxford American Handbooks in Medicine

The Oxford American Handbooks are pocket clinical books, providing practical guidance in quick reference, note form. Titles cover major medical specialties or cross-specialty topics and are aimed at students, residents, internists, family physicians, and practicing physicians within specific disciplines.

Their reputation is built on including the best clinical information, complemented by hints, tips, and advice from the authors. Each one is carefully reviewed by senior subject experts, residents, and students to ensure that content reflects the reality of day-to-day medical practice.

Key series features

- Written in short chunks, each topic is covered in a two-page spread to enable readers to find information quickly. They are also perfect for test preparation and gaining a quick overview of a subject without scanning through unnecessary pages.
- Content is evidence based and complemented by the expertise and judgment of experienced authors.
- The Handbooks provide a humanistic approach to medicine—it's more than just treatment by numbers.
- A "friend in your pocket," the Handbooks offer honest, reliable guidance about the difficulties of practicing medicine and provide coverage of both the practice and art of medicine.
- For quick reference, useful "everyday" information is included on the inside covers.

Published and Forthcoming Oxford American Handbooks

Oxford American Handbook of Clinical Medicine
Oxford American Handbook of Anesthesiology
Oxford American Handbook of Cardiology
Oxford American Handbook of Clinical Dentistry
Oxford American Handbook of Clinical Diagnosis
Oxford American Handbook of Clinical Examination and Practical Skills
Oxford American Handbook of Clinical Pharmacy
Oxford American Handbook of Critical Care
Oxford American Handbook of Emergency Medicine
Oxford American Handbook of Gastroenterology and Hepatology
Oxford American Handbook of Geriatric Medicine
Oxford American Handbook of Nephrology and Hypertension
Oxford American Handbook of Neurology
Oxford American Handbook of Obstetrics and Gynecology
Oxford American Handbook of Oncology
Oxford American Handbook of Ophthalmology
Oxford American Handbook of Otolaryngology
Oxford American Handbook of Pediatrics
Oxford American Handbook of Physical Medicine and Rehabilitation
Oxford American Handbook of Psychiatry
Oxford American Handbook of Pulmonary Medicine
Oxford American Handbook of Rheumatology
Oxford American Handbook of Sports Medicine
Oxford American Handbook of Surgery
Oxford American Handbook of Urology

Oxford American Handbook of
Clinical Examination and Practical Skills

Elizabeth A. Burns, MD, MA

Professor of Family Medicine
President and CEO
Michigan State University
Kalamazoo Center for Medical Studies
Kalamazoo, Michigan

Kenneth Korn, PA-C, ARNP

Adjunct Faculty, Physician Assistant Program
University of North Dakota
Grand Forks, North Dakota

and

Family Nurse Practitioner
Leon County Health Department
Florida Department of Health
Tallahassee, Florida

James Whyte, IV, ND, ARNP

Associate Professor
College of Nursing
Florida State University
Tallahassee, Florida

with

James Thomas

Tanya Monaghan

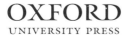

OXFORD
UNIVERSITY PRESS

OXFORD
UNIVERSITY PRESS

Oxford University Press, Inc. publishes works that further
Oxford University's objective of excellence
in research, scholarship and education.

Oxford New York

Auckland Cape Town Dar es Salaam Hong Kong Karachi
Kuala Lumpur Madrid Melbourne Mexico City Nairobi
New Delhi Shanghai Taipei Toronto

With offices in

Argentina Austria Brazil Chile Czech Republic France Greece
Guatemala Hungary Italy Japan Poland Portugal
Singapore South Korea Switzerland Thailand Turkey Ukraine Vietnam

Published by Oxford University Press Inc.
198 Madison Avenue, New York, New York 10016

www.oup.com

Oxford is a registered trademark of Oxford University Press.

First published 2011
UK version 2007

Library of Congress Cataloging-in-Publication Data

Oxford American handbook of clinical examination and practical skills / edited by
Elizabeth A. Burns, Kenneth Korn, James Whyte IV ; with James Thomas, Tanya
Monaghan.
p. ; cm.
Other title: Handbook of clinical examination and practical skills
Includes index.
ISBN 978-0-19-538972-2
1. Physical diagnosis—Handbooks, manuals, etc. I. Burns, Elizabeth A. (Elizabeth
Ann), 1950– II. Korn, Kenneth. III. Whyte, James, IV. IV. Title: Handbook of
clinical examination and practical skills.
[DNLM: 1. Clinical Medicine—methods—Handbooks. 2. Physical
Examination—Handbooks. WB 39]
RC76.O937 2011
616.07′54—dc22
2010027995

10 9 8 7 6 5 4 3 2 1

Printed in China
on acid-free paper through
Asia Pacific Offset

Preface (U.S.)

Although we would like to claim the idea for this text as our own, this is not the case; however, the belief in the text's adaptability for U.S. medical providers is. The first edition of this text was developed for use in the U.K., where a different model of health care exists.

In the United States, the primary care provider role was once the exclusive responsibility of the traditional, medical school–educated MD or DO. Primary care is no longer the realm of only one type of health-care provider. No longer is it the duty of only the physician to assess and care for the patient. Now, collaborative and collegial relationships exist among various disciplines. Cooperative-care models seek to provide optimal care. It is from this type of model that the U.S. authors elected to remove the term doctor from most areas of this text in preference to the term *health-care provider*.

Representing the varied disciplines now likely to serve as primary care providers, the U.S. team of authors illustrates the changing face of U.S. health care. The authors represent educators and practitioners from traditional allopathic medicine, nurse practitioner, and physician assistant disciplines.

This text is not offered as the quintessential text on physical examination; it is presented, as the title states, as a handbook of physical examination and practical skills. We also believe that as U.S. health care evolves, so will this text, with requisite changes and adaptations.

In this text, the important elements that will not change are those that comprise an appropriate exam and quality care. No matter which discipline the provider represents, quality is critical.

Elizabeth Burns, MD
Kenneth Korn, PA-C, ARNP
James White, ARNP
2010

* Out of great respect for the work of James Thomas and Tanya Monaghan, the U.S. authors chose to leave the following Preface and Acknowledgments by the U.K. authors unchanged.

Preface (U.K.)

There are very few people who, in the course of their daily work, can approach a stranger, ask them to remove their clothes, and touch their bodies without fear of admonition. This unique position of doctors, medical students, and other health care professionals comes with many strings attached. We are expected to act "professionally"and be competent and confident in all our dealings. This is hard to teach and hard to learn and many students are rightly daunted by the new position in which they find themselves.

We felt a little let down by many books during our time in medical school, and often found ourselves having to dip into several texts to appreciate a topic. This book, then, is the one text that we would have wanted as students covering all the main medical and surgical subspecialties. We anticipate it will be useful to students as they make the transition to being a doctor and also to junior doctors. We hope that it will be carried in coat pockets for quick glances as well as being suitable for study at home or in the library.

The first three chapters cover the basics of communication skills, history taking, and general physical examination. Chapters 4–14 are divided by systems. In each of these there is a section on the common symptoms seen in that system, with the appropriate questions to ask the patient, details of how to examine parts of that system, and important patterns of disease presentation. Each of these system chapters is finished off with an "elderly patient"page provided by Dr. Richard Fuller. Following the systems, there are chapters on paediatric and psychiatric patients—something not found in many other books of this kind. The penultimate chapter—practical procedures—details all those tasks that junior doctors might be expected to perform. Finally, there is an extensive data interpretation chapter which, while not exhaustive, tries to cover those topics such as ECG, ABG, and X-ray interpretation that may appear in a final OSCE examination.

Although we have consulted experts on the contents of each chapter, any mistakes or omissions remain ours alone. We welcome any comments and suggestions for improvement from our reader—this book, after all, is for you.

James Thomas
Tanya Monaghan
2007

Acknowledgments (U.S.)

The U.S. authors acknowledge the great work of the U.K. team in the development of a unique text. The combination of examination, procedures, and data interpretation into a single handbook-sized resource represents a new type of resource. It is recognized that this text is a resource with the potential for substantial enhancement. Your comments are welcome.

We would also like to thank Oxford University Press (U.S.) for the opportunity to be involved in this adaptation of this text, with special thanks to Andrea Seils and Staci Hou for their patience and assistance during this process.

Colleagues providing specialty review of the Americanization of the U.K. data and procedures also deserve special thanks.

As always, such projects represent time away from other responsibilities. We acknowledge and appreciate our co-workers and family for giving us the time to complete this project.

Finally, one last thank-you goes to the fine U.K. authors for those moments of humor while reviewing their text for "Britishisms."

Acknowledgments (U.K.)

We would like to record our thanks to the very many people who have given their advice and support through this project.

For contributing specialist portions of the book, we thank Dr. Tom Fearnley (pages relating to ophthalmology), Dr. Caroline Boyes (Chapter 16, The paediatric assessment) and Dr. Bruno Rushforth (ECG interpretation and other parts of Chapter 18). We also thank Heidi Ridsdale, senior physiotherapist at Leeds General Infirmary, for her help with the oxygen/airway pages and for providing all the equipment for the photographs. Dr. Franco Guarasci and Jeremy Robson read the NIV and inhaler pages, respectively, for which we are very grateful. We thank Senior Sister Lyn Dean of Ward 26 at the Leeds General Infirmary for reading parts of Chapter 17 (Practical procedures). Our thanks also go to Dr. Jonathan Bodansky, Mandy Garforth, and Mike Geall for providing the retinal photographs.

An extra special word of thanks is reserved for our models Adam Swallow, Geoffrey McConnell, and our female model who would like to remain anonymous. Their bravery and good humour made a potentially difficult few days very easy. They were a joy to work with. We thank the staff at the St James's University Hospital Medical Illustration Studio, in particular Tim Vernon, for taking the photographs.

We would also like to thank the staff at Oxford University Press, especially Catherine Barnes, for having faith in us to take this project on, and Elizabeth Reeve, for her seemingly endless patience, support, and guidance.

A special word of thanks is reserved for our official "friend of the book," Dr. Richard Fuller, who provided all the "elderly patient" pages. Aside from this, his steadfast and overtly biased support helped carry us through.

Finally, we would like to thank our good friend Dr. Paul Johns. He read through much of the text and provided invaluable advice and support from the very beginning. We wish Paul the very best with his own writing projects and hope to work with him in the future.

Our panel of readers was responsible for confirming the medical accuracy of the text. Most have performed far beyond our expectations, we are eternally grateful to them all.

Contents

How to use this book

The systems chapters

In each chapter, there are suggestions of what questions to ask and how to proceed depending on the nature of the presenting complaint. These are not exhaustive and are intended as guidance.

The history parts of the systems chapters should be used in conjunction with Chapter 2 in order to build a full and thorough history.

Practical procedures

This chapter (Chapter 18) describes those practical procedures that the health-care provider, whether a physician, physician assistant, nurse practitioner, or member of another health-care discipline, may be expected to perform. Some procedures should only be performed once you have been trained specifically in the correct technique by an experienced professional.

Each procedure has a difficulty icon as follows:

⚠ Requires no specific training, and all primary-care provider graduates should be competent to perform this procedure.

▶ Requires some skill. Providers with moderate experience should be able to perform this procedure with ease.

▶▶ More complex procedures that you may only come across in specialty practices and will not be required to perform without advanced training and experience.

Reality vs. theory

In describing the practical procedures, we have tried to be realistic. The methods described are the most commonly ones used across the profession and are aimed at helping the reader perform the procedure correctly and safely within a clinical environment.

There may be differences between the way a number of the procedures are described here and the way in which they are taught in a clinical skills laboratory. In addition, local hospitals and clinics may use different equipment for some procedures. Good practitioners should be flexible and make changes to their routine accordingly.

Data interpretation

A minority of the reference ranges described for some of the biochemical tests in the data interpretation chapter (Chapter 19) may differ slightly from those used by your local laboratory—this depends on the equipment and techniques used for measurement. Any differences are likely to be very small. Always check with, and be guided by, your local resources.

Detailed contents

Symbols and abbreviations

↑	increased
↓	decreased
↔	normal
~	approximately
📖	cross-reference
❗	warning
▶	important
ABC	airway, breathing, circulation
ABG	arterial blood gases
AC	acromioclavicular
ACE	angiotensin-converting enzyme
ACL	anterior cruciate ligament
ACLS	advanced cardiac life support
ACSM	American College of Sports Medicine
ACTH	adrenocorticotrophic hormone
AD	Alzheimer's disease
ADH	antidiuretic hormone
ADL	activities of daily living
ADP	adenosine diphosphate
AED	automated external defibrillator
AF	atrial fibrillation
AHA	American Heart Association
AITFL	antero-inferior tibio-fibular ligament
AMTS	Abbreviated Mental test Score
ANCOVA	analysis of covariance
ANOVA	analysis of variance
AP	anteroposterior
APH	antepartum hemorrhage
APL	antiphospholipid
ASD	atrial septal defect
ASL	American Sign Language
ATFL	anterior talofibular ligament
ATLS	advanced trauma life support
ATP	adenosine triphosphate

AV	atrioventricular
AVN	avascular necrosis
AVPU	Alert, Voice, Pain, Unresponsive (scale)
AXR	abdominal X-ray
BCC	basal cell carcinoma
BCG	bacillus Calmette-Guérin
bid	twice daily
BiPAP	bilevel positional vertigo
BMD	bone mineral density
BMI	body mass index
BMR	basal metabolic rate
BP	blood pressure
BPH	benign prostatic hyperplasia
bpm	beats per minute
BPV	benign positional vertigo
C	cervical
CABG	coronary artery bypass graft
CBC	complete blood count
CBRNE	chemical, biological, radiological, nuclear, & explosive
CC	chief complaint
CDC	Centers for Disease Control and Prevention
CEA	carcinoembryogenic antigen
CF	cystic fibrosis
CFS	chronic fatigue syndrome
CHD	coronary heart disease
CHF	congestive heart failure
CHO	carbohydrate
CIN	cervical intraepithelial neoplasm
CK	creatine kinase
CN	cranial nerve
CNS	central nervous system
COPD	chronic obstructive pulmonary disease
CP	cerebral palsy
CPAP	continuous positive airways pressure
CPK	creatine phosphokinase
CPR	cardiopulmonary resuscitation
CRF	corticotropin-releasing factor
CRP	C-reactive protein
CSF	cerebrospinal fluid
CT	computerized tomography

CTD	connective tissue disease
CVA	cerebrovascular accident
CVP	central venous pressure
CXR	chest X-ray
DEXA	dual-energy X-ray absorptiometry
DIP	distal interphalangeal
DKA	diabetic ketoacidosis
DM	diabetes mellitus
DO	detrussor overactivity
DOB	date of birth
DUB	dysfunctional uterine bleeding
DVT	deep venous thrombosis
EBP	epidural blood patch
ECG	electrocardiogram
ECRB	extensor carpi radialis brevis
ECRL	extensor carpi radialis longus
ECU	extensor carpi ulnaris
EDD	estimated date of delivery
EIA	exercise-induced asthma
EIB	exercise-induced bronchospasm
EJV	external jugular vein
EMG	electromyography
EMR	electronic medical record
ENMG	electoneuromyography
EPAP	expiration positive airways pressure
EPB	extensor polaris brevis
EPO	erythropoetin
ESR	erythrocyte sedimentation rate
ET	endotracheal
FCU	flexor carpi ulnaris
FDS	flexor digitorum superficialis
$FeCO_2$	expired air carbon dioxide concentration
FeO_2	expired air oxygen concentration
FEV_1	forced expiratory volume in 1 second
FH	family history
FHR	fetal heart rate
FMLA	Family Medical Leave Act
FPL	flexor policis longus
FRC	functional residual capacity
FSH	follicle-stimulating hormone

FVC	forced vital capacity
G	gauge
GALS	gait, arms, legs, spine
GBS	Guillain–Barré syndrome
GCS	Glasgow Coma Scale
GEJ	gastroesophageal junction
GERD	gastroesophageal reflux disease
GFR	glomerular filtration rate
GH	growth hormone
GI	gastrointestinal
GnRH	gonadotrophin-releasing hormone
hCG	human chorionic gonadotrophin
Hct	hematocrit
Hgb	hemoglobin
HDL	high-density lipoprotein
HIPAA	Health Insurance Portability & Accountability Act
HPI	history of present illness
HPV	human papillomavirus
HR	heart rate
HRT	hormone replacement therapy
HT	hormone therapy
HZV	herpes zoster virus
Hct	hematocrit
IA	intra-arterial
IBD	inflammatory bowel disease
IBS	irritable bowel syndrome
ICP	intracranial pressure
ICU	intensive care unit
ID	intradermal
IGF-1	insulin-like growth factor 1
IHD	ischemic heart disease
IHS	Indian Health Service
IHSS	idiopathic hypertrophic subaortic stenosis
IIH	idiopathic intracranial hypertension
IJV	internal jugular vein
ILI	influenza-like illness
IM	intramuscular
IMB	intermenstrual bleeding
IOC	International Olympic Committee
IPAP	inspiration positive airways pressure

IRMA	intraretinal microvascular abnormalities
ITB	ilio-tibial band
ITBS	ilio-tibial band syndrome
IUD	intrauterine device
IV	intravenous
IVP	intravenous pyelogram
JVP	jugular venous pressure
L	lumbar
LBBB	left bundle branch block
LBC	liquid-based cytology
LDH	lactate dehydrogenase
LDL	low-density lipoprotein
LEP	Limited English Proficiency
LFT	liver function test
LH	luetinizing hormone
LMA	laryngeal mask airway
LMN	lower motor neuron
LMP	last menstrual period
LP	lumbar puncture
LOC	loss of consciousness
LSB	left sternal border
LSE	left sternal edge
LV	left ventricle
LVH	left ventricular hypertrophy
MALT	mucosa-associated lymphoid tissue
MANOVA	multivariate analysis of the variance
MCL	medial collateral ligament
MCP	metacarpophalangeal
MC&S	microscopy, culture, and sensitivity
MDI	metered-dose inhaler
MI	myocardial infarction
MLF	medial longitudinal fasciculus
MMSE	Mini-Mental State Examination
MND	motor neuron disease
MPHR	maximum predicted heart rate
MRI	magnetic resonance imaging
MRSA	methicillin-resistant *Staphylococcus aureus*
MS	multiple sclerosis
MSH	melanocyte-stimulating hormone
MTP	metatarsophalangeal

MVA	motor vehicle accident
NG	nasogastric
NIV	noninvasive ventilation
NSAID	nonsteroidal anti-inflammatory drug
NYHA	New York Heart Association
OA	osteoarthritis
OCD	obsessive-compulsive disorder
OCP	oral contraceptive pill
OSHA	Occupational Safety & Health Administration
ORIF	open reduction and internal fixation
OTC	over the counter
PA	posterior–anterior
PCL	posterior cruciate ligament
PCOS	polycystic ovarian syndrome
PCP	primary care provider
PCR	polymerase chain reaction
PCS	post-concussion syndrome
PDA	patent ductus arteriosis
PE	pulmonary embolism
PFJ	patello-femoral
PID	pelvic inflammatory disease
PIP	proximal interphalangeal
PMH	past medical history
PMI	point of maximum impulse
PND	paroxysmal nocturnal dyspnea
PP	patient profile
PPH	postpartum hemorrhage
PPRF	parapontine reticular formation
PSIS	posterior superior iliac crest
PSYM	parasympathetic
PTFL	posterior talofibular ligament
PTH	parathyroid hormone
Q	cardiac output
q4h	every 4 hours
qid	4 times a day (quarter in die)
RAPD	relative afferent pupil defect
RBC	red blood count or cell
RICE	rest, ice, compression, elevation
ROM	range of motion
ROS	review of systems

RR	respiratory rate
RSE	right sternal edge
RV	residual volume; right ventricule
SA	sinoatrial
SAAG	serum/ascites albumin gradient
SANE	sexual assault nurse examiner
SAH	subarachnoid hemorrhage
SaO_2	oxygen saturation
SC	subcutaneous
SCC	squamous cell carcinoma
SH	social history
SI	stress incontinence
SIJ	sacroiliac joint
SLAP	superior labrum anterior to posterior
SLE	systemic lupus erythematosus
SLR	straight leg raise
SOB	shortness of breath
SPECT	single photon emission computer tomography
STD	sexually transmitted disease
STI	sexually transmitted infection
SQJ	squamo-columnar junction
SV	stroke volume
SVC	superior vena cava
SVT	sustained ventricular tachycardia
T	thoracic
T_3	triiodothyronine
T_4	thyroxine
TB	tuberculosis
TBG	thyroid-binding globulin
TBI	traumatic brain injury
TGA	transposition of the great arteries
TIA	transient ischemic attack
tid	three times daily
TPN	total parenteral nutrition
TSH	thyroid-stimulating hormone
TURP	transurethral resection of the prostate
UAP	unlicensed assistive personnel
UMN	upper motor neuron
UC	ulcerative colitis
UCL	ulnar collateral ligament

URI	upper respiratory infection
US	ultrasound
UTI	urinary tract infection
UV	ultraviolet
VEGF	vascular endothelial-derived growth factor
VF	ventricular fibrillation
VIN	vulval intraepithelial neoplasm
VIP	vasoactive intestinal polypeptide
VO_2	oxygen uptake
VRSA	vancomycin-resistant *Staphylococcus aureus*
VSD	ventricular septal defect
VT	ventricular tachycardia
WBC	white blood count
WHO	World Health Organization
WPW	Wolff–Parkinson–White (syndrome)

Important Notes

🄘 Write legibly on orders, or print or enter orders via computer.

🄘 Date, time, and sign all patient care orders.

🄘 Remember, all facilities should have an approved abbreviations list—follow it.

🄘 The official "Do Not Use" list of abbreviations is available at the Joint Commission Web site at: http://www.jointcommission.org.

Communication Skills

Introduction

Communication skills are notoriously hard to teach and describe. There are too many possible situations that you might encounter to be able to draw rules or guidelines. In addition, your actions will depend greatly on the personalities present—not least of which your own!

Using this chapter

Over the following pages, we present some general advice about communicating in different situations and to different people. We have not provided rules to stick to but rather have tried to give the reader an appreciation of the many ways in which the same situation may be tackled.

Ultimately, skill at communication comes from practice, self-knowledge and reflection, and a large amount of common sense.

Quite a bit has been written about communication skills in medicine and the health sciences. Most articles suggest a mix of accepted protocols and traditional approaches—this chapter is no different.

> The rule is: there are no rules.

Communication models

There are many models of the practitioner–patient encounter that have been discussed over the years at great length. These models are for the hardened student of communication. We mention them here so that the reader is aware of their existence.

Patient-centered communication

In recent years, there has been a significant change in the way health-care workers interact with patients. The biomedical model has fallen out of favor and instead, an appreciation has evolved that the patient has a unique experience of the illness. This experience involves the social, psychological, and behavioral effects of the disease. Some authors refer to this approach as the *biopsychosocial* model, which focuses on the patient in a more encompassing way.

The biomedical model
- The provider is in charge of the consultation and examination.
- Focus is on disease management.

The patient-centered model
- Power and decision-making are shared.
- Address and treat the whole patient.

Box 1.1 Key points in the patient-centered model

- Explore the disease and the patient's experience of it:
  - Understand the patient's ideas and feelings about the illness.
  - Appreciate the illness's impact on the patient's quality of life and psychosocial well-being.
  - Understand the patient's expectations of the encounter.
- Understand the whole person:
  - Family
  - Social and work environment
  - Beliefs
- Find common ground on disease management.
- Establish the doctor–patient relationship.
- Be realistic:
  - Priorities for treatment
  - Resources

Box 1.2 Confidentiality

As a doctor, health-care provider, or student, you are party to personal and confidential information. While Health Insurance Portability and Accountability Act (HIPAA) regulations must be followed, there are also times when confidentiality must or should be broken (📖 p. 26). The essence of day-to-day practice is:

Never tell anyone about a patient unless it is directly related to his or her care and you have permission.

This includes relatives, which can be very difficult at times, particularly if a relative asks you directly about something confidential.

You can reinforce the importance of confidentiality to relatives and visitors. If asked by a relative to speak about a patient, it is a good idea to approach the patient first and ask their permission, within full view of the relative. You can also seek permission from the patient in anticipation of such queries.

This rule also applies to friends outside of medicine. As care providers, we come across many amazing, bizarre, amusing, or uplifting stories on a day-to-day basis, but like any other kind of information, these should not be shared with anyone.

If you do intend to use an anecdote in public, at the very least you should ensure that there is nothing in your story that could possibly lead to the identification of the person involved. If you are in a small community, it is best to avoid sharing anything, lest you undermine your reputation as a professional.

Essential considerations

Attitudes
Patients are entrusting their health and personal information to you—they want someone who is confident, approachable, competent, and, above all, trustworthy.

Personal appearance
First impressions count—and studies have consistently shown that your appearance (clothes, hair, makeup) has a great impact on patients' opinion of you and their willingness to interact with you. Part of that intangible professionalism comes from your image.

The white coat is still part of medical culture for students and most providers. Fashions in clothing change rapidly, but some basic rules still apply:
- Neutralize any extreme tastes in fashion that you may have.
- Men and women should wear appropriate professional attire.
- Women may wear skirts or slacks but the length of the skirts should not raise any eyebrows.
- Necklines should not be revealing—no décolletage!
- The belly should be covered—no bare midriffs!
- The shoulders, likewise, should be covered.
- Shoes should be polished and clean.
- *Clean* surgical scrubs may be worn, if appropriate.
- Hair should be relatively conservatively styled and no hair should be over the face. Wear long hair tied up.
- Your name badge should be clearly visible, even if you don't like your picture.
- Stethoscopes are best carried or held in a coat pocket—worn at the neck is acceptable but a little pretentious, according to some views.
  - Try not to tuck items in your belt—use pockets or belt-holders for cell phones, keys, and wallets.

▶ Psychiatry, pediatrics, and a handful of other specialties require a different dress code, as they deal with patients who require differing techniques for bonding with the health-care professional.

Timing
If in a hospital setting, make sure that your discussion with a patient is not during an allocated quiet time or disturbing to the patient's roommate. You should also avoid mealtimes or when the patient's long-lost relative has just come to visit.

▶ If you plan to move the patient from the bed to an exam room, ask the supervising doctor (if not you) and the nursing staff, and let all concerned know where you have gone in case the patient is needed.

Setting
Students, doctors, and other medical providers tend to see patients on hospital floors filled with distractions that can break up the interaction.

Often such meetings are necessary during the course of the day. However, if you need to discuss an important matter that requires concentration from both of you, consider the following conditions:

- The room should be quiet, private, and free from disturbances.
- There should be enough seating for everyone.
- Chairs should be comfortable enough for an extended conversation.
- Arrange the seats close to yours, with no intervening tables or other furniture.

Box 1.3 Becoming a good communicator

Learning

As in all aspects of medicine, learning is a lifelong process. One part of this process, particularly for acquiring communication skills and at the beginning of your career, is **watching others**.

You should take every opportunity to observe provider–patient interactions.

▶ You should ask to be present during difficult conversations.

Instead of glazing over during clinic visits or on rounds, you should watch the interaction and consider if the behaviors you see are worth emulating or avoiding. Consider how you might adjust your future behavior.

Select the actions and words you like and use them as your own, building up your own repertoire of communication techniques.

Spontaneity vs. learned behaviors

When you watch a good communicator, you will see them making friendly conversation and spontaneous jokes, and using words and phrases that put people at ease. The conversation seems natural, relaxed, and spontaneous. Watching that same person interact with someone else can shatter the illusion as you see them using the same "spontaneous" jokes and other gambits from their repertoire.

This is one of the keys to good communication—an ability to judge the situation and pull the appropriate phrase, word, or action from your internal catalogue. If done well, it leads to a smooth interaction with no hesitations or misunderstandings. The additional advantage is that your mental processes are free to consider the next move, mull over what has been said, or assess findings, while externally you are partially on autopilot, following a familiar pattern of interaction.

During physical examination this ability is particularly relevant. You should be able to coax the wanted actions from the patient and put them at ease while considering findings and your next step.

It must be stressed, however, that this is *not* the same as lacking concentration—quite the opposite.

Essential rules

Avoid medical jargon

Medical personnel are so immersed in jargon that it becomes part of their daily speech. The patient may not understand the words or may have a different idea of their meaning.

Technical words such as *myocardial infarction* are in obvious need of avoidance or explanation. Consider also terms such as *exacerbate*, *chronic*, *numb*, and *sputum*—these may seem obvious in meaning to you but not to the patient.

You may think that some terms such as *angina* and *migraine* are so well known that they don't need explanation, but these are very often misinterpreted. Some examples of such words are given in Table 1.1.

Remember names

Forgetting someone's name is what we all fear; it is relatively easy to disguise by simple avoidance. However, using the patient's name will make you appear to be taking a greater interest in them. It is particularly important that you remember the patient's name when talking to family members. Getting the name wrong is embarrassing and can seriously undermine their confidence in you.

Aside from actually remembering the name, it is a good idea to have it written down and within sight—on a piece of paper in your hand, on the chart, or on the desk. It is a best practice to confirm the identity of the patient, using two identifiers (name, date of birth [DOB]), before you read results from the chart or electronic medical record (EMR). To be seen glancing at the name is forgivable; patients would rather have you double check than bluff your way through an interview.

Table 1.1 Some examples of differing interpretations of medical terms

Word	Your meaning	Patient's understanding
Acute	Rapid onset	Very bad, severe
Chronic	Long duration	Very bad, severe
Sick	Nauseated, vomiting	Unwell
Angina	Chest pain associated with ischemic heart disease	Heart attack, shortness of breath, palpitations
Migraine	Specific headache disorder	Any severe headache
Numb	Without sensation	Weak

Getting started

The start of an encounter is important but is fraught with potential difficulties. Like everything else in this chapter, there are no hard-and-fast rules. Issues you should take into consideration include the following:
- Are you using a language the patient can understand?
- Can the patient hear you?

Greeting

Beware of saying "good afternoon" or "good morning." These greetings can be inappropriate if you are about to break some bad news or if there is another reason for distress. Consider instead using a simple "hello."

Shaking hands

A traditional greeting, shaking hands will be readily accepted by most patients, but it can also present challenges (think of patients with severe arthritis of the hands). While physical contact always seems friendly and can warm a person to you, a handshake may be seen as overly formal by some and inappropriate by others. Consider using some other form of touch, such as a slight guiding hand on the patient's arm as they enter the room or a brief touch to the forearm. (See also 📖 p. 21.)

Introductions

This is a minefield! You may wish to alter your greeting depending on the circumstances—choose terms that suit *you*.

Title—patient

Older patients may prefer to be called "Mr." or "Mrs."; younger patients would find this odd. For female patients whose marital status you don't know, you can try using "Ms.," although some younger or married patients may find this term offensive.

Calling the patient by their first name may be considered too informal by some patients. A change to using the family name mid-way through the encounter may appear unfriendly or could indicate that something has gone wrong with the interaction.

There are no rules here; use common sense to judge the situation at the time. When unsure, the best option is always to ask.

> "Is it Mrs. or Miss Smith?" "How would you like to be addressed?"

Title—you

The title *doctor* has always been a status symbol and a badge of authority—within the health-care professions at least. Young doctors may be reluctant to part with the title so soon after acquiring it, but these days, when office visits are becoming two-way conversations between equals, patients may expect equity in the way they are addressed.

Many patients will simply call you "doctor" and the matter doesn't arise. We prefer using formality initially, then using first names if circumstances seem appropriate. Some elderly patients prefer—and expect—a certain level of formality, so each situation has to be judged.

Mid-level providers should follow the conventions of the health-care setting they are in. Formality is appropriate in many settings; however, most mid-level providers are more comfortable using first names.

Standing

Although this might be considered old-fashioned by some younger people, standing is a universal mark of respect. You should stand when a patient enters a room and take your seat at the same time as them. You should also stand as they leave, but if you have established a good rapport during the visit, this isn't absolutely necessary.

You may notice that patients stand when you enter the exam room. Put them at ease and acknowledge this gesture as well.

General principles

Demeanor
Give the patient your full attention. Appear encouraging with a warm, open manner. Use appropriate facial expressions—don't look bored!

Define your role
Along with the standard introductions, you should always make it clear who you are and what your role is. You might also wish to introduce your team members, if appropriate. In this era, when patients see so many health-care providers during the course of a hospitalization, it is helpful to write the team names down for them.

Style of questioning

Open questions vs. closed questions
Open questions are those for which any answer is possible:

> "What's the problem?"
> "How does it feel?"

These enable patients to give you the true answer in their own words. Be careful not to lead the patient or cut them off with closed questions.

Compare "How much does it hurt?" with "Does it hurt a lot?" The first question allows the patient to tell you how the pain feels on a wide spectrum of severity; the second one leaves the patient only two options and will not give a true reflection of the severity.

Multiple-choice questions
Often, patients have difficulty with an open question if they are not quite sure what you mean. A question about the character of pain, for example, is rather hard to formulate, and patients will often not know what you mean ("What sort of pain is it"; "What does it feel like, exactly?").

In these circumstances, you may wish to give them a few examples, but leave the list open-ended for them to add their own words. You must be very careful *not* to give the answer that you are expecting from them. For example, a patient whom you suspect has angina ("crushing" pain) you could ask the following:

> "What sort of a pain is it—burning, stabbing, or aching, for example?"

Clarifying questions
Use clarifying questions to get the full details:

> "When you say 'dizzy', what exactly do you mean?"

Reflective comments

Use reflective comments to encourage patients to continue and reassure them that you are following the story:

> "Yes, I see that."

Staying on topic

You should be directive but polite when keeping patients on the topic you want or moving them on to a new topic. Don't be afraid to interrupt them—some patients will talk for hours if you let them!

> "Before we move on to that, I would just like to get all the details of this dizziness."
> "We'll come to that in a moment."

Difficult questions

Recognize potentially offensive or embarrassing questions. Explain why it is necessary to ask these questions, to put the patient more at ease.

> "This may be an uncomfortable question, but I need to know…"

Eye contact

▶ Make eye contact and look at the patient when he or she is speaking.

Make a note of eye contact next time you are in conversation with a friend or colleague.

In normal conversations, the speaker usually looks away while the listener looks directly at the speaker. The roles then change when the other person starts talking, and so on.

In the medical situation, while the patient is speaking, you may be tempted to make notes, read the referral letter, look at a test result, or check the EMR—you should resist this urge and stick to the customary rules of eye contact.

Adjusting your manner

You would clearly not talk to another provider as you would to someone with no medical knowledge. In much the same way, you should try to adjust your manner and speech according to the patient's educational level. This is can be extremely difficult—you should not make assumptions about intellect or understanding solely on the basis of educational history. Even the most educated patient can have low health literacy.

A safe approach is to start in a relatively neutral way and then adjust your manner and speech according to what you see and hear in the first minute or two of the interaction, but be alert to whether this is effective and make changes accordingly. Understand that patients want to please and seem agreeable and may say "yes" when they really don't understand at all. Having patients explain what they heard back to you (teach back or "show me" method) is a good way to check their understanding.

Interruptions

Apologize to the patient if you are interrupted in your meeting with them.

Don't take offence or get annoyed

As well as being directly aggressive or offensive, people may be thoughtless in their speech or manner and cause offence when they don't really mean to. As a professional, you should rise above this situation.

Communicating with deaf patients

People who are hard of hearing may cope with this problem by using a hearing aid, lip-reading, or sign language. Whichever technique is used (if any), some simple rules should always apply:

- Speak clearly but not too slowly.
- Don't repeat a sentence if it is misunderstood—say the same thing in a different way.
- Write things down, if necessary.
- Use plain English and be succinct.
- Be patient and take the time to communicate properly.
- Check understanding frequently.
- Consider finding an amplifier—many geriatric floors or clinics will have one available.

Lip-readers

Patients who are able to lip-read do so by looking at the normal movements of your lips and face during speech. Exaggerating movements or speaking loudly will distort these movements and make it harder for them to understand you. In addition to the points above, when talking to lip-readers

- Maintain eye contact.
- Don't shout.
- Speak clearly but not too slowly.
- Do not exaggerate your oral or facial movements.

American Sign Language (ASL)

- ASL is not a signed version of English; it is a distinct language with its own grammar and syntax.
- For ASL users, English is a second language, so using a pen and paper may not be effective or safe for discussing complex topics or gaining consent.
- Seek an official interpreter, if possible, and follow the rules (📖 p. 14) on working with interpreters.

Cross-cultural communication

Cultural background and tradition may have a large influence on disease management. Beliefs about the origin of disease and prejudices or stigma surrounding the diagnosis can make dealing with the problem challenging.

Be aware of all possible implications of a person's cultural background. For example, a Muslim may not take anything by mouth in the daylight hours during Ramadan. This may have serious implications for medication management, particularly for chronic diseases such as diabetes or hypertension.

Even something as benign (to you) as eye contact may have important cross-cultural implications. For most individuals eye contact is desired, but for many Native American and Asian cultures, it carries negative connotations.

Above all, be aware of prejudice—yours and theirs. If you are not aware of cultural implications when seeing a patient of a different culture, ask for their input.

Interpreters

Federal and state laws require the use of interpreters for patients with Limited English Proficiency (LEP) and those with hearing disabilities. Health-care facilities have protocols to follow to meet the LEP regulations; they may have in-house or contract staff or use telephonic services. Official communicators are bound by a code of ethics, impartiality, and confidentiality; friends and relatives are not. It is often impossible to be sure that a relative is passing on all that is said in the correct way.

Sometimes, especially in urgent situations, the patient's children are used to interpret. This is clearly not advisable for a number of reasons. This places too much responsibility on the child, and the child may not be able to explain difficult concepts. Conversations about sex, death, or other difficult topics are unsuitable for children to take part in; if they do, this will impede optimal communication.

Using an official interpreter

Before you start
- Brief the interpreter on the situation, and clarify your role and the work of the department, if necessary.
- Allow the interpreter to introduce themselves to the patient and explain their role.
- Arrange seating so that the patient can see both the interpreter and health-care provider easily.
- Allow enough time (at least twice as long as normal).

During the exchange
- Speak to the patient, *not* the interpreter. This may be hard to do at first, but you should speak to and look at the patient at all times.
- Be patient—some concepts are hard to explain.
- Avoid complex terms and grammar.
- Avoid jargon.
- Avoid slang and colloquialisms that may be hard to interpret correctly.
- Check understanding frequently.
- The interpreter may also provide information on the patient's culture to assist in the communication.

Finishing off
- Check understanding.
- Allow time for questions.
- Take the time to debrief with the interpreter.

▶ If the conversation has been distressing, offer the interpreter support and let their employer know, if appropriate.

Written information
- If interpreting written information, read it out loud. The interpreter may not necessarily be able to translate written language as easily.
- Many state and federal health departments and charities provide written information in a variety of languages—some also provide recordings. You should be aware of what your locality has to offer.

Imparting information

There are some guidelines for imparting any information—good or bad—to a patient:

• Identify the topic for discussion.
• Identify the people present and ask if there is anyone else that they would like to be there.
• Establish previous experience and knowledge.
• Keep sentences and explanations short and simple.
• Repeat important information.
• Allow time for feedback and questions, and check understanding.
• Schedule time for follow-up.
• Be honest!

The importance of silence

In conversations with friends or colleagues, your aim is often to avoid silence, using filler noises such as "um" and "ah" while pausing.

In medical situations, by contrast, silences should be embraced and used to extract more information from the patient. Use silence in order to listen.

Practice is needed, as the inexperienced may find this situation uncomfortable. It is often useful, however, to remain silent once the patient has answered your question. You will usually find that the patient will start speaking again, and often provide useful and enlightening facts that you would otherwise not have gleaned.

Angry patients

With angry patients, use body language to take charge of the situation without appearing aggressive (📖 p. 21). Throughout the exchange, you should remain polite, avoiding confrontation, and resist becoming angry yourself.

• Look to your own safety first.
• Calm the situation, *then* establish the facts of the case. Anger is often secondary to some other emotion, such as loss, fear, or guilt.
• Acknowledge the patient's emotions through statements such as the following:
  • "I can see that this has made you angry."
  • "It's understandable that you should feel like this."
• Steer the conversation away from the area of unhappiness and toward the positive and plans, to move the situation forward.
• Don't incriminate colleagues—the patient may remember your throw-away comments, which could come back to haunt you. Avoid remarks like "he shouldn't have done that."
• Emphasize any grounds for optimism or plans for resolving the situation and putting things right.

Telephone and e-mail communication

The essential rule of confidentiality is that you must not impart personal information to anyone without the express permission of the patient concerned—except in a few specific circumstances (📖 p. 26).

You must not give out any confidential information over the telephone unless you are sure of the identity of the caller. All communication is best done face to face. This may cause difficulty if a relative calls to ask about the patient, but you should remain strict about this rule unless you have the expressed permission of the patient.

When discussing follow-up communication for test results, obtain the patient's permission to leave a message on an answering machine or as voice mail. Check to see if you have their correct phone number.

E-mail communications can be very problematic, especially if you do not have a secure, encrypted system. Most health-care institutions have their own policy regarding use of e-mail, so you should know what the rules are. Patient's e-mails should nonetheless be answered. Some providers will call the patient back, documenting the communication in the EMR or chart. Others will ask the patient to set up an appointment.

The use of social media (e.g., Facebook, Twitter) in medicine is still evolving. It is best not to use these for any patient information.

If telephone communication is essential but you are in doubt as to the caller's identity, you may wish to take their number, check it with your records, and then call them back.

Talking about sex

This can be a cause of considerable embarrassment for the patient and for the inexperienced professional. Sexual questions are inappropriate to ask in the presence of friends or relatives, so ask them to leave the room. Your aim is to put the patient at ease and make responses more forthcoming. Make no assumptions about a patient's sexual orientation.

- The key is to ask direct, clear questions and show no embarrassment.
- You should maintain eye contact.
- You should also show *no surprise* whatsoever, even if the sexual practices described differ from your own or from those that you would consider acceptable.
- Try to become familiar with sexual slang and sexual practices that you might not be familiar with.
  - A failure to understand slang may lead to an immediate barrier in the patient interview.
- In general, you should not use slang terms first. You may wish to consider mirroring the patient's speech as you continue the conversation.
- See 📖 p. 378 for details of taking the sexual history.

Breaking bad news

Students fear breaking bad news, and no one likes doing it. However, knowing that you have broken difficult news in a sensitive way and that you have helped the patient through a terrible experience can be one of the most uplifting aspects of working in health care.

Before you start
- Confirm all the information *for yourself* and ensure that you have all the information on hand, if necessary.
- Speak to the nursing staff to get background information on what the patient knows, their fears, and details of their relationship with any family or friends who may be present.

Choose the right place
- Pick a quiet, private room where you won't be disturbed.
- Ensure that there is no intervening desk or other piece of furniture.
- Arrange the chairs so that everyone can be seen equally.
- Hand your pager and cell phone to a colleague or turn it off.

Ensure that the right people are present
- Invite a member of the nursing staff to join you, particularly if they have already established a relationship with the patient.
  - Remember, it is usually the nursing staff that will be dealing with the patient and relatives after you leave, so they need to know exactly what was said.
- Would the patient like anyone in particular to be present?

Remember the general principles
See 📖 p. 6 and 📖 p. 9. Avoid using jargon, and speak slowly and clearly.

Establish previous knowledge
It is essential to understand what the patient already knows. The situation is very different for a patient who knows that you have been looking for cancer than that of a patient who thinks their cough is due to a cold.

> "What do you know so far?"
> "What have the other doctors told you?"

How much do they want to know?
This is key. Before you consider breaking bad news, you have to learn if the patient actually wants to hear it. Ask an open question, such as:

> "Have you thought about what might be causing these problems?"
> "Do you know why we've been doing these tests?"

You can also ask directly if they want to hear what you might have to say:

> "Are you the sort of person who likes to know all the available facts?"

Warning shots

If they do want to know, you should break the news in a step-wise fashion, delivering multiple "warning shots." This gives the patient a chance to stop you if they've heard enough or to ask for more information. Keep your sentences, short, clear, and simple. A conversation may go like this:

> **You:** I'm afraid the test results show that things are more serious than first thought.
> **Patient:** What do you mean more serious?
> **You:** Some of the cells look abnormal.
> **Patient:** Do you mean that I have cancer?
> **You:** Yes.

At any point, the patient may stop you, signaling that they don't want to hear more about it. Inexperienced practitioners sometimes feel that they ought to tell the patient the full story, but they must understand that many people would much rather not hear the words said aloud—this is their coping strategy and must be respected. More than likely, this will not be your only opportunity to speak with the patient.

> **You:** I'm afraid the test results show that things are more serious than first thought.
> **Patient:** Just tell me what we can do next.
> **You:** OK.

Allow time for information to sink in

You should allow time for each piece of information to sink in, ensuring that the patient understands all that has been said and repeating any important information.

Remember also that patients will not be able to remember the exact details of what you have said—you may need to reschedule at a later time to talk about treatment options or prognosis.

Honesty, above all else

Above all, you should be honest at all times. Never guess, predict, or lie.

The patient may break your pre-prepared flow of information, requiring you to think on your feet. Sometimes you simply can't abide by the rules above. If asked a direct question, you must be honest and straightforward. For example:

> **You:** I'm afraid the test results show …
> **Patient:** Just tell me, have I got cancer?
> **You:** Yes, I'm afraid you do.

Don't rush to the positive

When told of bad news, the patient needs a few moments to let the information sink in. After the "yes" in the previous examples, you should preferably wait in silence for the patient to speak next.

The patient may break down in tears, in which case they should be offered tissues and the support of relatives, if nearby.

If emotionally distressed, the patient will not be receptive to what you say next—you may want to give them some time alone with a relative or nurse before you continue to talk about prognosis or treatment options.

Above all, *you should not give false hope*. The moment after the bad news has been broken can be uncomfortable, and you must fight the instinctive move to positive,-sounding statements, such as "there are things we can do"; "on the plus side . . . "; "the good news is . . ."; or something similar.

Ending

Summarize the information given, check the patient's understanding, repeat any information as necessary, allow time for questions, and make arrangements for a follow-up appointment or a further opportunity to ask questions again.

Obviously, you shouldn't make promises that you can't keep. Don't offer to come back that afternoon if you're going to be in clinic!

> "Do you understand everything that we've discussed?"
> "Is there anything else that you would like to ask me?"
> "I'll plan to see you tomorrow morning. I'll be happy to come back in the meantime if you think of anything that you'd like to ask or if you need to talk. Just ask one of the nursing staff to page me."

Questions about time

"How long have I got?" is one of the most common questions asked, and the hardest to answer.
- As always, don't guess and don't lie.
- It's often impossible to estimate this. Giving a figure will almost always lead to you being wrong. If you don't know, it is perfectly acceptable to say so.
- Explain that it is impossible to judge, and ask if there is any date in particular that they don't want to miss—perhaps they want to experience Christmas or a relative's birthday.
- Don't assume that they are asking out of fear; some people are surprisingly practical and want to put their affairs in order before their death.

Box 1.4 Fear words

There are certain words that immediately generate fear, such as *cancer* and *leukemia*. You should use these if you are sure that the patient understands the full diagnosis and plan.

Beware, however, of avoiding these words and causing confusion by not giving the whole story.

You should also be aware of certain words that people will instinctively assume mean something more serious. For example, to most people a "shadow" on the lung means cancer. Don't then use the word when you are talking about pulmonary consolidation due to pneumonia!

Body language: an introduction

Body language is rarely given the place it deserves in the teaching of communication skills. There are over 600 muscles in the human body—90 in the face, of which 30 act purely to express emotion. Changes in your position or expression—some obvious, others subtle—can heavily influence the message that you are communicating.

We've all met someone and thought, "I didn't like him" or "she seemed trustworthy." Often these impressions of people are not built on what is said but the manner in which people handle themselves. You subconsciously pick up cues from the other person's body. Being good at using body language means having awareness of how the other person may be viewing you and getting your subconscious actions and expressions under conscious control.

If done well, you can influence the other person's opinion of you, make them more receptive to your message, or add particular emphasis to certain words and phrases.

Touching

Touching is one of the most powerful forms of nonverbal communication and needs to be managed with care.

- *Greeting:* Touch is part of greeting rituals in most cultures. It demonstrates that you are not holding a weapon and establishes intimacy.
- *Shaking hands:* There are many variations. The length of the shake and the strength of the grip impart a huge amount of information. For added intimacy and warmth, a double-handed grip can be used. For extra intimacy, one may touch the other's forearm or elbow.*
- *Dominance:* Touch is a powerful display of dominance. Touching someone on the back or shoulder demonstrates that you are in charge—this can be countered by mirroring the action back.
- *Sympathy:* The lightest of touches can be very comforting and is appropriate in the medical situation where another type of touch may be misread as dominance or intimacy (you shouldn't hug a patient you've just met!). Display sympathy by a brief touch to the arm or hand.

Open body language

A cluster of movements are associated with seeming *open*. The most significant part of this is the act of opening—signaling a change in the way you are feeling. Openness demonstrates that you have nothing to hide and are receptive to the other person. Openness encourages openness.

This can be used to calm an angry situation or when asking about personal information.

---

* Watch the first few minutes of the 1998 film "Primary Colors," which demonstrates the different uses of touch during handshakes.

▶ The key is to not have your arms or legs crossed in any way.

- **Arms open:** either at your side or held wide. Even better, hold your hands open and face your palms toward the other person.
- **Legs open:** this does not mean legs wide, rather, legs not crossed. You may hold them parallel. The feet often point toward something of subconscious interest to you—point them at the patient!

Emphasis

You can amplify your spoken words with your body, usually without noticing it. Actions include nodding your head, pointing, or other hand gestures. A gesture may involve your entire body.

Watch TV news anchors—often only their heads are in view, so they emphasize with nods and turns of their heads much more than one would during normal conversation.

- **Synchrony:** This is key. Time your points of the finger, taps of the hand on the desk, or other actions with the words you wish to emphasize.
- **Precision:** Signal that the words currently being spoken are worth paying attention to with delicate, precise movements. You could make an 'O' with your thumb and index finger or hold your hands such that each finger is touching its opposite counterpart—like a splayed prayer position.*

Eye level

This is a very powerful tool. In general, the person with a higher eye level is in control of the situation.

You can use this tactic to your advantage. When asking someone personal questions or when you want them to open up, position yourself such that your eyes are below theirs, meaning they have to look down at you slightly. This makes them feel more in control and comfortable.

Likewise, anger often comes from a feeling of lack of control—put the angry person in charge by lowering your eye level—even if that means squatting next to them or sitting when they are standing.

Conversely, you may raise your eye level to take charge of a difficult situation; looking down on someone is intimidating. Stand over a seated person to demonstrate that you are in charge.

Watch and learn

There is much that could be said about body language. You should watch others and yourself and consider what messages are being portrayed by nonverbal communication.

Stay aware of your own movements, and consider intentionally changing what would normally be subconscious actions to add to, or alter, the meaning of your speech.

---

* Many successful politicians are excellent users of body language. Pay attention to their campaign speeches and formal presentations as well as to their informal talks.

Written communication

Medical notes serve a number of purposes. The most important ones are as follows:
- They are a record of the patient's illness, treatments, and medical encounters, for use by other medical practitioners in the future.
- They are the only record of your actions—and the means by which you may be judged in case of future disputes.
- They are a record of events for the purposes of clinical audit.

How to write in the notes

Your entries in the notes should be tidy and legible. All entries should include the following:
- Date
- Time
- Medical information
- Signature (also print your name if your handwriting is illegible).
- Identity of the inscriber
- Contact number (pager and/or cell phone)
  Use black ink only (blue often doesn't photocopy easily and can fade).

What to write in the notes

- Everything that occurs should be recorded. If it isn't written down, it didn't happen!
- Remember especially to record discussions with relatives and the details of what the patient has been told of diagnoses.
- There are no specific rules on how things should be written—there are a number of conventions introduced throughout the book.
  In general, entries should be easily understood by another staff member.

Box 1.5 Standard examination drawings

The essential rule is that the record you make should be easily understood by another person. If it is hard to describe where the cut on the patient's foot is, draw it! There are a number of diagrams that, though not official, are widely used and accepted as standard.

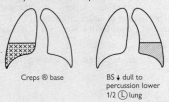

Creps ® base

BS ↓ dull to
percussion lower
1/2 Ⓛ lung

Chest

This is usually represented as a stylized version of the lungs seen from the front. You can then add symbols (e.g., BS—breath sounds) indicating your clinical finding.

Heart sounds

These are often represented as a version of a phonogram—see 📖 p. 171 for examples.

Abdomen

This is usually drawn as a hexagon, although the anatomical stickler may add the xiphoid process and the genitalia.

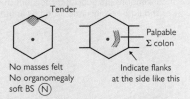

Tender

No masses felt
No organomegaly
soft BS Ⓝ

Palpable
Σ colon

Indicate flanks
at the side like this

Peripheral pulses and tendon reflexes

These are often indicated on stick-men. Be sure to make clear which are the left and right sides of the person.

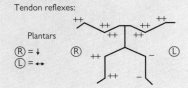

Tendon reflexes:

Plantars

Ⓡ = ↓
Ⓛ = ↔

Ⓡ

Ⓛ

Other body parts
You should feel free to make drawings to illustrate your findings.

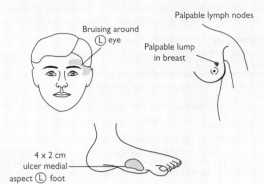

Law, ethics, and communication

No discussion of communication skills would be complete without mention of confidentiality, capacity, and consent. It is also worth knowing the four bioethical principles, about which much has been written elsewhere.

Four bioethical principles
- *Autonomy:* a respect for the individual and their ability to make decisions regarding their own health
- *Beneficence:* acting to the benefit of patients
- *Nonmalificence:* acting to prevent harm to the patient
- *Justice:* fairness to the patient and the wider community when considering the consequences of an action

Confidentiality

Confidentiality is closely linked to the ethical principles described above. Maintaining a secret record of personal information shows respect for the individual's autonomy and their right to control their own information. There is also an element of beneficence, whereas releasing the protected information may cause harm.

Breaking confidentiality

The rules surrounding the maintenance of confidentiality have already been mentioned (see 📖 p. 3). There are a number of circumstances in which confidentiality can, or must, be broken. The exact advice varies between different bodies; see Further Reading in this section. In general, confidentiality may be broken in the following situations:
- With the consent of the individual concerned
- If disclosure is in the patient's interest but consent cannot be gained
- If required by law
- When there is a statutory duty, such as reporting of births, deaths, and abortions, and in cases of certain communicable diseases
- If it is overwhelmingly in the public interest
- If it is necessary for national security or when prevention or detection of a crime may be prejudiced or delayed
- In certain situations related to medical research

Consent and capacity

There are three main components to valid consent. To be competent (or have capacity) to give consent, the patient
- Must understand the information that has been given
- Must believe that information
- Must be able to retain and evaluate the information to make a decision
  In addition, for consent to be valid, the patient must be free from any kind of duress.

▶ It should be noted that an assessment of capacity is valid for the specific decision at hand. It is not an all-or-nothing phenomenon—you cannot either have capacity or not. The assessment regarding competence must be made for each new decision faced.

Young people and capacity

- All persons aged 18 and over are considered to be a competent adult unless there is evidence to the contrary.
- People between 16 and 18 years of age may be treated as adults if they are covered by statutes regarding emancipated minors. However, the refusal of a treatment can be overridden by the courts.
- Children age 16 and younger are considered competent to give consent if they meet the three conditions mentioned previously. However, their decisions can be overridden by the courts or by people with parental responsibility.

Further reading

There are many articles on communication in the medical setting. A good summary of issues of communication, including cultural competency, Limited English Proficiency, and health literacy, can be found at the U.S. Department of Health and Human Services, Health Resources and Services Administration Web site. The online training module is entitled Unified Heath Communication: Addressing Health Literacy, Cultural Competency and Limited English Proficiency, at: http://www.hrsa.gov/healthliteracy/default.htm

HIPAA (Health Insurance Portability and Accountability Act)

Health records and personal communications have undergone a significant change since enactment of the Health Insurance Portability and Accountability Act (HIPAA) in 1996. This Act has dramatically affected issues of medical records, privacy, and security and transfer of information that are far beyond the scope of this text. Further information on this topic can be obtained at: http://www.hhs.gov/ocr/privacy

The history

History-taking

The *history* is a patient's account of their illness together with other relevant information you have gleaned from them. Like all things in medicine, there is a tried and tested standard sequence that you should conform to and is used by all providers.

It is good practice to make quick notes while talking to the patient that you can use to write a thorough history afterward—don't document every word they say, as this breaks up your interaction!

By the end of the history-taking you should have a good idea of a diagnosis or have several differential diagnoses in mind. The examination is your chance to confirm or refute these through the acquisition of more information.

History-taking is not a passive process. You need to keep your wits about you and gently guide the patient in giving you relevant information through use of all the communication skills described in Chapter 1.

The history should be broken down under the headings listed in Box 2.1 and recorded in the notes in this order—many people prefer to use the standard abbreviations instead of writing out the heading in full.

The outline shown in Box 2.1 is the standard method, although slight variations exist.

Many people list information on smoking and alcohol as part of the social history. We feel that these factors have such a significant impact on health that they are more appropriately placed as part of the past medical history, rather than as what the patient does in their spare time.

It is good practice in medicine to watch what other practitioners do and adapt the parts that you feel are done well to your own style, making them part of your own routine.

Box 2.1 The standard history framework

- Patient profile (PP)
- Chief complaint (CC)
- History of the present illness (HPI)
- Past medical history (PMH)
  - Allergies
  - Drug history
  - Alcohol
  - Smoking
- Family history (FH)
- Social History (SH)
  - Occupational History
- Review of Systems (ROS)

Using this book

This book is divided into chapters by organ system. Each chapter offers suggestions of how to proceed (see Boxes 2.2 and 2.3), depending on the nature of the presenting complaint, and notes on what you should especially ask about under each of the headings. These notes are not exhaustive and are intended as a guide to supplement a thorough history.

Box 2.2 Recording the history

Documentation is a vital part of all medical interactions.

The history should be recorded in the patient's notes according to the standard framework in Box 2.1, using the rules and procedures described in the section Written Communication in Chapter 1 (📖 p. 23).

Always remember: if it isn't written, it didn't happen!

Box 2.3 Collateral histories

There are many situations in which the patient may be unable to give a history (e.g., they are unconscious, delirious, demented, or dysphasic). In these situations, you should make an effort to speak to all who can help you fill in the gaps—regarding not only what happened to the patient but also their usual medication, functional state, living arrangements, and so on.

When taking a history from a source other than the patient, be sure to document clearly that this is the case and the reason(s) for the patient being unable to speak for themselves.

Useful sources of information include the following:
• Relatives, guardians, and cohabitants
• Close friends and roommates
• Primary care physician (PCP) or other members of the primary care team
• Pharmacist
• Staff at the nursing home or residential or other facility
• Ambulance personnel
• Anyone who witnessed the event.

Patient profile (PP)

• This is the essential identifying and biographic information required by the facility.
• Typically included in the PP will be the patient's name, address, and DOB.
• Other information included in the PP may include age, religion, nationality, marital status, and contact information as requested by the individual facility.

Chief complaint (CC)

- This is the patient's chief symptom(s) *in their own words.* It should generally be no more than a single sentence.
- If the patient has several symptoms, present them as a list that you can expand on later in the history.
- Ask the patient an open question, such as, "What's the problem?" or "What made you come to the office?" Each provider will have their own style. You should choose a phrase that suits you and your manner (one of the authors favors saying "tell me the story" after a brief introduction).

🔵 The question "What brought you here?" usually brings the response "an ambulance," "my feet," or "the taxi"—each patient being under the impression that they are the first to crack this joke. This question is thus best avoided.

▶ Remember, the CC is expressed *in the patient's words.* "Hemoptysis" is rarely a presenting complaint, but "coughing up blood" may well be!

History of the presenting illness (HPI)

Here you are asking about and documenting details of the presenting complaint. By the end of taking the HPI, you and readers of the record should have a clear idea about the nature of the problem and of exactly how and when it started, how it has progressed over time, and what impact it has had on the patient in their general physical health, psychology, and social and working lives. The HPI is best tackled in two phases.

First, ask an open question (as for the CC) and allow the patient to talk through what has happened for about 2 minutes. Don't interrupt! Encourage the patient with nonverbal responses and take discreet notes. This allows you to make an initial assessment of the patient in terms of education level, personality, and anxiety. Using this information, you can adjust your responses and interaction. It should also become clear to you exactly what symptom the patient is most concerned about.

In the second phase, you should revisit the whole story, asking more detailed questions. It may be useful to say, "I'd just like to go through the story again, clarifying some details." This is your chance to verify time-lines and the relation of one symptom to another. You should also clarify pseudo-medical terms (e.g., exactly what does the patient mean by "vertigo," "flu," or "rheumatism"?). Remember, this should feel like a conversation, not an interrogation!

▶ The standard features that should be determined for any symptom are shown in Box 2.4, along with additional features regarding pain (Box 2.5). A mnemonic for remembering the important factors in analyzing pain or a symptom is **O3PQRST**. This simple, alphabetically ordered pneumonic includes the significant factors: **O**nset, **P**revious occurrences, **P**rovoking factors, **P**alliative factors (including prescribed and home treatments attempted), **Q**uality (such as characteristics of

Box 2.4 For each symptom, determine

- The exact nature of the symptom
- The onset
  - Date it began
  - How it began (e.g., suddenly, gradually—over how long?)
  - If the symptom is long- standing, why is the patient seeking help now?
- Previous occurrences and frequency
  - Is the symptom constant or intermittent?
  - How long does it last each time?
  - What is the exact manner in which it comes and goes?
- Change over time
  - Is it improving or deteriorating?
- Exacerbating factors
  - What makes the symptom worse?
- Relieving factors
  - What makes the symptom better?
- Associated symptoms.

pain), **R**adiation (site of onset and any radiation), **S**everity, and **T**iming (duration; see Box 2.6).

See the rest of this book for guidance on tackling other, organ-specific presenting complaints.

At the end of the history of the presenting illness, you should have established a *problem list*. You should run through these items with the patient, summarizing what you have been told, and ask them if you have the information *correct* and if there is *anything further* that they would like to share with you.

Box 2.5 For pain, determine

- Site (where is the pain is worst—ask the patient to point to the site with one finger)
- Radiation (does the pain move anywhere else?)
- Character (i.e., dull, aching, stabbing, burning)
- Severity (scored out of 10, with 10 being the worst pain imaginable)
- Mode and rate of onset (how did it come on—over how long?)
- Duration
- Frequency
- Exacerbating factors
- Relieving factors
- Associated symptoms (e.g., nausea, dyspepsia, shortness of breath)

Box 2.6 Long-standing problems

If the symptom is long-standing, ask why the patient is seeking help now. Has anything changed? It is often useful to ask when the patient was last well. This may help focus their mind on the start of the problem, which may seem distant and less important to them.

Past medical history (PMH)

Some aspects of the patient's past illnesses or diagnoses may have already been covered. Here, you should obtain detailed information about past illnesses and surgical procedures.

   Ask the patient if they are receiving care for anything else or have ever been to the hospital before. Ensure that you get dates and a location for each event. Some conditions, listed in Box 2.7, you should ask patients about specifically. For each condition, ask the following:

• When was it diagnosed?
• How was it diagnosed?
• How has it been treated?

For operations, ask about any previous anesthesia problems.

   ⓘ Ask about immunizations. Have the patient provide as many specifics about types and dates of immunizations. Also ask about employment and insurance examinations. See Box 2.8 for gaining further clarification when taking the PMH.

Box 2.7 Specific conditions to include in PMH

• Diabetes
• Rheumatic fever
• Jaundice
• Hypercholesterolemia
• Hypertension
• Angina
• Myocardial infarction (MI)
• Stroke or transient ischemic attack (TIA)
• Asthma
• Tuberculosis (TB)
• Epilepsy
• Anesthetic problems
• Blood transfusions
• Childhood illnesses and sequelae

Box 2.8 Don't take anything for granted!

For each condition that the patient reports having, ask exactly how it was diagnosed (where? by whom?) and how it has been treated since then.

   For example, if the patient reports "asthma," ask who made the diagnosis, when the diagnosis was made, if they have ever had lung function tests, if they have ever seen a pulmonologist, and if they are taking any inhalers. Have they used any over-the-counter (OTC) treatments or alternative medications? Occasionally, patients will give a long-standing symptom a medical name, which can be very confusing. In this example, the patient's "asthma" could be how they refer to their wheeze that is due to congestive cardiac failure.

Allergies

Any allergies should be documented separately from the drug history because of their importance.

Ask if the patient has any allergies or is allergic to anything if they are unfamiliar with the term *allergies*. Be sure to probe carefully, as people will often tell you about their hay fever and forget about the rash they had when they took penicillin. Ask specifically if they have had any reactions to drugs or medication; don't forget to inquire about food or environmental allergies.

▶ If an allergy is reported, you should obtain the exact nature of the event and decide if the patient is describing a true allergy, intolerance, or simply an unpleasant side effect.

Drug history

Here you should list all the medications that the patient is taking, including the dosage and frequency of each prescription. If the patient is unsure about their medications, confirm the drug history with the prescribing provider or pharmacy. Take special note of any drugs that have been started or stopped recently.

You should also ask about compliance—does the patient know what dose they take? Do they ever miss doses? If they are not taking the medication, what's the reason? Do they have any compliance aids such as a pre-packaged weekly supply? It may also be valuable to ask if the patient is having any difficulty obtaining their medications.

The patient may consider some medications as not being drugs, so specific questioning is required. Don't forget to ask about the following:

• Eye drops
• Inhalers
• Sleeping pills
• Oral contraception
• OTC drugs (bought at a store or pharmacy), vitamin supplements
• Herbal remedies
• Illicit or "recreational" drug use

Alcohol

You should attempt to quantify, as accurately as possible, the amount of alcohol consumed per week, and establish if the consumption is spread out evenly over the week or concentrated in a smaller period. The CAGE questionnaire, long considered a standard in alcohol assessment, may be supplemented or possibly replaced by use of a single question: "How many times in the past year have you had X or more drinks in a day?," where X is 5 for men and 4 for women, and a response of 1 or more times has been validated and may prove to be valuable with certain populations (see Box 2.9).

In the United States and many European countries, alcohol is quantified as standard drinks. In the United States, a standard drink contains 0.54 ounces of alcohol (Box 2.10).

Healthy People 2010

Information on this initiative (Box 2.11) is available at: http://www.healthypeople.gov

Box 2.9 Alcohol consumption

Healthy People 2010 reports that males may be at risk for alcohol-related problems if they drink more than 14 drinks per week or more than 4 drinks per occasion. Likewise, females may be at risk if they drink more than seven drinks per week or three drinks per occasion.

Box 2.10 Alcohol amounts of common drinks

For typical strength alcoholic beverages the following contain approximately 0.54 ounces of ethanol.
• 12 ounces beer
• 5 ounces of wine
• 1.5 ounces of 80 proof distilled spirits

Box 2.11 Health People 2010

A target goal of Healthy People 2010 is to reduce the average annual alcohol consumption to 2 gallons per year from a 1997 baseline, when 2.18 gallons of ethanol was consumed per person age 14 years and older.

Smoking

Attempt to quantify the habit (Box 2.12) in pack-years: 1 pack-year is 20 cigarettes (1 pack) per day for 1 year (e.g., 40/day for 1 year = 2 pack-years; 10/day for 2 years = 1 pack-year).

Ask about previous smoking, as many patients will call themselves non-smokers if they gave up yesterday or are even on their way to the hospital or clinic!

Remember to ask about passive smoking. An inquiry such as, "Do you smoke in your house, in your car, or around your children?" may help to raise consciousness regarding health risks for children and the issue of influencing the child's future behavior.

🚫 Be aware of cultural issues—smoking is forbidden for Sikhs, for example, and they may take offence at the suggestion of smoking!

🚫 Beware of appearing judgmental.

Box 2.12 Haggling and the art of quantification

Smoking and alcohol histories are notoriously unreliable—alcohol especially so. The patient may be trying to please you or feel embarrassed about openly admitting their true consumption. Gaining an accurate account of consumption can sometimes feel like haggling. There are two steps in this process.

First, appear nonjudgmental and resist acting surprised *in any way*, even in the face of liquor or tobacco consumption that you may consider excessive and unwise.

Second, if the patient remains reticent ("I smoke a few"), suggest a number, but start very high ("Shall we say 60 a day?") and the patient will usually give you a number nearer the true amount ("Oh no, more like 20"). If you start low, the same patient may only admit to half that amount.

Family history (FH)

The FH details the following:
- Makeup of the family, including age and gender of parents, siblings, children, and extended family, as relevant
- Health of the family

You should ask about any diagnosed conditions in other living family members. Stating a "laundry list" of common conditions will help the patient understand conditions that you are most concerned about. You should also document the age and cause of death for all deceased first-degree relatives and for other family members if you feel it is appropriate.

It may help to draw a family tree (genogram), as shown in Box 2.13. These diagrams are particularly useful in pediatric assessments, families with multiple health problems that demonstrate familial propensities, and families with hereditary conditions.

Box 2.13 Family trees

Conventionally, males are represented by a square (□) and females by a circle (○). The patient you are talking to is called the *propositus, proband,* or *index* and is indicated by a small arrow (↗).

Horizontal lines represent marriages or other relationships resulting in a child. Vertical lines descend from these, connecting to a horizontal line from which the children "hang." You can add ages and causes of death.

Family members who have died are represented by a diagonal line drawn through their circle or square (Ø, ⌀), and those with the condition of interest are represented by shaded shapes (●, ■).

Example 1 Our patient is an only child and has no children, his parents are alive, but all his grandparents have died of different causes.

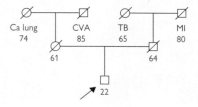

Box 2.13 (Cont'd.)

Example 2 Our patient suffers from colon cancer and has no children. She has a brother who is well. Her parents are both alive and her mother has colon cancer. Of her grandparents, only her paternal grandfather is alive. Her maternal grandfather died of colon cancer.

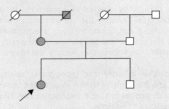

Example 3 Our patient has epilepsy, as does her father. She has 3 children, 2 boys and a girl. One of the boys also has epilepsy.

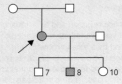

Social history (SH)

This is your chance to document the details of the patient's personal life that are relevant to the working diagnosis, the patient's general well-being, and recovery or convalescence. The SH will help in understanding the impact of the illness on the patient's functional status.

This is a vital part of the history but is often given only brief attention. The disease and, indeed, the patient do not exist in a vacuum but are part of a community that they interact with and contribute to. Without these details, it is impossible to take a holistic approach to the patient's well-being. Establish the following:

- Marital status
- Sexual orientation
- Occupation (or previous occupations if retired)
  - You should establish the *exact* nature of the job if it is unclear—does it involve sitting at a desk, carrying heavy loads, or traveling?
- Other people who live at the same address
- Type of accommodation (e.g., house, apartment—and on what floor)
- Does the patient own their accommodation or rent it?
- Are there any stairs? How many?
- Does the patient have any aids or adaptations in their house (e.g., rails near the bath)?
- Does the patient use any walking aids (e.g., cane, walker, scooter)?
- Does the patient receive any help on a daily basis?
  - Who from (e.g., family, friends, social services)?
  - Who does the laundry, cleaning, cooking, and shopping?
- Does the patient have relatives living nearby?
- What hobbies does the patient have?
- Does the patient own any pets?
- Has the patient been abroad recently or spent any time abroad in the past?
- Does the patient drive?

Review of systems (ROS)

Prior to the exam, you should perform a screening of the other body systems relevant to the chief complaint. When conducting the comprehensive exam, review of all systems is necessary and use of a cranial–caudal approach to the review may be most appropriate.

The review of systems often proves to be more important than you expect. You may find symptoms that the patient had forgotten about or identify secondary, unrelated problems that can be addressed as part of the review. Not only is the finding of unexpected symptoms important, the absence of particular symptoms may be of even greater significance, therefore, *always document significant negatives*.

The questions asked will depend on any previous discussion(s). If you have discussed chest pain in the history of presenting complaint, there is no need to ask about it again.

Ask the patient if they have any of the following symptoms:

General symptoms
• Weight change (loss or gain), change in appetite (loss or gain), fever, lethargy, malaise

Skin symptoms
• Lumps, bumps, sores, ulcers, rashes, itch

Sensory symptoms
• Vision problems hearing deficits

Respiratory symptoms
• Cough, sputum, hemoptysis, shortness of breath, wheeze, chest pain

Cardiovascular symptoms
• Shortness of breath on exertion, paroxysmal nocturnal dyspnea, chest pain, palpitations, ankle swelling, orthopnea, claudication

Gastrointestinal symptoms
• Dysphagia, indigestion, abdominal pain, nausea, vomiting, a change in bowel habit, constipation, diarrhea, rectal blood loss

Genitourinary symptoms
• Urinary frequency, polyuria, dysuria, hematuria, nocturia, menstrual problems, impotence

Neurological symptoms
• Headaches, dizziness, tingling, weakness, tremor, faint, seizures, convulsions, epilepsy, blackouts or other loss of consciousness

Psychological symptoms
• Depression, anxiety, sleep disturbances

Endocrine symptoms
• Intolerance to heat or cold

Musculoskeletal symptoms
• Aches, pains, stiffness, swelling

The elderly patient

Obtaining a history from older people might be regarded as no greater task than that for any other patient; however, cognitive decline, deafness, and acute illness can make this difficult. Taking a good history from older people is a skill that you will find useful in all other situations.

While the history is key for making diagnoses, it is also an opportunity for much more—your first interaction with an older patient sets important first impressions. A skillful history not only reaps diagnostic rewards but also marks you as a competent provider who can gain trust, reassure, and communicate well with patients in any challenging situation.

Key points

Learn to listen

It can be tempting to ask lots of questions to obtain every fact in the history, particularly if you are rushed. Doing this will not only frustrate and offend your patient (because you clearly don't listen) but will also risk your missing important facts.

Instead, learn to stay quiet—and listen in detail to the history of the presenting complaint, which may only be 3–4 minutes, but gives your patient a chance to be heard (see Box 2.14). Seemingly irrelevant detail is often useful when patients have the chance to put it in context. It often saves you time, as other key information may emerge, and you can better focus the history.

Problem lists

Patients with chronic illness or multiple diagnoses may have more than one strand to their acute presentation. Consider breaking the history of the presenting complaint down into a problem list, e.g., 1) worsening heart failure; 2) continence problems; 3) diarrhea; 4) falls. This can often reveal key interactions between diagnoses that you might not have thought about.

Drug history

Remember to consider polypharmacy and that patients may not remember all the treatments they take. Be aware that more drugs mean more side effects and less compliance, so ask which are taken and why—(older) people are often quite honest about why they omit tablets.

Many elderly individuals use supplements or alternative remedies that may interfere with your prescribed treatments, so ask about them! Eye drops, sleeping pills, and laxatives are often regarded non-medicines by patients, so be thorough and ask about each separately. Avoid precipitating delirium due to acute withdrawal of benzodiazepines.

Finally, remember the cost of medications and the impact they have on an individual on a fixed income.

Functional history

A comprehensive functional history is a cornerstone of your history-taking in older people—we make no apologies for reminding you about this throughout this book. Diseases may not cured or modified, but their key component—the effects on patients and their lives—might be easily transformed through manipulation of activities of daily living.

Remember to ask about support systems for the patient at home—have things resulted in a crisis for the patient because a caregiver is ill? Be polite and ask tactfully about finances and available services. Are social service benefits, such as home health and meals-on-wheels, available? Many patients do not realize that they might be eligible, so precede your questions with an explanation that, if desired, information about resources or referral may be provided.

Social history

SH is exactly that and should complement the functional history. Occupation (other than retired) can be of value when one is faced with a new diagnosis of pulmonary fibrosis or bladder cancer and may give your patient a chance to sketch out more about their lives. Inquire about family—don't assume that a relative may be able to provide help, as they may live far away; the patient may still have a spouse, but be separated.

Chat with patients about their daily lives—interests and pursuits can help distract an ill patient, give hope for the future, and act as an incentive for recovery and meaningful rehabilitation.

Box 2.14 A note on narratives

- Akin to learning to listen is recognition that many patients might not deliver their histories in a style that fits the traditional pattern described in this chapter. Pushing (older) patients through histories is not recommended. Older people will often discuss events and preferences with a constituted story, and it is important to recognize the value of this. Narrative analysis at its most simple—i.e., your ability to listen and interpret—is a vital skill for all clinicians. Listening to stories allows you to understand patients' preferences, hopes, and fears.

- Remember also that older patients often have different views about what they want from their doctors. Their "agendas" may differ hugely from what you think treatment plans should be, but they may not make their views known, through fear of offending you. If you are unsure, always ask—learning to involve your patients in key decisions about their care will make you a better clinician.

The pediatric patient

Obtaining a history about or from children may present additional challenges, depending on who is available to provide the history and how active the child is.

Key points

Learn to listen

Remember to listen to the child in addition to the caregiver. Again, it can be tempting to ask lots of questions to obtain every fact in the history. Doing this may result in missed opportunities to observe the patient–caregiver interaction.

The child who is given appropriate attention during the history may feel more engaged and be more cooperative during the exam. Instead of having the child be quiet, remember to solicit the input of your youthful patient. It gives them a chance to be heard. It can even save time, as key information may emerge from the unexpected source—the child.

Drug history

Remember that parental practices may put children at risk. Ask about the use of OTC medications and alternative treatments. This is often an overlooked area when dealing with children.

Social history

Don't assume that a relative bringing the child in for an exam may be able to provide all the needed information. The child may be the subject of a shared-custody agreement, or the noncustodial parent, who has minimal information about the child, may be bringing the child in. Remember to ask about formal and informal support for the patient and family during illness.

Ask tactfully about the availability of parental benefits, including sick time, as many parents do not realize that they might be eligible for such benefits as leave time under the Family and Medical Leave Act (FMLA).

Chat with the child about their daily activities. Understanding the child's perceptions about their illness as well as their life in general may give important clues to the best ways to provide care. Having the child discuss interests and practices can help in providing treatment and supporting parental relationships.

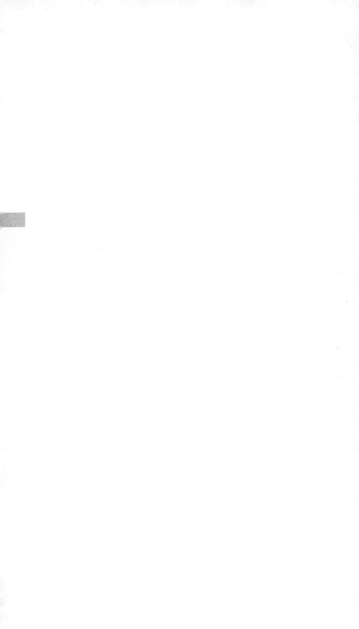

General examination

Approaching the physical examination

General conduct

Medical professionals are in a position of trust. It is generally assumed that, as a medical professional, you will act with professionalism, integrity, and honesty, as well as respect for the dignity and privacy of your patient.

In no part of the patient encounter is this more evident than during the physical examination. People you may have only just met will take off their clothes and allow you to look at and touch their bodies—something that would be completely unacceptable to many people in any other situation. They will, of course, be more comfortable with this if you have established an appropriate rapport during the history-taking phase of the visit.

Communication does not stop at the end of taking the history, as additional historical information should be elicited during the physical examination. The manner in which you conduct yourself during the examination can be the difference between an effective examination and a formal complaint. It is essential that cultural and religious norms be taken into consideration in the context of the physical examination.

This is not to say that you should shy away from examining the patient for fear of acting inappropriately and causing offense. In particular, you should not avoid examining members of the opposite sex, especially their intimate body parts, as there should be no sexual undertones in the relationship whatsoever.

The examiner must project a self-confident and empathetic persona throughout thee examination. Further, the use of consistent verbal and nonverbal communication should ensure that no misunderstandings occur. You should, of course, be sure that you have a chaperone present—another student, doctor, nurse, or other health-care professional—whenever you perform any intimate examination. Ideally, the chaperone should be of the same gender as the patient.

Format of the examination

Examination techniques may seem overstructured and unnaturally formulaic at first, but these routines ensure that no part of the examination is missed.

The right approach

One important rule is that you should always stand at the patient's right-hand side. This gives them a feeling of control over the situation (most people are right-handed). All the standard examination techniques are formulated with this orientation in mind.

Systems examinations

The physical examination can be accomplished through a body systems approach, which is the format of this book.

Often you will need to examine several systems simultaneously by integrating examination techniques in an integrated manner. For example, you may wish to examine the patient's thorax with a view to the cardiovascular and respiratory systems, listening for heart and breath sounds during the auscultation phase of the exam, rather than completing the heart exam and then returning to examine the chest and respiratory system.

Examination framework

Each system-based examination is divided into the following categories:
- Inspection (looking)
- Palpation (feeling)
- Percussion (tapping)
- Auscultation (listening)

In addition, there may be special tests and other added categories; you will meet these as you go through this book.

Using this book

- Each chapter in this book is based around one body system and describes the standard examination format for that system only.
- At the beginning of each encounter, you should consider the topics covered in this chapter before moving to the more specific examination.
- You should not consider these examination routines to be entirely separate entities. If examining several systems at once, you should combine these frameworks to create a single, fluid routine.

First impressions

Diagnosis at first sight

From the first moment you set eyes on the patient, you should be forming impressions of their general state of health. It takes experience and practice to pick up on all of the possible clues, but much can be gained by combining common sense with medical knowledge. Ask yourself the following:

- Did the patient walk in unassisted?
- Does the patient appear comfortable or distressed?
- Does the patient appear well or ill?
- Is there a recognizable syndrome or facies?
- Does the patient appear well nourished and hydrated ?

You will note many of these features subconsciously, but you must work to make yourself consciously aware of them.

Bedside clues

In a hospital setting, there may be additional clues as to the patient's state of health in the objects around them. In other circumstances, look at objects they are carrying or that are visible in their pockets. Examples include oxygen tubing, inhalers, insulin syringes, a glucose meter, or cigarettes.

Vital signs

It is also essential that vital signs be assessed at an early stage. These usually include the following:

- Temperature
- Blood pressure
- Pulse
- Oxygen saturation
- Respiratory rate
- Level of pain

Consciousness level

If necessary, a rapid and initial assessment of a patient's level of consciousness can be made using the Alert, Voice, Pain, Unresponsive (AVPU) scale (Box 10.9 📖 p. 332) or the Glasgow Coma Scale (GCS) (Box 10.10 📖 p. 332).

Preparing for the examination

Before commencing a formal examination, introduce yourself, explain what you would like to do, and obtain verbal consent.

- Ensure that the patient has adequate privacy to undress.
- Make sure that you will not be disturbed.
- Check that the examination couch or bed is draped or covered by a clean sheet or disposable drape.
- If the patient is accompanied, ask them if they would like their companion to remain in the room during the exam.
- Check that any equipment you will require is available (light source, cotton ball, reflex hammer, stethoscope, etc.).
- When ready, the patient should be positioned supine with the head and shoulders raised to 45°.

Color

The color of the patient, or parts of the patient, can give clues to their general state of health and to particular diagnoses. Look especially for evidence of pallor, central or peripheral cyanosis, jaundice, and abnormal skin pigmentation.

Pallor (paleness)

Facial pallor is often a sign of severe anemia and is especially noticeable on inspecting the palpebral conjunctiva, nail beds, and palmar skin creases.

Ask the patient to look upward and gently draw down their lower eyelid with your thumb—the conjunctiva should be red or pink.

However, pallor is an unreliable sign in patients suffering shock or in those with vascular disease. Peripheral vasoconstriction or poor blood flow causes pallor of the skin and conjunctiva, even in the absence of blood loss.

Cyanosis

See also 📖 p. 191. *Cyanosis* refers to a bluish discoloration of the skin and mucous membranes and is due to the presence of at least 2.5 g/dL of deoxygenated hemoglobin in the blood.

In *central cyanosis*, the tongue appears blue from an abnormal amount of deoxygenated blood in the arteries. This may develop in any lung disease in which there is a ventilation/perfusion mismatch, such as chronic obstructive pulmonary disease (COPD), cor pulmonale, and massive pulmonary embolus (PE). It will also occur in right-to-left cardiac shunts. Finally, polycythemia and hemoglobinopathies (such as methemoglobinemia) may give the appearance of cyanosis due to abnormal oxygen carriage.

Peripheral cyanosis is bluish discoloration at the extremities (fingers, toes) only. It is usually due to a decrease in blood supply or a slowing of the peripheral circulation. The latter commonly arises with exposure to cold, reduced cardiac output, or peripheral vascular disease.

Note that one cannot have central cyanosis without also demonstrating peripheral cyanosis. Peripheral cyanosis, however, can occur alone.

Jaundice

Jaundice (icterus) refers to a yellow pigmentation of those tissues in the body that contain elastin (skin, sclerae, and mucosa) and occurs from an increase in plasma bilirubin (visible at >35 µmol/L).

It is best appreciated in fair-skinned individuals in natural daylight. Jaundice should not be confused with carotenemia, which also causes a yellow discoloration of the skin, but the sclerae remain white.

During the examination, expose the sclera by gently holding down the lower lid and asking the patient to look upward. It is important that the examiner consider the possibility that in patients with black or brown skin, hyperpigmented areas on the sclera are often nonpathological and are associated with the presence of melanin in the tissue of the sclera.

Other abnormalities of coloration

You will see other distinctive color patterns throughout this book; a list here would be lengthy and probably unnecessary.

These include the classic slate-gray appearance of hemachromatosis, silver-gray coloration in argyra (silver poisoning), hyperpigmented skinfold pigmentation seen in Addison's disease, and nonpigmented patches of vitiligo (📖 p. 83).

Temperature

- Record the patient's temperature using either a mercury or electronic thermometer. The recording will depend on the site of measurement.
- Normal oral temperature is usually considered to be 98.6°F, with a range of 97.5° to 99.5°F. Rectal temperature is 1.0°F higher and axillary temperature is 1.0°F lower.
- There is also a diurnal variation in body temperature, with peak temperatures occurring between 6 and 10 PM and the lowest temperatures between 2 and 4 AM.

High temperature

The febrile pattern of most diseases also follows this diurnal variation. Sequential recording of temperature may show a variety of patterns that can be helpful in the diagnosis of disease.

For example, *persistent pyrexia* may be a sign of malignant hyperthermia, a drug fever (e.g., halothane, succinylcholine), typhus, or typhoid fever.

Intermittent pyrexia can be suggestive of lymphomas and pyogenic infections, such as milliary TB.

A *relapsing high temperature* occasionally occurs in patient with Hodgkin's disease and is characterized by 4–5 days of persistent fever that then returns to baseline before rising again.

Also note any rigors (uncontrollable shaking), which may accompany high fever and are often characteristic of biliary sepsis or pyelonephritis.

Low temperature

Hypothermia is a core (rectal) temperature of <95.0°F and occurs usually from exposure to cold (e.g., near-drowning) or secondary to an impaired level of consciousness (e.g., following excess alcohol or drug overdose) or in the elderly (e.g., myxedema).

Patients may be pale with cold, waxy skin and stiff muscles; consciousness is often reduced. Patients typically lose consciousness at temperatures <81°F.

Hydration

When assessing hydration status, you may already have obtained clues from the history. For example, a patient may have been admitted with poor fluid intake and may be thirsty. Sepsis, bleeding, or bowel obstruction and vomiting can also cause a person to become dehydrated.

Examination

- Begin with looking around the patient for any obvious clues, including fluid restriction signs, urinary catheter bag, or nutritional supplements.
- Inspect face for sunken orbits (sign of moderate–severe dehydration).

Mucous membranes

- Inspect the tongue and mucous membranes for moisture.
  - Dehydration will cause these surfaces to appear dry.

Skin turgor

- Assess by gently pinching a fold of skin on the forearm, holding for a few moments, and letting go.
  - With normal hydration, the skin will promptly return to its original position, whereas in dehydration, skin turgor is reduced and the skin takes longer to return to its original state.
  - ❶This sign is unreliable in elderly patients, whose skin may have lost its normal elasticity.

Capillary refill

- Test by raising the patient?s thumb to the level of the heart, pressing hard on the pulp for 5 seconds and then releasing. Measure the time taken for the normal pink color to return.
  - Normal capillary refill time should be <2 seconds; a prolongation is indicative of poor blood supply to the peripheries.

Pulse rate

- A compensatory tachycardia may occur in dehydration or in fluid overload.

Blood pressure

- Check lying and standing blood pressure (📖 p. 50) and look for low blood pressure on standing, which may suggest dehydration (along with many other diagnoses).

Jugular venous pressure (JVP)

- See 📖 p. 146. Assess height of the JVP, which is one of the most sensitive ways of judging intravascular volume.
  - The JVP is low in dehydration but raised in fluid overload (e.g., pulmonary edema). The latter commonly causes fine basal inspiratory rales (📖 p. 198).

Edema

- Edema is another useful sign of fluid overload (consider right heart failure, constrictive pericarditis, hypoalbuminemia). Remember to test for both ankle and sacral edema (📖 p. 55).

Edema

Edema refers to fluid accumulation in the subcutaneous tissues and implies an imbalance of the Starling forces (intravascular pressure or reduced intravascular oncotic pressure), causing fluid to seep into the interstitial space.

Edema will occur in hypoproteinemic states (especially nephrotic syndrome, malnutrition, and malabsorption) and severe cardiac and renal failure (see Box 3.1).

Examination

In ambulatory patients, palpate the distal shaft of the tibia for edema by gently compressing the area for up to 10 seconds with the thumb. If the edema is pitting, the skin will show an indentation where pressure was applied, which refills slowly.

► If edema is present, note its upper level. Edema may also involve the anterior abdominal wall and external genitalia.

When a person with edema lies down, fluid moves to the new dependent area, causing sacral edema. This can be checked for by asking the patient to sit forward, exposing the lower back and sacral region, and again applying gentle pressure with your fingertips.

Box 3.1 Some causes of leg swelling

Local causes
- Cellulitis (usually unilateral)
- Ruptured baker's cyst (usually unilateral)
- Occlusion of a large vein—i.e., thrombophlebitis, deep venous thrombosis (DVT), extrinsic venous compression
- Chronic venous insufficiency—pigmentation induration, inflammation, lipodermatosclerosis
- Lipomatosis
- Gastrocnemius rupture—swelling and bruising around the ankle joint and foot

Systemic causes
- Congestive heart failure
- Hypoproteinemia (nephrotic syndrome, liver cirrhosis, protein-losing enteropathy, kwashiorkor)
- Hypothyroidism
- Hyperthyroidism
- Drugs (e.g., corticosteroids, nonsteroidal anti-inflammatory drugs [NSAIDs], vasodilators)

Lymphedema
This is non-pitting edema associated with thickened and indurated skin. It can be idiopathic or secondary to proximal lymphatic obstruction, such as post-surgery, in metastatic cancer, or with chronic infection.

Nutritional status

The nutritional status of the patient may be an important marker of disease and is often overlooked in physical examination. The following are simple clinical measures that can be easily undertaken to assess a patients overall nutritional status.

General physical appearance

- Note the patient's overall body habitus: are they fat or thin ? Do they appear to have recently lost or gained weight ? (See Boxes 3.2 and 3.3.)
- Weight loss can lead to muscle wasting, seen as skeletal prominence, especially cheek bones and heads of humerus and major joints, rib cage, and the bony landmarks of the pelvis.

Body weight and height

All patients should be weighed with accurate scales and have their height recorded (ideally using a stadiometer).

Body mass index

The body mass index (BMI) is a useful estimate of body composition and related health risk.

$$BMI = \frac{weight\ (kg)}{[height\ (m)^2]}$$

The World Health Organization (WHO) has classified BMI as follows:
- 19–25 = normal
- 25–30 = overweight
- 30–40 = obese
- >40 = extreme or morbid obesity

Regional fat distribution

A central distribution of body fat (waist–hip circumference ratio >1.0 in men, >0.9 in women) is associated with a higher risk of morbidity and mortality.

Skin-fold thickness

Skin-fold thickness is another useful method of assessing body composition and is usually measured at the triceps halfway between the olecranon and acromial processes. This is measured using specialist calipers.

The examiner should pinch a fold of skin and subcutaneous tissue between the thumb and first finger and then apply the calipers to the skin-fold. Three measurements are normally taken and the average calculated (normal values are 20 mm in men and 30 mm in women).

Mid-arm circumference

An additional method for estimating body fatness at the bedside is to measure mid-arm muscle circumference.

As with skin fold thickness, use the midpoint between the tip of the olecranon and acromial processes as the standard measurement point. With the arm in flexed right-angle position, take three tape measurements at this point before calculating the average. Standard age and sex charts are available.

Box 3.2 Some conditions associated with malnutrition

- Any very ill patient
- Malignancy
- Metabolic disease (e.g., renal failure)
- Gastrointestinal disease (especially small bowel)
- Sepsis
- Trauma
- Post-surgery
- Psychosocial problems (e.g., depression, anorexia nervosa, social isolation)
- Dementia

Box 3.3 Some conditions associated with obesity

- Simple obesity ('biopsychosocial')
- Genetic, e.g., Prader–Willi, Lawrence–Moon–Biedl syndrome
- Endocrine (e.g., Cushing's syndrome, hypothyroidism)
- Drug induced (e.g., corticosteroids)
- Hypothalamic damage due to a tumor or trauma

Lymph nodes

An examination of the lymph nodes forms a portion of the routine exam for most body regions. As there is no need to percuss or auscultate, examination involves inspection followed by palpation. Normally, lymph nodes should be nonpalpable. Lymphadenopathy occurs when various health states result in enlargement of lymphoid tissues (see Box 3.4).

There are a great many lymph nodes that are not accessible to the examining hand—for example, within the mediastinum or the intestinal mesentery.

Several groups of lymph nodes are accessible for the purposes of physical examination. In the head and neck, these are located along the anterior and posterior aspects of the neck and on the underside and angle of the jaw (see Fig. 3.1). In the upper limb and trunk, lymph nodes are located in the epitrochlear (Fig. 3.2) and axillary (Fig. 3.3) regions, and in the lower limbs nodes can be examined in the inguinal (Fig. 3.4) and popliteal regions.

▶ Remember that the liver and spleen are often enlarged in the presence of generalized lymphadenopathy These should be examined as on 📖 p. 233 (Liver) and 📖 p. 234 (Spleer), respectively.

Inspection

Large nodes are often clearly visible on inspection, particularly if the enlargement is asymmetrical. If nodes are infected, the overlying skin may be red and inflamed.

Palpation

Lymph nodes should be palpated using the most sensitive part of your hands—the fingertips.

Head and neck

The nodes should be palpated with the patient in an upright position and the examiner standing behind—similar to examination of the thyroid gland (📖 p. 60).

Axillae

To examine the nodes at the *right* axilla:
• The patient should be sitting comfortably and you should stand at their right-hand side.
• Support their right arm abducted to 90° with your right hand.
• Examine the axilla with your left hand.

To examine the nodes at the *left* axilla:
• Perform the same maneuver as for the right, but on the opposite side.

Inguinal

With the patient lying supine, palpate their inguinal region along the inguinal ligament—the same position as when feeling for a hernia (📖 p. 243) or the femoral pulse (📖 p. 151).
• There are two chains of superficial inguinal lymph nodes—a horizontal chain that runs just below the inguinal ligament, and a vertical chain that runs along the saphenous vein.

Epitrochlear nodes

Place the palm of your right hand under the patient's slightly flexed right elbow and feel with your fingers in the groove above and posterior to the medial epicondyle of the humerus.

Popliteal

This is best examined by passively flexing the knee and exploring the fossa with the fingers of both hands—much like feeling for the popliteal pulse (📖 p. 157).

Findings

Similar to the considerations when examining a lump (📖 p. 88), during palpation of lymph nodes, the following features should be assessed:

- *Site:* Important diseases, such as both acute and chronic infections and metastatic carcinoma, will cause localized lymphadenopathy, depending on the site of primary pathology. It is often helpful to draw a diagram detailing exactly where the enlarged node is.
- *Number:* How many nodes are enlarged ? Make a diagram and detail the palpable nodes clearly and carefully.
- *Size:* Normal nodes are not palpable. Palpable nodes, therefore, are enlarged. You should measure their length and width.
- *Consistency:* Malignant lymph nodes feel unusually firm or hard and irregular. Enlarged nodes secondary to infection may feel rubbery.
- *Tenderness:* Painful, tender nodes usually imply infection.
- *Fixation:* Nodes fixed to surrounding tissue are highly suspicious of malignancy. Matted glands may occur in tuberculous lymphadenopathy.
- *Overlying skin:* Inflamed nodes may cause redness and swelling in the overlying skin. Spread of a metastatic carcinoma into the surrounding tissue may cause edema and surface texture changes.

Box 3.4 Some causes of generalized lymphadenopathy

- Hematological malignancies (e.g., lymphoma, acute, and chronic lymphatic leukemia)
- Infections
  - Viral (e.g., HIV, infectious mononucleosis, cytomegalovirus [CMV])
  - Bacterial (e.g., tuberculosis, syphilis, brucellosis)
- Infiltrative diseases (e.g., sarcoidosis, amyloidosis)
- Autoimmune diseases (e.g., systemic lupus erythematosus [SLE], rheumatoid arthritis)
- Drugs (e.g., phenytoin causes a pseudolymphoma)

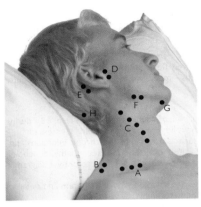

A = Supraclavicular
B = Posterior triangle
C = Jugular chain
D = Preauricular
E = Postauricular
F = Submandibular
G = Submental
H = Occipital

Fig. 3.1 Cervical and supraclavicular lymph nodes.

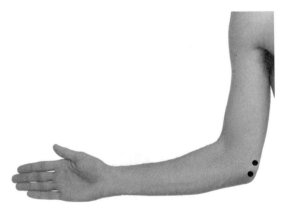

Fig. 3.2 Epitrochlear lymph nodes.

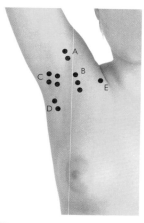

A = Lateral
B = Pectoral
C = Central
D = Subscapular
E = Infraclavicular

Fig. 3.3 Axillary lymph nodes.

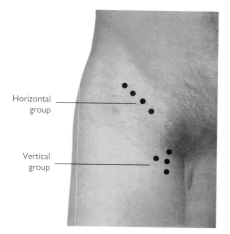

Horizontal group

Vertical group

Fig. 3.4 Inguinal lymph nodes.

Hands

Examination of the hands is an important part of all examination routines and may provide a large number of diagnostic clues. The examination of the hands, even if only through a handshake, is an almost universal part of every exam.

You will note the various 'hand signs' relevant to the body systems throughout the book.

Preparation
Begin by exposing the forearms up to the elbows and asking the patient to place their hands on a pillow on their lap with you sitting opposite.

Bedside clues
Make a point of looking around the room or the patient for any functional aids or adaptations.

Inspection
- *Dorsum:* ask the patient to hold their hands out flat, palms down.
- *Palm:* next, ask the patient to turn their hands over.
- It is often possible to make a spot diagnosis with inspection of the palmar and dorsal surfaces as many diseases cause characteristic hand changes (e.g., rheumatoid arthritis, systemic sclerosis, psoriasis, ulnar nerve palsy).
- *Skin color:* take note of the color (e.g., palmar erythema, vasculitis, digital ischemia, purpura) and consistency of the skin.
- Note that pathological palmar erythema can also be found on the thenar and hypothenar eminences and also continues along the digits.
- *Discrete lesions:* are there any discrete lesions present ? Examine as described as in Chapter 4.
- *Muscles:* look at the small muscles of the hand and the larger muscles of the forearm and make note of any wasting or fasciculation.
- *Joints:* make a point of looking at each joint in turn:
- Distal interphalangeal (DIP).
- Proximal interphalangeal (PIP).
- Metacarpophalangeal (MCP).
- Wrist.
- *Bony deformities:* look for evidence of swelling or deformities.
- *Nails:* the nails should be inspected carefully. See Box 3.7 for important nail signs not to be missed.

Box 3.5 Dupuytren's contracture
Dupuytren's fasciitis causes progressive thickening and contracture of fibrous bands on the palmar surface of the hand. This leads to a progressive fixed flexion of the fingers—usually the fourth and fifth digits.

Dupuytren's is more common in men than in women. the cause is unknown. it may be familial, sporadic, and has been associated with alcoholism, use of anticonvulsant drugs, and diabetes.

Box 3.6 Some finger joint deformities

- **Swan neck:** fixed flexion at the DIP and extension at the PIP joints—associated with rheumatoid arthritis (📖 p. 365).
- **Boutonniere:** fixed extension at the DIP and flexion at the PIP joints—associated with rheumatoid arthritis (📖 p. 365).
- **Z-shaped thumb(Hitchhiker's Thumb):** flexion at the MCP joint of the thumb with hyperextension at the interphalangeal joint—associated with rheumatoid arthritis (📖 p. 365).
- **Ulnar deviation:** a feature of rheumatoid arthritis and other conditions, the fingers are deviated medially (toward the ulnar aspect of the forearm) at the MCP joints.
- **Wrist subluxation:** deviation (either ulnar or radial) at the wrist.
- **Heberden's nodes:** swelling (due to osteophytes) at the DIP joints—a feature of osteoarthritis (📖 p. 367).
- **Bouchard's nodes:** similar to Heberden's nodes but at the PIP joints—a feature of osteoarthritis (📖 p. 367).

Box 3.7 Some important nail/finger-tip signs

- Important signs to look for are described elsewhere in this book:
- Leukonychia, koilonychia, Muehrcke's lines, blue lanulae = 📖 p. 81.
- Xanthomata, Osler's nodes, Janeway lesions = 📖 p. 156.
- Splinter hemorrhages, pitting, onycholysis, Beau's lines, paronychia, onychomycosis = 📖 p. 81.

Clubbing

Also described on 📖 p. 191. This is ↑ curvature of the nails. Early clubbing is seen as a softening of the nail bed but this is very difficult to detect. Progression leads to a loss of the angle at the base of the nail (the Lovibond angle) and eventually to gross curvature and deformity.

Objectively check for clubbing by putting the patients nails back-to-back as in Fig. 8.2. Clubbing leads to a loss of the diamond-shaped gap (Schamroth's sign).

Causes of clubbing

The full list of causes is huge. The diseases to be aware of are:
- *Pulmonary:* chronic interstitial lung diseases, chronic lung infections (e.g., bronchiectasis), cystic fibrosis, lung abscess, asbestosis, fibrosing alveolitis, lung cancer.
- *Cardiac:* cyanotic congenital heart disease, infective endocarditis.
- *Other:* liver cirrhosis, inflammatory bowel disease.

Palpation

- Palpate any abnormalities identified on inspection.
- ❶ Ask the patient if there is any tenderness and palpate those areas last.

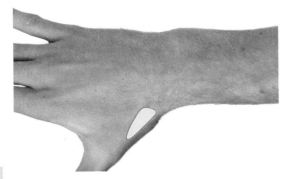

Fig. 3.5 The anatomical snuff box formed by the tendons of the extensor pollicis brevis and abductor pollicis longus laterally and the tendon of the extensor pollicis longus medially.

- Pay attention to areas of temperature change.
- It is worth remembering to palpate the anatomical snuff box (Fig. 3.5).
  - At the base of the anatomical snuff box are the scaphoid and trapezium bones. Tenderness here may be the only sign of scaphoid damage. Pathology here is easily missed.

Movement

Before assessing movement, always ask the patient if they have pain anywhere in the hands. If allowed to continue, test passive and then active movements in all joints.

Passive movements

As in Chapter 11, move each joint and assess range of movement, any crepitus and whether there is any pain.

Active movements

▶ The examination here overlaps with that in Chapter 11.

- Ask the patient to open and close their hands quickly to test for signs of myotonic dystrophy (hand will be slow to relax).
- **Wrist extension:** test with the 'prayer sign' maneuver them with fingers extended as in Fig. 3.6. Ask the patient to place their hands, palm to palm, in front of.
- **Wrist flexion:** test with the 'reverse prayer' position. Ask the patient to place their hands back to back in front of them with fingers extended (Fig. 3.7).
- **Finger flexion:** ask the patient to make a fist.
- **Finger extension:** as the patient straighten their fingers out. Also tested with the prayer and reverse prayer positions.

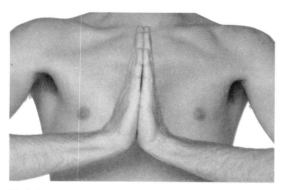

Fig. 3.6 The prayer position.

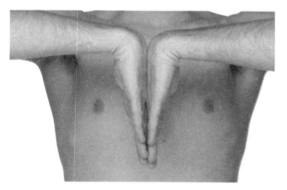

Fig. 3.7 The reverse prayer position.

- **Dorsal interossei:** (ulnar nerve). These can be assessed by asking the patient to spread the fingers apart (abduction) and resist your attempts to push them together.
- **Palmar interossei:** (ulnar nerve). These can be tested by asking the patient to hold a piece of paper between their fingers and resisting your attempts to pull it free.
- **Abductor pollicis brevis:** (median nerve). Ask the patient to put their hand out, palm upwards, and then point their thumb at the ceiling. You should then try to push the thumb back towards the hand whilst they resist you.

• *Opponens pollicis:* (median nerve). This can be assessed by asking the patient to put thumb and little finger together in an 'O' and again instructing the patient to try to stop you pulling them apart.

Sensation

Test modalities of light touch, pin prick (pain), vibration, and joint position sense in both peripheral nerve (ulnar, median, radial) and dermatomal distributions. Examining the hands neurologically is detailed on 📖 p. 312.

Pulses

Palpate both radial and ulnar pulses (📖 p. 157).

Elbows

• Always examine the elbows to elicit any clues as to the cause of joint pathology.
• For example, there may be rheumatoid nodules, psoriatic plaques, xanthomata or scars.

Function

Testing function is a vital part of any hand examination and should not be overlooked. Ask the patient to:
• Write their name.
• Pour a glass of water.
• Fasten and unfasten a button.
• Pick a coin up from a flat surface.

Box 3.8 Allan's test

This is a test of hand perfusion.
• Ask the patient to make a fist.
• Next, occlude both radial and ulnar arteries by applying pressure over them for 5 seconds.
• Ask the patient to open the palm—which should now be white.
• Release the pressure from the radial artery and look at the color of the palm. If perfusion is adequate, it should change from pale to pink.
• Repeat for the ulnar artery.

Box 3.9 Some more eponymous signs at the hand

Tinel's sign

A test for nerve compression. Commonly used at the wrist to test for median nerve compression in carpal tunnel syndrome.

- Percuss the nerve over the site of possible compression (at the wrist, gently tap centrally near the flexor palmaris tendon).
- If the nerve is compressed, the patient will experience tingling in the distribution of the nerve on each tap.

Froment's sign

A test of ulnar nerve function. Ask the patient to grasp a piece of paper between their thumb and forefinger. Alternatively, ask them to make a fist. If there is ulnar nerve damage, the thumb will be unable to adduct so will flex instead (see Fig. 10.23, 📖 p. 317).

Finkelstein's test

Ask the patient to flex the thumb then flex and ulnar deviate the wrist. Pain is indicative of De Quervain's tenosynovitis (tendons of abductor pollicis longus and extensor pollicis brevis).

Recognizable syndromes

Some physical (especially facial) characteristics are so typical of certain congenital, endocrine, and other disorders that they immediately suggest the diagnosis.

The following are the physical features of certain conditions that can be appreciated on first inspection—enabling a 'spot diagnosis'. Most of these conditions have many other features which are not detailed here.

Down's syndrome (trisomy 21)

- *Facies:* oblique orbital fissures, epicanthic folds, hypertelorism (widely spaced eyes), conjunctivitis, lenticular opacities, small low set ears, flat nasal bridge, mouth hanging open, protruding tongue (large, heavily fissured).
- *Hands:* single palmar crease (not pathogneumonic), short broad hands, curved little finger, hyperflexible joints with generalized hypotonia.
- *Other:* mental deficiency, wide gap between first and second toes, short stature, dementia of Alzheimer type, hypothyroidism.

Turner's syndrome (45 XO)

- *Facies:* micrognathia (small chin), epicanthic folds, low set ears, fish-like mouth, hypertelorism, ptosis, strabismus.
- *Neck:* short, webbed neck, redundant skin folds at back of neck, low hairline.
- *Chest:* shield-like chest, widely spaced nipples.
- *Upper limbs:* short fourth metacarpal or metatarsal, hyperplastic nails, lymphoedema, ↑ carrying angle of the elbow.

Marfan's syndrome

Autosomal dominant condition caused by defects in fibrillin gene (ch15q).

- *Facies:* long, narrow face, high-arched palate, lens dislocation, heterochromia of iris, blue sclera, myopia.
- *Limbs:* tall stature, armspan > height, hyperextensibility of joints, recurrent dislocations.
- *Hands:* elongated fingers and toes (arachnodactyly).
- *Chest:* funnel or pigeon chest, pectus excavatum, kyphoscoliosis, aortic incompetence.
- *Other:* cystic disease of the lungs (spontaneous pneumothorax, bullae, apical fibrosis, aspergilloma and bronchiectasis), inguinal or femoral hernias.

Tuberous sclerosis

Also known as Bourneville's disease of the skin. Autosomal dominant condition localized to chromosomes 16 and 9.

- *Skin:* adenoma sebaceum (angiofibromata—papular, salmon-colored eruption on centre of the face, especially at the nasolabial folds), Shagreen patches (flesh-colored, lumpy plaques found mostly on the lower back), ungal fibromata (firm, pink, periungal papules growing out

from nail beds of fingers and toes), hypopigmented 'ash-leaf' macules
(trunk and buttocks), café-au-lait macules and patches.

Neurofibromatosis—type 1

Also known as von Recklinghausen's disease—autosomal dominant.
- *Skin:* neurofibromata (single, lobulated or pedunculated, soft, firm,
  mobile, lumps or nodules along the course of nerves), Cafe-au-
  lait spots (especially in the axillae), axillary freckling.
- *Other:* kyphoscoliosis, nerve root involvement or compression, muscle
  wasting, sensory loss (Charcot's joints), plexiform neuroma, lung cysts.

Peutz–Jegher's syndrome

- *Skin:* sparse or profuse small brownish-black pigmented macules on
  lips, around mouth and on buccal mucosa, hands and fingers.

Oculocutaneous albinism

Marked hypomelaninosis (pale skin), white hair or faintly yellow blonde.
Nystagmus, photophobia, hypopigmented fundus, translucent iris (pink).

Myotonic dystrophy

- *Facies:* myopathic facies (drooping mouth and long, lean, sad, sleepy
  expression), frontal balding in men, ptosis, wasting of facial muscles
  (especially temporalis and masseter), cataracts.
- *Other:* wasting of sternomastoids, shoulder girdle and quadriceps,
  areflexia, myotonia (percussion in tongue and thenar eminence, delay
  before releasing grip), cardiomyopathy, slurred speech, testicular
  atrophy, diabetes, intellect and personality deterioration in later stages.

Parkinson's disease

- *Facies:* expressionless, unblinking face, drooling, titubation,
  blepharoclonus (tremor of eyelids when eyes gently closed).
- *Gait:* shuffling, festinant gait with reduced arm swing.
- *Tremor:* pill-rolling tremor, lead-pipe rigidity, cog-wheel rigidity,
  glabellar tap positive (📖 p. 325) small, tremulous, untidy hand writing
  (micrographia).

Osler–Weber–Rendu syndrome

Also known as hereditary hemorrhagic telangiectasia (HHT).
- *Facies:* telangiectasia (on face, around mouth, on lips, on tongue,
  buccal mucosa, nasal mucosa), telangiectasia may also be found
  on fingers. Associated with epistaxis, GI, iron deficiency anemia,
  hemoptysis.

Systemic sclerosis/CREST syndrome

- *Face/hands:* telangiectasia and pigmentation, pinched nose, perioral
  tethering, tight, shiny and adherent skin, vasculitis, atrophy of finger
  pulps, calcinosis (fingers), Raynaud's phenomenon.

Vitamin and trace element deficiencies

Fat soluble vitamins

Vitamin A (retinol)
- Found in dairy produce, eggs, fish oils, and liver.
- Deficiency causes night blindness, xerophthalmia, keratomalacia (corneal thickening) and follicular hyperkeratosis.

Vitamin D (cholecalciferol)
- Found in fish liver oils, dairy produce, and undergoes metabolism at the kidneys and the skin using UV light.
- Deficiency causes rickets (in children) and osteomalacia (in adults). Proximal muscle weakness may be evident.

Vitamin E (alpha-tocopherol)
- Widely distributed, green vegetables, and vegetable oils.
- Deficiency causes hemolytic anemia (premature infants) and gross ataxia.

Vitamin K (K_1 = phylloquinine K_2 = menaquinone)
- Widely distributed but particularly in green vegetables. Synthesized by intestinal bacteria.
- Deficiency causes coagulation defects seen as easy bruising and hemorrhage.

Water soluble vitamins

Vitamin B_1 (thiamine)
- Found in cereals, peas, beans, yeast, and whole-wheat flour. It is an essential factor in carbohydrate metabolism and transketolation reactions.
- Deficiency causes dry beri-beri (sensory and motor peripheral neuropathy), wet beri-beri (high output cardiac failure and edema), Wernicke–Korsakoff syndrome.

Vitamin B_2 (riboflavin)
- Found in whole-wheat flour, meat, fish, and dairy produce. It is a coenzyme in reversible electron carriage in oxidation–reduction reactions.
- Deficiency gives angular stomatitis (fissuring and inflammation at the corners of the mouth), inflamed oral mucous membranes, seborrhoeic dermatitis, and peripheral neuropathy.

Vitamin B_3 (niacin)
- Found in fish, liver, nuts, and whole-wheat flour.
- Deficiency causes pellagra): dermatitis, diarrhea, dementia.

Vitamin B_6 (pyridoxine)
- Widespread distribution, also synthesized from tryptophan.
- Deficiency causes peripheral neuropathy, convulsions, and sideroblastic anemia. Deficiency may be provoked by a number of commonly used

drugs (e.g., isoniazid, hydralazine, penicillamine) and is also seen in alcoholism and pregnancy.

Vitamin B₁₂ (cyanocobalamin)

- Causes of a deficiency are numerous and include partial or total gastrectomy, Crohn's disease, ileal resection, jejunal diverticulae, blind loop syndrome, and tapeworm.
- Deficiency causes megaloblastic anemia, peripheral neuropathy, subacute combined degeneration of the spinal cord depression, psychosis, and optic atrophy.

Vitamin B₉ (folic acid)

- Deficiency can be caused by poor diet, malabsorption states, celiac disease, Crohn's disease, gastrectomy, drugs (e.g., methotrexate, phenytoin), excessive utilization (e.g., leukemia, malignancy, inflammatory disease).
- Consequences of deficiency include megaloblastic anemia, and glossitis.

Vitamin C (ascorbic acid)

Deficiency causes scurvy (perifoillicular hemorrhage, bleeding swollen gums, spontaneous bruising, corkscrew hair, failure of wound healing), anemia, and osteoporosis.

Trace elements

Copper

- Deficiency results in hypochromic and microcytic anemia, Wilson's disease, impaired bone mineralization, Menks' kinky hair syndrome (growth failure, mental deficiency, bone lesions, brittle hair, anemia).
- Usually caused by copper malabsorption.

Zinc

Deficiency causes achondromatosis enterpathica (infants develop growth retardation, hair loss, severe diarrhea, candida and bacterial infections), impaired wound healing, skin ulcers, alopecia, night blindness, confusion, apathy, and depression.

Magnesium

Severe deficiency can cause cardiac arrhythmias, paraesthesia and tetany.

Iodine

Severe deficiency can cause cretinism (children), hypothyroidism, and goiter.

The elderly patient

Many individuals perceive a comprehensive physical examination to be an intrusive event that is best avoided if possible. However, for older people, in whom the 'typical' presentations of illness may be subtle or unusual, a thorough physical examination is a cornerstone of assessment.

The value of a thorough physical examination can be underestimated by healthcare professionals, but may be highly regarded as a therapeutic benefit by patients. This general overview complements the system-based chapters that follow, but the key message is repeated throughout—to reinforce the value of a comprehensive, holistic and unrushed examination.

General points

Use your eyes
A key question in your mind should be 'is the patient unwell ?'. Learn not to overlook key indices such as hypothermia (see below) and delirium which point to an acutely unwell patient.

Seek additional diagnoses
Multiple illnesses are a typical feature of old age—seemingly incidental findings (to the presenting condition) are common, so look out for skin lesions which are often malignant, new/isolated patches of 'psoriasis' (Bowen's disease ?), asymptomatic peripheral arterial disease etc.

Talk to your patient
During the examination. As indicated, it is often of huge therapeutic benefit, of reassurance, engendering trust, and potentially gaining additional history—especially if an incidental lesion is discovered.

Key points

Observations
It is essential that observations be recorded and acted upon. Detailed documentation is essential so that all members of the healthcare team are made aware of the findings of the assessment, and actions taken on behalf of the patient to address one's findings.
- Many patients may run low blood pressures, often as a consequence of medications—a small drop from this point is easily overlooked, but may be the only sign of a myocardial infarction.
- Recognize the limits of temperature/ or fever in the elderly—seriously ill older people may actually be hypothermic.

Hydration
may be difficult to assess—reduction in skin turgor through changes in elasticity with age, dry mucous membranes (e.g., through mouth breathing), or sunken eyes (muscle wasting, weight loss) are useful in younger patients, but less reliable in elders.

A useful alternative is axillary palpation—are they sweating ?

Skin and nail health
asteatosis and varicose eczema are common, but easily overlooked.

- Look out for typical lesions in atypical places—squamous cell carcinomas are notorious in this respect.
- Learn to look at footwear/toenails—is there onychomycosis ?

Nutrition
Signs of weight loss are often obvious—ill-fitting clothes and dentures are good examples.

Joints
Remember to look and examine—is the patient's mobility worse, or the reason for falling acute (pseudo) gout ?

Mini Mental Status Examination
Should be mandatory for the majority of patients.

Gait (where possible)
Akin to the mental status examination, should be undertaken whenever possible. See the Chapter 10 (📖 p. 321) for a brief description of the 'get up and go' test.

Box 3.10 Geriatric giants

So described by Bernard Isaacs, one of the key figures of contemporary geriatric medicine. Isaacs described five 'giants'
- Immobility
- Instability
- Incontinence
- Intellectual impairment
- Iatrogenic illness

These are not 'diagnoses', so avoid reaching them—but extremely common presentations of illness in older people, for which an underlying cause (or causes!) should be sought.

Skin, hair, and nails

Applied anatomy and physiology

The skin, nails, hairs, glands, and associated nerve endings make up the integumentary system.

Skin

The skin acts as a physical, biochemical, and immunological barrier between the outside world and the body. It also has a role in temperature regulation, synthesis of vitamin D, prevention of water loss, antigen presentation, and sensation.

It is important to remember that the skin also has an important psychosocial function. When we look at another person, we are in fact looking at their skin. As our skin represents our outward appearance to the world, unsightly blemishes or lesions can have a significant impact on a person's self-esteem, despite their small size.

The skin is made up of 3 layers—epidermis, dermis, and hypodermis.

Epidermis

This is the outermost layer and is formed of a modified stratified squamous epithelium. Almost 90% of epithelial cells are keratinocytes. These cells are produced in the basal layer and then rise to the surface as more are produced below and the outer cells are shed. The time from forming in the basal layer to shedding is usually about 3 months.

Melanocytes reside in the basal layer and secrete melanin into surrounding keratinocytes via long projections. This, along with the underlying fat and blood, gives the skin its color. In this way, skin tone is determined by the size and number of melanin granules, not by the number of melanocytes.

Dermis

Below the epidermis lies a layer of connective tissue consisting of collagen, elastic fibers, and ground substance. This is where the skin appendages, muscles, nerves, and blood vessels lie.

Hypodermis

Also known as the subcutaneous layer or the superficial fascia, this consists of adipose tissue and serves for lipid storage and provides insulation. It also contributes to the body contours and shape.

Glands

After infancy, sebaceous glands become active again at puberty and secrete sebum, a mixture of fatty acids and salts, directly onto the skin or into the necks of hair follicles. This waterproofs and lubricates the skin and hair. These glands are particularly numerous in the upper chest, back, face, and scalp.

Sweat glands secrete a mixture of water, electrolytes, urea, urate, ammonia, and mild acids. Eccrine sweat glands are found all over the body surface, besides the mucosa. Apocrine sweat glands are found in the axillae and pubic regions, secrete a more viscous sweat, and are under autonomic control. They do not function until puberty.

Hair

Hairs are formed by follicles of specialized epidermal cells buried deep in the dermis. Humans are covered with hair, apart from the palms, soles, inner surface of the labia minora, prepuce, and glans penis. Most hair is fine, unpigmented, *vellous* hair and not easily seen. *Terminal* hair is coarser, pigmented, and seen on the scalp, beard, and pubic regions.

Growth is cyclical with each follicle shedding its hair and then regrowing. A cycle lasts ~4 years for scalp hair. Pregnancy can have widely variable effects on hair appearance, growth, loss, texture and strength.

Nails

These are sheets of keratin that are continuously produced by the matrix at the proximal end of the nail plate. This can often be seen as the small, lighter, crescent-shaped area just before the cuticle. Nails grow at ~0.1 mm/day, toenails growing slower than fingernails.

Dermatological history

Patients with a skin condition may describe a variety of complaints. However, whether they talk of a rash, spots, growth, lump, ulcer, itch, or pain, the following guide should be used.

The history should help you establish the time course and behavior of the complaint as well as any possible precipitating or exacerbating factors.

▶ Don't waste time listening to the patient describe what the rash looks like—you're about to examine it yourself!

History of presenting illness

- When was the problem first noticed?
- How have things changed since? Has it been a continuous or intermittent problem?
- Where did it start?
- Has it spread—is it still spreading?
- If spreading, is it spreading from the edge or appearing in crops?
- What is the distribution of the problem?
- Is there any discharge, bleeding, or scale?
- Is there pain, itch, or altered sensation?
- Has it started to resolve?
- Are there any obvious factors that either trigger or relieve the problem? Ask especially about the following:
  • UV light (sunlight)
  • Foods
  • Temperature
  • Contact with any other substances
- What has it been treated with—was the treatment effective?
- Are there any systemic symptoms such as fever, headache, fatigue, anorexia, weight loss, or sore throat?

PMH

- Are there previous skin problems?
- Does the patient have diabetes, connective tissue disease, inflammatory bowel disease, asthma?
- What does the patient use on their skin—e.g., soaps, creams, cleansers, aloe or other plant products?

Allergies

Remember to ask about the *nature* of any allergic reaction.

Drug history

- Which drugs is the patient taking and for how long?
- Did the start of any therapy coincide with the start of the skin complaint? (Remember, there can be a delay of months before a rash becomes apparent.)
- Remember to ask about topical and over-the-counter drugs and alternative treatments and herbal products.

FH
Ask especially about atopy, eczema, psoriasis, and skin cancers.

SH
- Occupation?
- Hobbies? Include pets and any pets of close friends or relatives.
- Living conditions—how many share the house or living space?
- Recent travel? Were appropriate vaccinations received before leaving?
- Insect bites?
- Has the patient been exposed to venereal disease or HIV? Consider a full sexual history—see Chapters 12 and 14.

▶ Remember, venereology was considered a predecessor to dermatology and is still combined with dermatology in some countries. Sir William Osler's famous quote "He who knows syphilis, knows medicine" is reflective of the long-standing relationship of venereology and dermatology.

Psychosocial impact
Be aware of the psychological and social function of the skin. Ask what effect the condition has had on the patient in this regard and consider whether this aspect of the condition needs to be formally addressed.

Hair and nail symptoms

Hair loss

Alopecia is the loss of hair (see Box 4.1) and should be treated in much the same way as any other symptom, noting the following:

- Mode of onset (sudden/gradual)
- Associated symptoms
- Pain
- Rash
- Family history of hair loss

Note also:

- Regions of hair loss (scalp, body, face)
- A recognizable pattern of hair loss?
  - Male-pattern baldness is at the frontal and temporal areas of the scalp and at the crown.
  - Hair loss at the very front of the scalp can be caused by pulling back of hair when styling, particularly in women.

Abnormal hair growth

Facial hair growth is common in postpubertal women, but many find this distressing. If the patient reports abnormal hair growth, treat as any other symptom but remember to ask about the following:

- FH of a similar problem
- Menstrual cycle—when was the last menstrual period? Are they usually regular or erratic?
- Symptoms of virilization (if female)—e.g., voice change, clitoromegaly
- Prescription or OTC drug use or use of any supplements?

Box 4.1 Important hair disorders and signs

- *Male-pattern baldness* commonly occurs from the second decade. Hair is lost first from the temporal regions, frontal area, and the crown.
- *Alopecia areata* is associated with autoimmune disorders and occurs in the second or third decade. Sharply defined, noninflammatory bald patches appear on the scalp. There may be exclamation-mark hairs thinner at the base. This also affects the eyebrows and beard. Nails may be slow growing and show pitting.
- *Alopecia totalis* is loss of hair from all areas of the scalp.
- *Alopecia universalis* is loss of all body hair.
- *Telogen effluvium:* Normally, hairs grow and shed at different times and different rates. A severe illness, high fever, pregnancy, and, more commonly, child-birth may synchronize all the hair follicles, causing them to shed at the same time, about 3 months later. This gives a brief total hair loss that grows back.
- *Scarring alopecia:* Inflammatory lesions causing hair loss include lichen planus, burns, and infection.

Nail symptoms

These should be treated as any other dermatological condition, but you should remember to direct your questions toward finding other conditions that involve nails (e.g., psoriasis, eczema, fungal infections) (see also Box 4.2).

Box 4.2 Important nail disorders and signs

See also Chapter 3 (📖 p. 63).

- *Splinter hemorrhages* are tiny, longitudinal streak hemorrhages under the nails caused by microemboli or trauma. They can be a normal finding in manual workers.
- *Pitting* involves tiny indentations in the surface of the nail. It is a feature of psoriasis and less commonly eczema, lichen planus, and alopecia areata.
- *Onycholysis* is is premature lifting of the nail.
- *Leukonychia* is white discoloration of the nail. It is a sign of low albumin or chronic ill health.
- *Beau's lines* are transverse depressions in the nail. They coincide with arrested nail growth during a period of acute illness.
- *Paronychia* is infection of the skin adjacent to the nail, causing pain, swelling, redness, and tenderness.
- *Koilonychia* is spooning (concave indentation) of the nail. It is associated with severe iron deficiency.
- *Clubbing:* See Chapter 8, Fig. 8.2 (📖 p. 192).
- *Onychomycosis* is fungal nail infection causing the nail to become thickened, opaque, crumbly, and yellow. It often occurs with onycholysis and may be indistinguishable from psoriatic nail changes.

Examining the skin

Avoid focusing on the area identified by the patient—the whole organ needs to be examined.

After explaining the examination and asking permission, ask the patient to undress to their underwear and lie back comfortably on the exam table or bed, and cover them with a sheet. Ensure that the room is warm and private and that you have adequate lighting, preferably in the form of an adjustable light source. You should consider having an assistant to help with and chaperone the exam.*

The examination in dermatology consists largely of a careful, thorough inspection along with an accurate description using recognized dermatological terms.

General inspection of the skin

Begin by scanning the whole surface of the skin for any abnormal lesions. This can be done in any order, but it will help you to build a pattern that you can consistently remember that does not miss any areas!

Remember to inspect those areas that are usually hidden:
- Inner thighs
- Undersurfaces of female breasts
- External genitalia
- Axilla
- Gluteal cleft (between the buttocks)

⓵ Remember also to inspect the mucosal surfaces of the mouth, nails, hair, and scalp.

Skin color
Skin color varies widely between individuals but should always be even in distribution, with normal variation for sun-exposed surfaces.

Inspecting a lesion
Inspect each lesion carefully and note the following:
- Grouped or solitary? Pattern if grouped (see Figs. 4.2. and 4.3. , 📖 p. 86)
- Distribution and location
  - Symmetrical or asymmetrical?
  - Peripheral?
  - In only light-exposed areas?
  - Dermatomal?
- Color
- Shape
- Size
- Surface
- Edge
- Nature of the surrounding skin

* The presence of chaperones is controversial–attitudes vary between geographic areas and institutions. It is considered prudent advice that providers have a chaperone present when performing a sexually sensitive examination. In practice, male providers performing an examination on a female and females performing an examination on a male should consider having a chaperone present; the need for a chaperone in other situations can be judged at the time.

For each of the previous points, describe it as accurately as you can using dermatological terms. However, if a lesion is pear shaped, it is perfectly acceptable to call it just that!

When noting the distribution, bear in mind the type of clothing (or lack of) is usually at that site and what other objects or substances that part of the body would come into contact with. (Consider especially belt buckles, watches, gloves, and jewelry.)

Palpation

Each lesion should be felt (remember to ask for, and be granted, permission first). It is rare to catch an infection from touching a rash or lesion, and it's even rarer to see a dermatologist wearing gloves. Each situation should be judged at the time—obviously, gloves should be worn if there is bleeding or exudate present or if you are examining the genitalia.

For each lesion, note the following:

- Tenderness (watch the patient's face)
- Consistency
- Temperature
  - Use the back of your hand (inflamed lesions are usually hot)
- Depth and height
- Mobility
  - What skin layer is the lesion in? Is it attached to any underlying or nearby structures?
  - Can it be moved in all directions or only in one or two?
  - Does it move with movement of underlying muscle or tendons?

Beyond the lesion

The skin condition must be seen in the context of the whole patient, and other organ systems should be examined as necessary. Remember to palpate regional lymph nodes if appropriate (See Chapter 3, Lymph Nodes, 📖 p. 58).

Box 4.3 Koebner's phenomenon

This is the tendency for certain rashes or lesions to form at the site of skin trauma, including surgical scars.

Box 4.4 Some common skin color abnormalities

- **Jaundice:** a yellow tinge to the skin; best appreciated at sclera
- **Carotenemia:** a yellow–orange tinge to the skin that is similar to that of jaundice but the sclera are spared
- **Hemochromatosis:** slate-gray skin coloration
- **Addison's disease:** darkened scars and skin creases on the palms and soles–also darkening of mucosa
- **Albinism:** a lack of pigmentation with white skin and pink irises
- **Vitilgo:** autoimmune phenomenon resulting in patchy loss of skin color

Describing a lesion

A careful description often clinches the diagnosis in dermatology. All lesions should be documented in accepted dermatological terms (Figs. 4.1, 4.2, and 4.3. and Box 4.5)

(a)
Flat, nonpalpable changes in skin color

Macule
Flat, nonpalpable change in skin color <0.5 cm diameter.
Freckles are pigmented macules

Patch
Flat, nonpalpable change in skin color >0.5 cm diameter

Elevation due to fluid in a cavity

Vesicle
Fluid below the epidermis <0.5 cm diameter

Bulla
Large, fluid-filled lesion below the epidermis >10 cm diameter

Blister
Fluid below the epidermis >0.5 cm diameter

Pustule
Visible collection of pus in the subcutis

Elevation due to solid masses

Papule
A raised area <0.5 cm diameter

Plaque
A raised area >2 cm diameter

Nodule
A mass or lump >0.5 cm diameter

Wheal
Dermal edema

Callus
Hyperplastic epidermis, often found on the soles, palms or other areas of excessive friction and use

Loss of skin

Erosion
Partial epidermal loss
Heals without scarring

Ulcer
Full-thickness skin loss
(see p. 90)
Atrophy
Thinning of the epidermis
Loss of tissue (epidermis/dermis + /or subcutis)

Fissure
A linear crack

Fig. 4.1 (a) Primary lesions.

(b)

Scale
A small thin piece of horny epithelium resembling that of a fish

Crust (scab)
Dried exudate is a crust of blood/plasma

Excoriation
A scratch mark

Lichenification
Thickening of the epidermis with exaggerated skin markings (bark-like) usually due to repeated scratching

(c)

Telangiectasia
Easily visible superficial blood vessels

Spider nevus
A single telangiectatic arteriole in the skin

Purpura
A rash caused by blood in the skin—often multiple petechiae

Petechia
microhemorrahge 1–2 mm diameter

Ecchymosis
A 'bruise,'. Technically a form of purpura

Erythema
A reddening of the skin due to local vasodilatation

Fig. 4.1 (b) Secondary lesions. (c) Vascular lesions.

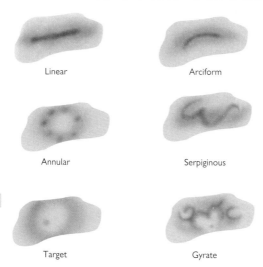

Linear

Arciform

Annular

Serpiginous

Target

Gyrate

Fig. 4.2 Descriptive terms for lesion shapes and patterns of grouped lesions.

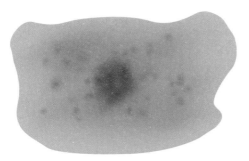

Fig. 4.3 Confluence of grouped lesions. Note how the smaller lesions coalesce to form a larger lesion.

Box 4.5 Malignant melanoma

This is an invasive malignant tumor of melanocytes, occurring mostly in white adults, and is more common in women. Malignant melanoma can be present on any skin surface but is most frequently seen on the trunk of men and women and the legs of women. It can also be found in the eyes, ears, oral and genital mucosa, and internal sites.

You should be alert to the possibility of a malignant mole if the patient describes a newly presenting pigmented lesion.

The system most commonly used to assist in diagnosis of malignant melanoma is the ABCD of the American Cancer Society.

ABCD
- A: asymmetry
- B: irregular border
- C: irregular color
- D: diameter >6 mm

Inclusion of an E, for *evolving*, is used by the American Academy of Dermatology. Recent additions to the traditional ABCD warning signs for malignant melanoma include the "Ugly Duckling sign" or "funny-looking mole."

For more information from the American Cancer Society, go to http://www.cancer.org

For more information from the American Academy of Dermatology, go to http://www.aad.org

Examining a lump

Any raised lesion or lump should be inspected and palpated as described previously. Note position, distribution, color, shape, size, surface, edge, nature of the surrounding skin, tenderness, consistency, temperature, and mobility.

When examining a lump, there are some points to pay particular attention to.

Which layer is the lump in?

- Does it move with the skin? (epidermal or dermal)
- Does the skin move over the lump? (subcuticular)
- Does it move with muscular contraction? (muscle/tendon)
- Does it move only in one direction? (tendon or nerve)
  - If the lesion belongs to a nerve, the patient may feel pins and needles in the distribution of the nerve when the lump is pressed.
- Is it immobile? (bone)

Additional characteristics to consider

- *Consistency:* e.g., stony, rubbery, spongy, soft (Remember, the consistency does not always correlate with the composition—a fluid-filled lump will feel hard if it is tense.)
- *Fluctuation:* Press one side of the lump—the other sides may protrude.
- If the lump is solid, it will bulge at the opposite side only.
- *Fluid thrill:* This can only be elicited if the fluid-filled lesion is very large. Examine by tapping on one side and feeling the impulse on the other, much as you would for ascites (see Chapter 9, 📖 p. 240).
- *Translucency:* Darken the room and press a lit penlight to one side of the lump—it will glow, illuminating the whole lump in the presence of water, serum, fat, or lymph. Solid lumps will not transilluminate.
- *Resonance:* This is only possible to test on large lumps. Percuss as you would any other part of the body (see Chapter 8, 📖 p. 196) and listen (and feel) if the lump is hollow (gas-filled) or solid.
- *Pulsatility:* Can you feel a pulse in the lump? Consider carefully if the pulse is transmitted from an underlying structure or if the lump itself is pulsating.
  - Use two fingers and place one on either side of the lump.
  - If the lump is pulsating, it will be expansile and your fingers will move up and outward, away from each other.
  - If the pulse is transmitted from a structure below, your fingers will move upward but not outward (see Chapter 9, 📖 p. 238).
- *Compressibility:* Attempt to compress the lump until it disappears. If this is possible, release the pressure and watch for the lump reforming. Compressible lumps may be fluid-filled or vascular malformations. Note that this is not reducibility.
- *Reducibility:* This is a feature of hernias. Attempt to reduce the lump by maneuvering its contents into another space (e.g., back into the abdominal cavity). Ask the patient to cough and watch for the lump reforming.

Auscultation

You should always listen with a stethoscope over any lump; you could gain important clues regarding its origin and contents. Listen especially for the following:

- Vascular bruits
- Bowel sounds

Examining an ulcer

Ulcers should be examined just like any other skin lesion, noting the position, distribution, color, shape, size, surface, edge, nature of the surrounding skin, tenderness, consistency, and temperature.

If the shape of the ulcer or its position is unusual or difficult to describe, make a drawing!

Some of the following characteristics particular to ulcers need to be considered.

Base

If the base of the ulcer can be seen (i.e., not covered with mucus, blood, or crust), it should be carefully examined and described. Ulcers usually have either slough or granulation tissue at the base. Look especially for bone, tendons, and blood vessels.

Edge

Look carefully at the edge—it may help to make a quick drawing of the edge in cross-section. Some typical edges are described as follows (also see Fig. 4.4):

- **Sloping:** These ulcers are usually shallow and a sloping edge implies that it is healing (e.g., venous ulcers).
- **Punched out:** This is full-thickness skin loss and typical of neuropathic ulceration and vasculitic lesions.
- **Undermined:** These extend below the visible edge, creating a lip. This is typical of pyoderma gangrenosum and infected ulceration such as TB.
- **Rolled:** Here the edge is mounded but neither everted or undermined and implies proliferation of the tissues at the edge of the ulcer. Basal cell carcinoma typically has a rolled edge that is often described as pearly in color with thin overlying vessels.
- **Everted:** The tissues at the edge of the ulcer are proliferating too fast, creating an everted lip. This is typical of neoplastic ulceration.

Depth

Determine what layer (of skin or underlying tissues) the ulcer extends to. If possible, estimate the depth in mm.

Discharge

Any discharge (e.g., serous fluid, pus, blood) from the ulcer should be examined and noted. If there is an overlying scab or crust (dried discharge or scale), this should be carefully removed in order to examine the base of the ulcer.

(a)

(b)

(c)

(d)

(e)

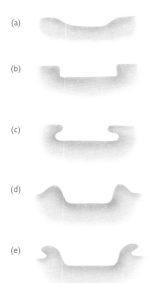

Fig. 4.4 Representation of some ulcer edges. (a) sloping; (b) punched out; (c) undermined; (d) rolled; (e) everted.

Box 4.6 Leg ulcers

Leg ulcers are often a result of mixed venous and arterial disease. However, one pathology may predominate, giving the findings below.

Venous ulceration

Venous hypertension causes fibrin to be laid down at the pericapillary cuff (lipodermatosclerosis), interfering with the delivery of nutrients to the surrounding tissues. There may be brown discoloration (hemosiderin deposition), eczema, telangiectasia, and, eventually, ulcer formation with a base of granulation tissue and a serous exudate. Venous ulcers occur at the medial or lateral malleoli especially. These ulcers will often heal with time and care.

Arterial ulceration

Along with other symptoms and signs of leg ischemia (Chapter 7, 📖 p. 178), there may be loss of hair, and toenail dystrophy. Chronic arterial insufficiency may lead to deep, sharply defined, and painful ulcers that will not heal without intervention to restore blood supply. Arterial ulcers appear especially on the foot or mid-shin.

The elderly patient

While the skin may be regarded as the largest organ of the body, it is sadly the one most often overlooked in any assessment of a patient. Many of the functional changes in aging skin make it increasingly susceptible to injury, with delayed resolution of wounds and consequent ↑ in infection risk.

Systemic illnesses often manifest in skin and nail changes, and astute assessment can resolve challenging diagnoses—e.g., erythema ab igne as a manifestation of hot water bottle use for abdominal pain and underlying pancreatic cancer or late-onset icthyosis associated with lymphoma.

For acutely ill older people, being alert to the existence and development of pressure ulcers can significantly reduce pain and immobility as well as delays in their recovery.

History

Symptoms
These should be taken seriously. While it is tempting to dismiss pruritus if there is no visible skin lesion, doing so risks missing a range of important diagnoses, including iron-deficiency anemia and liver disease.

Attributing symptoms to age-related changes in the skin should be a diagnosis of exclusion by generalists (and avoid the term *senile pruritus*—older people find it offensive). Always remember that many systemic diseases may first manifest through skin changes.

Pre-existing conditions
Carefully documenting the presence of (and treatment plan for) pressure ulcers is the obligation of medical and nursing staff. Do not shirk this responsibility—it is important to plan pressure care as critically as any other intervention. You should be particularly thorough if there is diabetes mellitus.

Medications
It is important to ask about new changes in drugs and to carefully document what an allergy or intolerance consists of—contact the patient's primary provider if needed. In the presence of infusion or injection sites, it is always important to evaluate the integrity of the site.

Functional history
Are overgrown toenails really a sign of self-neglect, or are they more likely due to poor vision, arthritis, poor handgrip, or neuropathy? Consider asking about diet, particularly in continuing-care and nursing home residents.

Examination

General
An assessment of pressure areas is critical—ask about and look for sore heels (and prescribe heel pads if needed). Is the skin frail, intact, marked, or broken? Asteatosis is extremely common, especially in states of dehydration. Prescribing emollients will earn the thanks of your patients (who may be uncomfortable and itching) and colleagues.

Edema
Avoiding hurting your patient—palpate gently. Is the edema gravitational; are there signs of venous insufficiency or hypoalbuminemia? Avoid rushing instantly to the diagnosis of heart failure.

Gravitational eczema
This is often linked with edematous change, as above. Look for pigment change and ensure that emollients are prescribed. For patients who may receive compression bandaging or hosiery, check peripheral pulses carefully. Carefully describe any ulceration present.

ECG electrodes
If you perform an electrocardiogram (ECG), remove the electrodes immediately afterward. Frail skin is easily torn and ulcerated when attempts at removal are made the next day, merely from the thoughtlessness of the person recording the ECG.

Skin malignancies

Common presentations
We all spend significant amounts of time examining and talking to our patients. Don't overlook the typical ulceration of a basal cell carcinoma around the eye or nasal region and the ears.

If you suspect a skin cancer, explore the patient's previous occupation or lifestyle. Most importantly, if lesions are suspicious, biopsy them or refer for further evaluation.

Atypical presentations
Atypical presentations of common problems in atypical sites are legion, so be thoughtful and carefully examine areas where patients might not look or be able to see (e.g., scalp, back, calves). Examine nails particularly carefully for signs of systemic disease or subungual melanoma.

Be careful about rushing to a diagnosis of psoriasis in a new, isolated plaque. This is more likely to be Bowen's disease, so seek expert review. New onset of diffuse psoriasis-like type plaques in the mature patient with no history of psoriasis may actually represent lesions of tertiary syphilis.

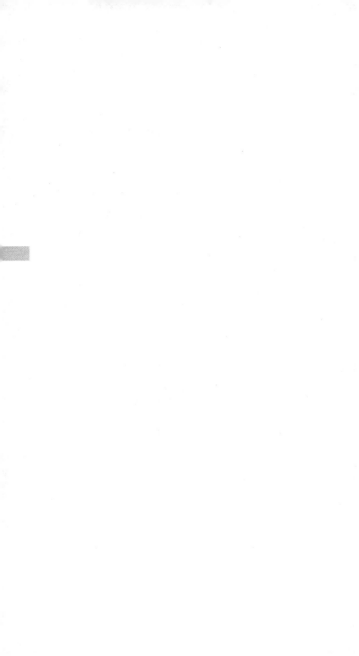

Endocrine system

Applied anatomy and physiology

The *endocrine system* is a complex, delicately balanced arrangement of hormonal feedback loops designed to coordinate organ functions. It maintains the internal environment (homeostasis), controls the storage and utilization of energy substrates, regulates growth and reproduction, and controls the organ responses to external stimuli.

The major glands that make up the human endocrine system are the hypothalamus, pituitary, thyroid, parathyroids, adrenals, pineal, and reproductive glands, which include the ovaries and testes (Fig. 5.1). The pancreas and the digestive system have endocrine components secreting insulin, glucagons, gastrin, and somatostatin.

The following is a very brief overview of those aspects of the endocrine system that may have an impact on the history and examination. Readers wanting more extensive information on endocrine physiology are advised to consult a more traditional physiology text.

The hypothalamopituitary axis

The *hypothalamus* is a collection of specialized cells located in the lower central part of the brain and, along with the pituitary gland sitting just below the optic chiasm, forms the primary link between the endocrine and nervous systems. Neurons in the hypothalamus control the pituitary gland by producing chemical releasing factors that either increase or suppress hormone secretion.

This part of the brain is also important in the regulation of satiety, metabolism, and body temperature.

The releasing factors produced in the hypothalamus reach the pituitary via a short portal system running down the pituitary stalk (infundibulum). The *pituitary gland* is a pea-shaped structure lying in a bony walled cavity, the sella turcica, in the sphenoid bone at the base of the skull. It has an anterior lobe that develops from an outgrowth of ectoderm called the *hypophyseal (Rathke's) pouch* in the roof of the mouth and a posterior lobe that is directly linked to the hypothalamus.

Anterior pituitary hormones

- *Growth hormone (GH)* stimulates general body growth and regulates aspects of metabolism.
- *Thyroid-stimulating hormone (TSH)* controls the production of thyroid hormones by the thyroid gland.
- *Follicle stimulating hormone (FSH)* and *luteinizing hormone (LH)* together act on the secretion of estrogen and progesterone from the ovaries, maturation of oocytes, and secretion of testosterone and production of spermatozoa in the testes.
- *Prolactin* initiates milk production in mammary glands.
- *Adrenocorticotrophic hormone (ACTH)* stimulates the adrenal cortex to produce glucocorticoids.
- *Melanocyte stimulating hormone (MSH)* enhances skin pigmentation.

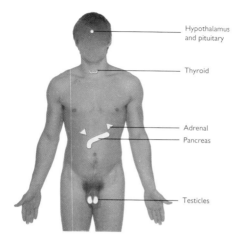

Hypothalamus and pituitary

Thyroid

Adrenal
Pancreas

Testicles

Fig. 5.1 The major endocrine glands of the body.

Posterior pituitary gland

Hormones released here are actually produced in the hypothalamus but travel down axons in the pituitary stalk to be stored ready for release. They include anitdiuretic hormone (ADH) and oxytocin.
- *Oxytocin* acts principally to stimulate contraction of smooth muscle cells in the uterus during childbirth and around glandular cells of the mammary glands to cause milk ejection.
- *ADH (vasopressin)* is secreted by neurosecretory cells in the hypothalamus in response to increased blood osmotic pressure, dehydration, and loss of blood volume. It acts to conserve body water.

Thyroid

The thyroid gland is made up of the isthmus and two lateral lobes. The isthmus overlies the second and third rings of the trachea, while the lobes extend from either side of the thyroid cartilage downward.

TSH stimulates the release of T_4 (thyroxine) and T_3 (triiodothyronine). T_3 is considered the active hormone, as it is about 2–4 times more potent than T_4, which can be considered a prohormone. Around 80% of circulating T_3 is derived from the deiodination (removal of iodine) of T_4. This takes place in peripheral tissue—the remaining 20% is secreted directly by the thyroid gland. Most circulating T_3 and T_4 is bound to proteins, including albumin and thyroid-binding globulin (TBG).

The effects of thyroid hormones are multiple, including increased baseline metabolism, O_2 utilization, energy turnover, and heat production.

Presenting symptoms in endocrinology

As hormones have an impact on every body system, it is necessary to cover all areas of general health in history-taking.

This section outlines some of the more important presenting symptoms in endocrine disease that should not be missed (if clinical suspicion of endocrine dysfunction is high), but it is by no means exhaustive.

Appetite and weight changes

Many people do not routinely weigh themselves but may have noticed the consequences of weight change—e.g., their clothes becoming looser or tighter (see Box 5.1, □ p. 100).

Lethargy

Lethargy or fatigue is a difficult symptom to pin down. Ask the patient how the tiredness affects their daily life. What are they able to do before needing to rest, and has this changed?

Fatigue may be a feature of undiagnosed diabetes mellitus, Cushing's syndrome, hypoadrenalism, hypothyroidism, or hypercalcemia.

Consider depression and chronic disease of any other kind (e.g., anemia, chronic liver and renal problems, chronic infection, and malignancy).

Bowel habit

See □ p. 312. Constipation is a common feature of hypercalcemia and hypothyroidism. Hyperthyroidism and Addison's disease may produce diarrhea.

Urinary frequency and polyuria

See □ p. 108. Common endocrine causes are diabetes mellitus and diabetes insipidus. Hyperglycemia caused by Cushing's syndrome can also result in polyuria. Polyuria may also be seen in the presence of hypercalcemia.

Thirst and polydipsia

Consider diabetes mellitus, diabetes insipidus, and hypercalcemia.

Sweating

↑ Perspiration may be seen during episodes of hypoglycemia as well as in hyperthyroidism and acromegaly and is associated with the other adrenergic symptoms of a pheochromocytoma.

Pigmentation

Localized loss of pigmentation may be due to *vitiligo*—an inherited autoimmune disorder associated with other endocrine immune diseases such as hypo- or hyperthyroidism, Addison's disease, and Hashimoto's thyroiditis.
- ↑ *pigmentation:* Addison's disease, Cushing's syndrome
- ↓ *pigmentation:* generalized loss of pigmentation in hypopituitarism

Hair distribution

Hirsutism, or excessive hair growth, in a female may be due to endocrine dysfunction. Consider polycystic ovarian syndrome, Cushing's syndrome, congenital adrenal hyperplasia, acromegaly, and virilizing tumors.

Hypogonadism, or adrenal insufficiency, leads to decreased adrenal androgen production and loss of axillary and pubic hair in both sexes.

Skin and soft tissue changes

Endocrine disorders cause many soft tissue changes:
- **Hypothyroidism:** dry, coarse, pale skin with xanthelasma formation, and, classically, loss of outer 1/3 of the eyebrows
- **Hyperthyroidism:** thyroid achropathy is seen only in hyperthyroidism due to Grave's disease. It is finger clubbing and new bone formation at the fingers. There is also *pretibial myxedema*—reddened edematous lesions on the shins (often the lateral aspects).
- **Hypoparathyroidism:** generally dry, scaly skin
- **Diabetes mellitus:** xanthelasma, ulceration, repeated skin infections, necrobiosis *lipoidica diabeticorum*—shiny, yellowed lesions on the shins
- **Acromegaly:** soft tissue overgrowth with skin tags at the axillae and anus, doughy-looking hands and fingers, *acanthosis nigricans*—velvety black skin changes at the axilla. (Acanthosis nigricans can also be seen in Cushing's syndrome, polycystic ovarian syndrome and insulin resistance.)

Headache and visual disturbance

Visual field defects, cranial nerve palsies, and headache may be caused by space-occupying lesions within the skull. Pituitary tumors classically cause a bitemporal hemianopia by impinging on the optic chiasm (□ p. 266).

Blurred vision is rather nonspecific, but consider osmotic changes in the lens due to hyperglycemia.

Alteration in growth

Hypopituitarism, hypothyroidism, growth hormone deficiency, and steroid excess may present with short stature. Tall stature may be caused by growth hormone excess or gonadotrophin deficiency.

Growth hormone excess in adults (acromegaly) causes soft tissue overgrowth. Patients may notice an increase in shoe size, glove size, or facial appearance (do they have any old photographs for comparison?).

Changes in sexual function

Altered menstrual pattern in a female may be an early symptom suggestive of pituitary dysfunction. See □ Chapter 14 for more detail.

In men, hypogonadism may result in loss of libido and an inability to attain or sustain an erection (see □ Chapter 12). Remember to look for nonendocrine causes of sexual dysfunction, such as alcoholism, spinal cord disease, or psychological illness (see □ Chapters 11 and 15).

Flushing

Flushing may be a symptom of carcinoid tumor or menopause.

Ask about the nature of the flushing, any aggravating or relieving factors, and, importantly, any other symptoms at the time, such as palpitations, diarrhea, or dizziness. Remember to take a full menstrual history (see □ Chapter 14).

The rest of the history

A full history should be taken (📖 Chapter 2). In a patient with endocrine symptoms, you should pay special attention to the following (see also Box 5.1).

Drug history

As ever, a detailed medication history should be sought. Remember to ask especially about the following:

- Over-the-counter medicines
- Hormonal treatments—including oral contraceptive pill, and local and systemic steroids
- Amiodarone
- Lithium
- Herbal or other alternative remedies

Past medical history

- Any previous thyroid or parathyroid surgery
- Any previous Iodine [131] (radioiodine) treatment or other antithyroid drugs
- Gestational diabetes
- Hypertension
- Any previous pituitary or adrenal surgery

Family history

Ask especially about the following:

- Type 2 diabetes (Box 5.2).
- Related autoimmune disorders (pernicious anemia, celiac disease, vitiligo, Addison's disease, thyroid disease, type 1 diabetes)
  - Many patients will only have heard of these disorders if they have a family member who suffers from them.
- Congential adrenal hyperplasia (CAH)
- Tumors of the MEN syndromes (Box 5.3)

Box 5.1 Weight, appetite, and endocrine disorders

- ↑ *Appetite*, ↓ *weight:* thyrotoxicosis, uncontrolled diabetes mellitus
- ↑ *Appetite*, ↑ *weight:* Cushing's syndrome, hypoglycemia, hypothalamic disease
- ↓ *Appetite*, ↓ *weight:* gastrointestinal disease, malignancy, anorexia, Addison's disease, diabetes mellitus
- ↓ *Appetite*, ↑ *weight:* hypothyroidism

Box 5.2 Diabetic history

As with other diseases, you should establish when the diagnosis was made (and how) and the course and treatment of the disease. Additional questions relating to disease monitoring and diabetic complications that you should ask patients with diabetes are as follows:

- When was it first diagnosed?
- How was it first diagnosed?
- How was it first managed?
- How is it managed now?
- If on insulin, when was that first started?
- Are they compliant with a diabetic diet?
- Are they compliant with their diabetic medication?
- How often do they check their blood sugar?
- What readings do they normally get (if possible, ask to see their monitoring booklet)?
- What is their latest Hb_A1_C (many will know this)?
- Have they ever been admitted to hospital with diabetic ketoacidosis (DKA)?
- Do they go to a podiatrist?
- Have they experienced any problems with their feet? Do they use any moisturizers or cream on their feet?
- Do they participate in a retinal screening program?
- Have they needed a referral to an ophthalmologist?
- In the newly diagnosed diabetic, ask about a history of weight loss (will differentiate type 1 and type 2 diabetes).

Box 5.3 MEN syndromes

These are multiple endocrine neoplasias (MEN) that display autosomal dominant inheritance.

- **MEN 1:** the "3 Ps: **p**arathyroid hyperplasia (100%), **p**ancreatic endocrine tumors (40–70%), **p**ituitary adenomas (30–50%)
- **MEN 2:** medullary cell thyroid carcinoma (100%), pheochromocytoma (50%), and the following:
  - **MEN 2a:** parathyroid hyperplasia (80%)
  - **MEN 2b:** mucosal and bowel neuromas, marfanoid habitus

General examination

It is not possible to perform an examination of the endocrine system in the same way that you examine other organ systems. Usually, an endocrine examination is focused—looking for signs to confirm or refute differential diagnoses that you have developed during history-taking or examining the function of one or more specific glands (e.g., thyroid).

You may, however, perform a quick screening general examination of a patient's endocrine status. Combine this with the examination described in 📖 Chapter 3.

Hands and arms

Check size, subcutaneous tissue, length of the metacarpals, nails, palmar erythema, and sweating, tremor. Note also skin thickness (thin skin in Cushing's, thick skin in acromegaly) and look for signs of easy bruising.

Assess pulse and blood pressure—lying and standing. Test for proximal muscle weakness (📖 p. 343).

Axillae

Note any skin tags, loss of hair, abnormal pigmentation, or acanthosis nigricans.

Face and mouth

Look for hirsutism, acne, plethora, or skin greasiness. Look at the soft tissues of the face for prominent glabellas (above the eyes) and enlargement of the chin (macrognathism). In the mouth, look at spacing of the teeth and if any have fallen out. Note any buccal pigmentation and tongue enlargement (macroglossia). Normally, the upper teeth close in front of the lower set; reversal of this is termed *prognathism*.

Eyes and fundi

See 📖 p. 110–113.

Neck

Note any swellings or lymphadenopathy (📖 p. 60). Examine the thyroid. Palpate the supraclavicular regions and note any excessive soft tissue.

Chest

Inspect for any hair excess or loss, breast size in females, and gynecomastia in males. Note the nipple color, pigmentation, or galactorrhea.

Abdomen

Inspect for central adiposity and obesity, purple striae, and hirsutism. Palpate for organomegaly. Look at the external genitalia to exclude any testicular atrophy in males or virilization (e.g., clitoromegaly) in women.

Legs

Test for proximal muscle weakness (📖 p. 343) and make note of any diabetes-related changes (📖 p. 108 and p. 109 respectively).

Height and weight

Calculate the patient's BMI (📖 p. 56).

Box 5.4 Signs of tetany

Trousseau's sign

Inflate a blood pressure cuff just above the systolic pressure for 3 minutes. When hypocalcemia has caused muscular irritability, the hand will develop flexor spasm.

Chvostek's sign

Gently tap over the facial nerve (in front of the tragus of the ear). The sign is positive if there is contraction of the lip and facial muscles on the same side of the face.

Examining the thyroid

The patient should be sitting upright on a chair or the edge of a bed.

Inspection

Look at the thyroid region. If the gland is quite enlarged (goiter), you may notice it protruding as a swelling just below the thyroid cartilage. The normal thyroid gland is usually neither visible nor palpable.

Thyroid gland

The gland lies ~2–3 cm below the thyroid cartilage and has two equal-sized lobes connected by a narrow isthmus.

If a localized or generalized swelling is visible, ask the patient to take a mouthful of water and then swallow—watch the neck swelling. Also ask the patient to protrude their tongue and watch the neck swelling.

- The thyroid is attached to the thyroid cartilage of the larynx and will move up with swallowing.
- Other neck masses, such as an enlarged lymph node, will hardly move.
- Thyroglossal cysts will not move with swallowing but will move upward with protrusion of the tongue.

The rest of the neck

- Carefully inspect the neck for any obvious scars (thyroidectomy scars are often hidden below a necklace and are easily missed).
- Look for the JVP and make note of dilated veins, which may indicate retrosternal extension of a goiter (see Box 5.5).
- Redness or erythema may indicate suppurative thyroiditis (Box 5.6).

Palpation

Thyroid gland

Always begin palpation from behind the patient. Place a hand on either side of their neck, which should be slightly flexed to relax the sternomastoids. ➊ Explain what you are doing.

- Ask if there is any tenderness.
- Place the middle three fingers of either hand along the midline of the neck, just below the chin.
- Gently walk your fingers down until you reach the thyroid gland.
  - The central isthmus is almost never palpable.
- If the gland is enlarged, determine if it is symmetrical.
- Are there any discrete nodules?
- Assess the size, shape, and mobility of any swelling.
- Repeat the examination while the patient swallows.
  - Ask them to hold a small amount of water in their mouth, then ask them to swallow once your hands are in position.
- Consider the consistency of any palpable thyroid tissue.
  - Soft: normal
  - Firm: simple goiter
  - Rubbery hard: Hashimoto's thyroiditis
  - Stony hard: cancer, cystic calcification, fibrosis, Riedel's thyroiditis
- Feel for a palpable thrill, which may be present in metabolically active thyrotoxicosis.

The rest of the neck

Palpate cervical lymph nodes, carotid arteries (to check for patency—can be compressed by a large thyroid), and the trachea for deviation.

Percussion

- Percuss downward from the sternal notch.
- In retrosternal enlargement, the percussion note over the manubrium of the sternum is dull, in contrast to the normal resonance.

Auscultation

Apply the diaphragm of the stethoscope over each lobe of the thyroid gland and auscultate for a bruit.

- A soft bruit is indicative of increased blood flow characteristic of the hyperthyroid goiter seen in Grave's disease.
  - You may need to occlude venous return within the internal jugular vein (IJV) to rule out a venous hum.
  - Listen over the aortic area to ensure that the thyroid bruit is not an outflow obstruction murmur conducted to the root of the neck.

Box 5.5 Pemberton's sign

This signifies thoracic inlet obstruction (e.g., retrosternal goiter).

- Ask the patient to raise both arms above the head.
  - Patients with inlet obstruction may develop signs of venous compression (facial plethora, cyanosis, dizziness, syncope).
- Look at neck veins for congestion and listen for stridor.

Box 5.6 Assessing thyroid status: examination

- Observe the patient's composure (relaxed, agitated, fidgety?).
- Measure heart rate and note if patient is in atrial fibrillation.
- Inspect hands for erythema, warmth, and thyroid acropachy (phalangeal bone overgrowth similar to pulmonary osteopathy).
- Feel the palms—are they sweaty or dry?
- Look for peripheral tremor—ask patient to stretch out arms with fingers out straight and palms down. Resting a piece of paper on back of the hand can make a tremor more obvious.
- Inspect the face.
  - Exophthalmos, proptosis (📖 p. 106)
  - Hypothyroid features (📖 p. 114)
- Examine the eyes (📖 p. 106).
- Examine thyroid and neck (📖 p. 104).
- Test tendon reflexes at the biceps and ankle (📖 p. 302).
- Test for proximal myopathy by asking the patient to stand from a sitting position.
- Look for pretibial myxedema.

Eye signs in thyroid disease

Examination

Inspection
- Look at the patient's eyes from the front, side, and above.
- Note whether the sclera is visible above or below the iris and whether the eyeball appears to sit forward (proptosis—best seen from above).
- Note health of the conjunctiva and sclera, looking especially for any ulceration or conjunctivitis.
- Ensure that both eyes can close (failure is a medical emergency).

Visual fields
It is wise to perform a quick screening test of the visual fields (📖 p. 264 and 265).

Eye movements
Test eye movements in all directions (📖 p. 276).

Lid lag(von Graefe's sign)
- Hold your finger high and ask the patient to look at it and follow it with their eyes as it moves (keeping their head still).
- Quickly move your hand downward—in this way the patient is made to look upward and then quickly downward.
- Watch the eyes and eyelids—do they move smoothly and together?
  - If lid lag is present, the upper eyelid seems to lag behind movement of the eye, allowing white sclera to be seen above the iris as the eye moves downward.

Findings

Proptosis
This is protrusion of the globes as a result of an increase in retro-orbital fat, edema, and cellular infiltration (see Box 5.7). It can be formally assessed using Hertel's exophthalmometer.

Exophthalmos
This is more severe form of proptosis. Sclera becomes visible below the lower edge of the iris (the inferior limbus). In very severe cases, the patient may not be able to close their eyelids and can develop the following:
- Corneal ulceration
- Chemosis (edema of the conjunctiva and sclera caused by obstruction of the normal venous and lymphatic drainage)
- Conjunctivitis

Lid retraction
The upper eyelid is retracted such that you are able to see white sclera above the iris when the patient looks forward.

This condition is caused by increase tone and spasm of levator palpebrae superioris as a result of thyroid hormone excess (Dalrymple's sign).

Lid lag
This is caused by sympathetic overstimulation of the muscles supplying the upper eyelid, seen in thyroid hormone excess.

Box 5.7 Eye signs of thyrotoxicosis and Graves disease

A common misconception is that proptosis and exophthalmos are caused by thyrotoxicosis, but this is not the case. Proptosis and exophthalmos may be seen in 50% of patients with Graves disease, and thyrotoxicosis may occur in Graves disease. However, proptosis may persist once thyroid hormone levels have normalized.

Eye signs of thyrotoxicosis
- Lid retraction
- Lid lag

Eye signs of Graves disease (Graves ophthalmopathy)
- Periorbital edema and chemosis
- Proptosis/exophthalmos
- Ophthalmoplegias (particularly of upward gaze)
- Lid retraction and lid lag *only* when thyrotoxicosis is present
  Visual blurring may indicate optic neuropathy, therefore, fundoscopy
(📖 p. 268) should be performed.

Examining the patient with diabetes

As diabetes has an impact on every body system, you can make the examination of a diabetic patient complex or simple depending on the circumstances (Box 5.8).

In diabetes clinics, a quick screening examination is performed looking for major complications, particularly those involving the feet.

In general, you should be alert to cardiovascular disease, renal disease, retinal disease, peripheral neuropathy, especially sensory, health of insulin injection sites, the diabetic foot, secondary causes of diabetes (e.g., acromegaly, Cushing's syndrome, hemochromatosis), and associated hyperlipidemia.

The diabetic foot

The combination of peripheral vascular disease and peripheral neuropathy can lead to repeated minor trauma to the feet, resulting in ulceration and infection, which are very slow to heal. Chronic infection and other foot complications are a major cause of morbidity and mortality in the diabetic patient (see Box 5.8 for examination).

Box 5.8 Important points for a thorough diabetic examination

Inspection
- Hydration, weight, facies associated with a known endocrine disease, pigmentation (hyperpigmentation or patchy loss)
- Legs
- Muscle wasting, hair loss, skin atrophy, skin pigmentation, leg ulceration (especially around pressure points and toes), skin infections

Injection sites
- Inspect and palpate for fat atrophy, fat hypertrophy, or local infection

Associated skin lesions
- Necrobiosis lipoidica diabeticorum—look on the shins, arms, and back for sharply demarcated oval plaques with a shiny surface, yellow waxy atrophic centers, and brownish-red margins with surrounding telangiectasia. Also look for granuloma annulare.

Hyperlipidemia
- Eruptive xanthoma, tendon xanthoma, xanthelasma

Neurological examination
- Visual acuity, fundoscopy, peripheral sensory neuropathy—evidence of injury, ulceration, and Charcot joint formation. Test muscle strength and examine feet.

Cardiovascular examination
- Ideally, a conduct a full cardiovascular examination, including lying and standing blood pressure measurements.

Box 5.9 Framework for diabetic foot examination

Inspection
- Color
- Ulceration
- Dryness
- Callous formation
- Infection
- Evidence of injury—are shoes rubbing?
- Charcot's joints (grossly abnormal and dysfunctional joints due to repeated minor trauma and poor healing from a loss of pain sensation)

Neurology
- 10 g monofilament test (see below)
- Light touch sensation, pain sensation, vibration sense, and joint position sense (proprioception)

Circulation
- Peripheral pulses (dorsalis pedis and posterior tibial)
- Temperature
  - Capillary filling time.

Using a 10 gram monofilament
Small, thin plastic filaments are used for testing peripheral sensation in the diabetic foot. They are designed such that it bends under approximately 10 grams of pressure.
- Apply filament to the patient's skin at spots shown in Fig. 5.2a.
- Press firmly so that the filament bends (Fig. 5.2b).
- Hold the filament against the skin for ~1.5 seconds and ask the patient if they can feel it.
- The filament should not slide, or stroke or scratch the skin.
- Do not press on ulcers, calluses, scars, or necrotic tissue.
  - The patient's feet are at risk if they cannot feel the monofilament at any of the sites.

(a)   (b)

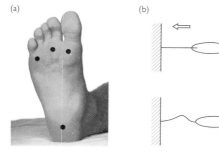

Fig. 5.2 (a) Sites to test with a 10 g monofilament in the diabetic patient. (b) Apply the monofilament to the skin with enough force to make it bend.

The fundus in endocrine disease

Diabetes mellitus

Diabetes mellitus (DM) is the most common cause of blindness in people between ages 25 and 74 worldwide. Early diagnosis and treatment of diabetic retinopathy can eliminate >95% of diabetic blindness. For this reason, it is essential for all diabetics to undergo an annual eye examination.

Mechanisms of damage

The precise metabolic mechanisms underlying the retinal changes seen in diabetes are still unclear. There may be a role for aldose reductase, the enzyme responsible for the conversion of glucose to sorbitol. High levels of sorbitol are found in the lens, pericytes, and Schwann cells of diabetic patients and are thought to lead to cell damage. A great deal of the damage may be caused by the release of vascular endothelial-derived growth factor (VEGF) in response to retinal ischemia.

The changes seen in the fundus of diabetic patients arise from common microvascular lesions. These include the following:

• Microaneurysms
• Hemorrhages—dot and blot
• Hard exudates—lipid precipitated out of the plasma
• Cotton wool spots—represent ischemia and occur from interruption of axoplasmic flow in the nerve fiber layer
• Intraretinal microvascular abnormalities (IRMA)
• Venous beading
• Neovascularization

Classification of diabetic retinopathy

A simple classification system exists and is detailed below.

Background diabetic retinopathy

Microaneurysms, hard exudates, and hemorrhages are present (Fig. 5.3). It may be extensive and widespread in severe disease.

Pre-proliferative retinopathy

Ischemia is demonstrated by cotton wool spots; venous beading may also be present.

Proliferative

New retinal vessel formation occurs (Fig. 5.4). This may progress to vitreous bleeding, traction, retinal detachment, and blindness.

Maculopathy

Pathology affecting the macula causes catastrophic visual loss:

• Exudates and hemorrhages in the macular area (Fig. 5.5)
• ▶The patient may have reduced visual acuity with no abnormality seen on fundoscopy.

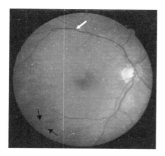

Fig. 5.3 Retinal photograph showing background diabetic retinopathy. White arrow shows a microaneurysm, black arrows show hemorrhages.

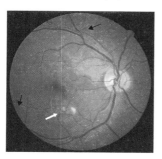

Fig. 5.4 Retinal photograph showing proliferative diabetic retinopathy. White arrow shows new vessels growing into an ischemic area (cotton wool spot). Dot hemorrhages (black arrows) are also apparent.

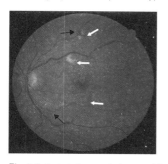

Fig. 5.5 Retinal photograph showing diabetic maculopathy. Thin white arrows show hard exudates; black arrows show hemorrhages—both within the macula. New vessels are growing into the macula (thick white arrow).

Further ocular manifestations of diabetes

While a great deal of focus is placed on retinal changes seen in diabetes, it is also worth noting that diabetic patients are predisposed to a number of other sight-threatening conditions (see Box 5.10 for prevention).

Glaucoma

- Open angle
- Neovascular secondary to rubeosis iridis—new vessel formation on the iris and interruption of the drainage angle (Fig. 5.6)

Cataract

Cataract treatment can be very difficult (Fig. 5.7). Generally, diabetic retinopathy should be treated first before contemplating cataract surgery.

Optic neuropathy

- Acute ischemic optic neuritis
- Diabetic optic neuropathy

Cranial nerve palsy

See cranial nerve examination in 📖 Chapter 10 for the common palsies associated with diabetes.

Box 5.10 Avoiding visual loss in diabetes

Management of the diabetic eye requires a multidisciplinary approach involving the primary care provider, diabetes physician, diabetes center staff, optician, ophthalmologist, and, not least of all, the patient.

Ocular examination at the time of diagnosis and yearly screening thereafter coupled with tight control of weight, blood pressure, cholesterol, and blood glucose can help the patient to avoid the devastating consequences of diabetic eye disease.

Hypertensive retinopathy

This is classified into mild, moderate, and severe forms to better correlate with the duration of systemic hypertension and associated risk of coronary artery and cerebrovascular disease (see Fig. 5.8 for treatment).

Appearance—mild

- Generalized or focal arteriolar narrowing of the retinal arterioles
- Opacity of the retinal artery walls—so-called silver/copper wiring
- Arteriovenous (AV) nicking—the retinal arteries cross the veins at a more perpendicular angle and impinge on the surface of the vein.

Appearance—moderate

- Retinal hemorrhage.
- Cotton wool spots—small areas of ischemia with resulting disruption of axoplasmic flow in the nerve fiber layer of the retina
- Hard exudates
- lipid exudates
- Microaneurysms

Appearance—severe

- All the above plus optic disc swelling

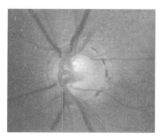

Fig. 5.6 Retinal photograph showing close-up of the optic disc in glaucoma. Note how the disc is sunken—the vessels appear to disappear into it (left side of picture).

(a)   (b)

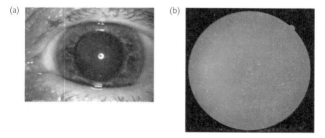

Fig. 5.7 Cataract. (a) External appearance. (b) Fundoscopy becomes very difficult or impossible.

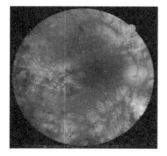

Fig. 5.8 Retinal photograph showing proliferative diabetic retinopathy treated with laser therapy. Note the multiple rounded scars on the retina.

Important presenting patterns

Hypothyroidism

Causes
These include dietary iodine deficiency, autoimmune thyroiditis (Hashimoto thyroiditis), lymphocytic thyroiditis (10% of postpartum women), drugs (amiodarone, interferon alpha, thalidomide, dopamine, lithium), radioactive iodine treatment, surgical thyroid injury, external irradiation (e.g., for head and neck neoplasms or breast cancer), and pituitary adenoma.

Symptoms
Symptoms include tiredness, weight gain, anorexia, cold intolerance, poor memory, depression, ↓ libido, goiter, puffy eyes, brittle hair, dry skin, arthralgia, myalgia, muscle weakness, constipation, and menorrhagia.

Signs
A croaking voice, mental and physical sluggishness, and pseudodementia "myxedema madness" can be present.

Inspection
- Coarse, cool dry skin (look for yellowish tint of carotenemia "peaches and cream" complexion), palmar crease pallor, peripheral cyanosis, puffy lower eyelids, loss of outer 1/3 of eyebrows, thinning of scalp hair, tongue swelling, xanthalasma

Cardiovascular and chest
- Mild hypertension, pericarditis, pleural effusion, low cardiac output, cardiac failure, bradycardia, small-volume pulse

Neurological
- Carpal tunnel syndrome, peripheral neuropathy, cerebellar syndrome, proximal muscle weakness, myotonia, muscular hypertrophy, delayed ankle jerks, bilateral neural deafness (seen in congenital hypothyroidism)

Hyperthyroidism

Causes
These include Graves disease, chronic thyroiditis (Hashimoto thyroiditis), sub acute thyroiditis (de Quervain thyroiditis), postpartum thyroiditis, drugs (iodine-induced, amiodarone), bacterial thyroiditis, postviral thyroiditis, idiopathic, toxic multinodular goitre, malignancy (toxic adenoma, TSH-producing pituitary tumors).

Symptoms
Symptoms include weight loss, ↑ appetite, irritability, restlessness, muscle weakness, tremor, breathlessness, palpitations, sweating, heat intolerance, itching, thirst, vomiting, diarrhea, eye complaints (Graves ophthalmopathy), oligomenorrhea, loss of libido, and gynecomastia.

Signs
Irritability and weight loss can occur.

Inspection
- Onycholysis, palmar erythema, tremor, sweaty palms, thyroid acropachy, hyperkinesis, gynecomastia, pretibial myxedema, Graves ophthalmopathy

Cardiovascular and chest
- Resting tachycardia, high cardiac output, systolic flow murmurs

Neurological
- Proximal myopathy, muscle wasting, hyperreflexia in legs

Polycystic ovarian syndrome (PCOS)

PCOS is caused by abnormal metabolism of androgens and estrogen with abnormal control of androgen production.

Symptoms

These include oligomenorrhea with an ovulation and erratic periods, and infertility. Some patients present with hirsutism.

Signs

Obesity (50%), male-pattern hair growth, male-pattern baldness, increased muscle mass, deep voice, clitoromegaly, and acanthosis nigricans are among the signs of PCOS.

Glucocorticoid excess (Cushing's syndrome)

Causes

Causes include high ACTH production from a pituitary adenoma and ectopic ACTH (e.g., small cell lung cancer). Primary hypercortisolemia caused by adrenal hyperplasia, adrenal tumor (adenoma or carcinoma), use of exogenous steroids, ectopic (CRF) production (very rare), depression, and alcohol use can also contribute to excessive glucocorticoid levels.

Symptoms

These include weight gain (central or upper body), change in appearance, menstrual disturbance, thin skin with easy bruising, acne, excessive hair growth, muscle weakness, ↓ libido, depression, and insomnia.

Signs

There are supraclavicular fat pads, moon face, thoracocervical fat pads ("buffalo hump"), centripetal obesity, hirsutism, thinning of skin, easy bruising, purple striae, poor wound healing, skin infections, proximal muscle weakness (shoulders and hips), ankle edema, hypertension, fractures due to osteoporosis, hyperpigmentation (if raised ACTH), and glycosuria.

Hypoadrenalism (Addison's disease)

Causes

These include autoimmune adrenalitis (up to 80% of U.S. cases), tuberculosis, metastatic malignancy, amyloidosis, hemorrhage, infarction, bilateral adrenalectomy, and HIV.

Symptoms

Anorexia, weight loss, tiredness, nausea, vomiting, diarrhea, constipation, abdominal pain, confusion, erectile dysfunction, amenorrhea, dizziness, syncope, myalgia, and arthralgia can occur.

Signs

These include skin pigmentation (especially on sun-exposed areas, mucosal surfaces, axillae, palmar creases, and in recent scars), cachexia, loss of body hair, postural hypotension, low-grade fever, and dehydration.

Growth hormone excess (acromegaly)

Causes

Pituitary tumor (>95%), hyperplasia due to GHRH excess (very rare), and tumors in the hypothalamus, adrenal, or pancreas are possible causes.

Symptoms

These include headache, diplopia, change in appearance, enlarged extremities, deepening of the voice, sweating, tiredness, weight gain, erectile dysfunction, dysmennorrhea, galactorrhea, snoring, arthralgia, weakness, numbness, paresthesia, polyuria, and polydipsia.

Signs

These include prominent supraorbital ridges, a large nose and lips, protrusion of the lower jaw (prognathism), interdental separation, macroglossia, spade-like hands, doughy soft tissue, thick oily skin, carpal tunnel syndrome, hirsutism, bitemporal hemianopia (if pituitary tumor impinges on optic chiasm), cranial nerve palsies (particularly III, IV, and VI), and hypertension.

Prolactinoma

This is a pituitary tumor (the most common hormone-secreting tumor).

Symptoms

Symptoms depend on the patient's age, sex, and degree of prolactinemia. In females there is oligomenorrhea, vaginal dryness, dyspareunia, and galactorrhea. In males there is ↓ libido, erectile dysfunction, infertility, and galactorrhea. If prolactinoma occurs before puberty in males, they may have a female body habitus and small testicles.

Signs

Visual field defects (bitemporal hemianopia), cranial nerve palsies (III, IV, and VI), and galactorrhea can occur. Males may have small testicles and a female pattern of hair growth.

Hypercalcemia

Causes

Common causes include hyperparathyroidism and malignancy (PTHrp production or metastases in bone). Less common causes are vitamin D intoxication, granulomatous disease, familial hypocalciuric hypercalemia. Rarely, hypercalcemia results from certain drugs (e.g., bendrofluazide), hyperthyroidism, or Addison's disease.

Symptoms

These depend largely on the underlying cause. Mild hypercalcemia is asymptomatic. Higher levels may cause nausea, vomiting, drowsiness, confusion, abdominal pain, constipation, depression, muscle weakness, myalgia, polyuria, headache, and coma.

Signs

Often there are signs of the underlying cause. There are no specific signs of hypercalcemia.

Hypocalcemia

Causes

These include hypoalbuminemia, hypomagnesemia, hyperphosphatemia, surgery to the thyroid or parathyroid glands, parathyroid hormone (PTH) deficiency or resistance, and vitamin D deficiency.

Symptoms

Depression, paresthesia around the mouth, and muscle spasms occur.

Signs

Carpopedal spasm (flexion at the wrist and the fingers) occurs when blood supply to the hand is reduced by inflating a sphygmomanometer cuff on the arm (Trousseau's sign). There is also nervous excitability—tapping a nerve causes the supplied muscles to twitch (Chvostek's sign—tapping the facial nerve at the parotid gland about 2 cm anterior to the tragus of the ear causes the facial muscles to contract).

Ear, nose, and throat

Applied anatomy and physiology

Following is a brief review of anatomy relevant to clinical examination.

Ear

The ear is involved in both balance and hearing and is divided into the external, middle, and inner ear.

The external ear is composed of the pinna (auricle), external auditory meatus, and the lateral wall of the tympanic membrane.

The auricle is divided into the antihelix, helix, lobe, tragus, and concha (see Fig. 6.2, 📖 p. 133) and is composed of fibrocartilage. The ear lobe is adipose only.

The tympanic membrane is a thin, gray, oval, semitransparent membrane at the medial end of the external acoustic meatus ~1 cm in diameter. It detects air vibrations (sound waves). These tiny movements are then transmitted to the auditory ossicles.

The middle ear lies in the petrous part of the temporal bone and is connected to the nasopharynx via the Eustachian tube. It connects with the mastoid air cells.

The tympanic cavity contains three tiny bones (ossicles: the malleus, incus, and stapes) that transmit vibrations to the cochlea and two small muscles (stapedius and tensor tympani). The chorda tympani branch of the facial nerve passes through here before it exits the skull.

The inner ear (vestibulocochlear organ) is involved in the reception of sound and maintenance of balance. It consists of a series of interconnecting bony-walled, fluid-filled chambers (vestibule, semicircular canals, and cochlea). Within the bony labyrinth is a further series of interconnecting membranous chambers (membranous labyrinth: saccule, utricle, cochlear duct, and semicircular ducts).

The vestibule and semicircular canals contain the peripheral balance organs. These have connections to the cerebellum and are important in the maintenance of posture and fixed gaze. The sensory impulses are conducted by the cochlear and vestibular divisions of cranial nerve VIII.

Nose and paranasal sinuses

The main functions of the nose and nasal cavities are olfaction, respiration, and air filtration.

The upper 1/3 of the external nose is bony; the rest is cartilaginous. The inferior surface holds the anterior nares (nostrils), which are separated from each other by the bony and cartilaginous nasal septum. The lateral wall of each cavity supports a series of three ridges called *turbinates* (superior, middle, and inferior).

The paranasal sinuses are air-filled extensions of the nasal cavity. They are named according to the bones in which they are located: frontal, ethmoid, sphenoid, and maxilla (see Fig. 6.1). Their purpose is thought to include protection of intracranial structures and the eyes from trauma, an aid to vocal resonance, and reduction of skull weight.

Mouth and throat

The oral cavity comprises the lips, the anterior 2/3 of the tongue, hard palate, teeth, and alveoli of the mandible and maxilla.

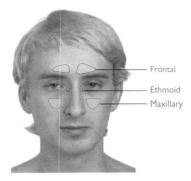

Frontal

Ethmoid

Maxillary

Fig. 6.1 Surface anatomy of the facial sinuses.

The tongue is involved with mastication, taste, swallowing (deglutination) and articulation.

Two sets of teeth develop within a lifetime. The first set is deciduous (milk teeth). The incisors are the first to erupt at ~6 months of age; the rest follow within 3 years. In the permanent set, the first molar or central incisor erupts first (~6 years), the second molar erupts at ~11 years of age; the third molar emerges at ~18 years (wisdom teeth).

The pharynx is divided into three parts: nasopharynx, oropharynx, and hypopharynx. The nasopharynx lies posterior to the nose and superior to the soft palate. The oropharynx lies posterior to the oral cavity, extending from the soft palate to the epiglottis, and contains the tonsils. The hypopharynx lies posterior to the larynx, extending from the epiglottis to the inferior border of cricoid cartilage, where it is continuous with the esophagus.

The larynx lies at the level of the bodies of C3–C6 vertebrae. It connects the inferior part of the pharynx with the trachea. It functions to prevent food and saliva from entering the respiratory tract and as a phonating mechanism for voice production. It is supported by a framework of hyaline cartilage connected by ligaments.

The thyroid cartilage is the largest of the laryngeal cartilages and can be seen as the Adam's apple. The nervous supply of the larynx is from cranial nerve X (sensory and motor).

The epiglottis is attached to the thyroid cartilage and occludes the laryngeal inlet during swallowing.

Salivary glands

The main salivary glands are the parotid, submandibular, and sublingual. The sublingual glands are the smallest; their ducts open onto the floor of the mouth, as do the ducts of the submandibular glands. The parotid glands are the largest ones. The parotid ducts cross the masseter muscles and open into the oral cavity opposite the upper second molar teeth.

Symptoms of ear disorders

Otalgia

Earache (otalgia) is common in both children and adults and may be oto-logical (local) or nonotological (referred) in cause (Box 6.1).

Take a standard pain history, as on 🕮 p. 34.

Ask about associated discharge, hearing loss, previous ear operations, use of Q-tips, trauma, swimming, and air travel.

▶ Remember that the ear has a sensory supply from cranial nerves V, IX, and X and from the second and third cervical nerves, so otalgia may be referred from several other areas.

Otorrhea

This is discharge from the external auditory meatus. Ask about other ear symptoms, when the discharge began, and any precipitating or exacerbat-ing factors. Ask especially about the nature of the discharge:

• Watery: eczema, cerebrospinal fluid (CSF)
• Purulent: acute otitis externa
• Mucoid: chronic suppurative otitis media with perforation
• Mucopurulent or blood-stained: trauma, acute otitis media, cancer
• Foul-smelling: chronic suppurative otitis media ± cholesteatoma

Hearing loss

Deafness or total hearing loss is unusual. Hearing loss is usually described as being mild, moderate, or profound. Hearing loss may be conductive, sensorineural, mixed, or nonorganic.

Conductive hearing loss may be due to pathology of the ear canal, ear-drum, or middle ear (Box 6.2). Sensorineural hearing loss is caused by disease in the cochlea or the neural pathway to the brain.

Box 6.1 Some causes of otalgia

Otological
• Acute otitis externa
• Acute otitis media
• Perichondritis
• Furunculosis
• Trauma
• Neoplasm
• Herpes zoster

Nonotological causes (referred)
• Cervical spine disease
• Tonsillitis
• Dental disease
• Temporomandibular joint disease
• Neoplasms of the pharynx or larynx

Box 6.2 Some causes of hearing loss

Conductive
- Cerumen
- Otitis externa, if ear is full of debris
- Middle ear effusion
- Trauma to ossicles
- Otosclerosis
- Chronic middle ear infection (current or previous)
- Tumors of the middle ear

Sensorineural
- Presbycusis
- Vascular ischemia
- Noise exposure
- Inflammatory or infectious diseases (e.g., measles, mumps meningitis, syphilis)
- Ototoxicity
- Acoustic tumors (progressive unilateral hearing loss, but may be bilateral)

Take a full history as in 📖 Chapter 2. In particular, note the following:
- **CC:** As well as the usual questions, establish the following:
- Time and speed of onset
  - Is it partial or complete?
  - Are both ears affected or just one?
  - Is there associated pain, discharge, or vertigo?
- **PMH:** especially tuberculosis and septicemia
- **FH:** Hearing loss may be inherited (e.g., otosclerosis).
- **Drug history:** Certain drugs, particularly those toxic to the renal system, affect the ear (e.g., aminoglycosides, some diuretics, cytotoxic agents). Salicylates and quinine show reversible toxicity.
- **SH:** occupation and leisure activities should not be overlooked. Prolonged exposure to loud noise (e.g., heavy industrial machinery) can lead to sensorineural hearing loss. The Occupational Safety and Health Administration (OSHA) requires ear protection or limited exposure at levels of 90 dB or greater.
  - ⓘ OSHA mandated limits are available at http://www.osha.gov.

Nonorganic hearing loss
ⓘ Diagnose only after fully excluding an organic cause. In such cases, there may be a discrepancy between the history and clinical and audiometric findings.

Tinnitus

This is the perception of abnormal noise in the ear or head and may be caused by almost any pathology in the auditory apparatus (Box 6.3).

As well as taking the full standard history, ask the patient about the character of the tinnitus, associated hearing loss, how the tinnitus bothers them (i.e., whether sleep or daily living is affected), and any previous history of ear disease.

Rushing, hissing, or buzzing tinnitus is most common and is usually associated with a hearing loss. It is caused by pathology in the inner ear, brainstem, or auditory cortex (although it can sometimes appear with conductive hearing loss).

Pulsatile tinnitus is caused by noise transmitted from blood vessels close to the ear. These include the internal carotid artery and internal jugular vein (the latter can be diagnosed by abolition of the noise by pressure on the neck). Occasionally, pulsatile tinnitus can be heard by an observer, by using a stethoscope over the ear or neck.

Cracking and popping noises can be associated with dysfunction of the Eustachian tube or rhythmic myoclonus of the muscles in the middle ear or attached to the Eustachian tube.

▶ Remember to distinguish tinnitus from complex noises (e.g., voices, music) that may constitute auditory hallucinations and point to a psychiatric diagnosis.

Injury to the ear

- Trauma may be self-inflicted, especially in children; foreign bodies inserted in the ear can damage the meatal skin or the eardrum.
- Head injuries can cause temporal bone fractures, with bleeding from the ear. Fracture may be associated with dislocation of the ossicles or may pass through the labyrinth, causing severe vertigo and complete deafness.
- Temporary or permanent facial nerve palsy may also occur.

Deformity of the ear

- This may be either congenital or acquired (usually traumatic).
- There may be complete or partial absence of the pinna (anotia or microtia), accessory auricles (anterior to the tragus) or a preauricular

---

Box 6.3 Some causes of tinnitus

- Presbycusis
- Noise-induced hearing loss
- Menière's disease
- Ototoxic drugs, trauma
- Any cause of conductive hearing loss
- Acoustic neuromas

Pulsatile tinnitus

- Arterial aneurysms
- Arteriovenous malformations
- Glomus tumors of the middle ear

sinus. Protruding ears may cause social embarrassment and can be surgically corrected.
- Small auricles are seen in Down syndrome, often with a rudimentary or absent lobule.

Dizziness

The term *dizziness* can mean different things to different people and must be distinguished from light-headedness, presyncope, and simple unsteadiness. Two features of dizziness suggest that it arises from the vestibular system:
- Vertigo (a hallucination of movement, most commonly rotational)
- Dizziness related to movement or position change

Both of these symptoms can occur together, separately in time, or alone in different people. Disequilibrium (unsteadiness or veering) may accompany vestibular dizziness.

Important points from the history

Obtain a precise history, aiming to establish whether or not the dizziness is due to vestibular disease (Boxes 6.4 and 6.5). Ask about the following:
- Nature and severity of the dizziness
- Whether it is persistent or in intermittent attacks
- Duration of attacks (seconds, hours, or days)
- Pattern of events since the onset
- Relation to movement or position, especially lying down
- Associated symptoms (e.g., nausea, vomiting, hearing change, tinnitus, headaches)
- History, including alcohol or drug use
- Other ear problems or previous ear surgery

Peripheral vestibular lesions

Vertigo caused by vestibular problems is most commonly rotational but may be swaying or tilting. Whether it is movement of the person or surroundings is irrelevant.

Any rapid head movement may provoke the dizziness, but dizziness provoked by lying down, rolling over, or sitting up is generally specific to benign paroxysmal positional vertigo.

Box 6.4 Some otological causes of dizziness

- Benign paroxysmal positional vertigo
- Menière's disease
- Vestibular neuronitis
- Trauma (surgery or temporal bone fracture)
- Perilymph fistula
- Middle ear infection
- Otosclerosis
- Syphilis
- Ototoxic drugs
- Acoustic neuromas

Central vestibular lesions

These are not always easy to distinguish on the history, with vertigo being less evident. Gait disturbances, along with other neurological signs and symptoms, might suggest the presence of a central vestibular lesion.

Box 6.5 Some nonotological causes of dizziness and disequilibrium

- These are often more disequilibrium than dizziness.
- Aging (poor eyesight and proprioception)
- Cerebrovascular disease
- Parkinson's disease
- Migraine
- Epilepsy
- Demyelinating disorders
- Hyperventilation
- Drugs (e.g., cardiovascular, neuroleptic drugs, alcohol)

Symptoms of nasal disorders

Nasal obstruction

As well as the full history (📖 Chapter 2), establish the following:
- Is the nose blocked constantly or intermittently?
  - Constant: long-standing structural deformity such as deviated septum, nasal polyps, or enlarged turbinates
  - Intermittent: allergic rhinitis or common cold
- Unilateral or bilateral obstruction?
- Associated nasal discharge
- Relieving or exacerbating factors
- Use of nose drops or any other nasal substance (e.g., "huffing," glue-sniffing, or drug-snorting)
- ▶ Don't miss a previous history of nasal surgery.

Nasal discharge

Ask about the specific character of the discharge, which is often very helpful in deciding etiology. See Box 6.6.

The terms *catarrh* and *postnasal drip* should be reserved only for complaints of nasal discharge flowing backward into the nasopharynx.

Epistaxis

This is a nasal hemorrhage, or nosebleed. The anterior septum, known as Kiesselbach's plexus or Little's area, is the point of convergence of the anterior ethmoidal artery, the septal branches of the sphenopalatine and superior labial arteries, and the greater palatine artery. This is a common site of bleeding.

Epistaxis is most commonly due to spontaneous rupture of a blood vessel in the nasal mucous membrane.

Explore the possible causes (Box 6.7) during history-taking.

Box 6.6 Some causes of nasal discharge

- *Watery or mucoid:* allergic or infective (viral) or vasomotor rhinitis
  - A unilateral copious watery discharge may be due to CSF rhinorrhea.
- *Purulent:* infective rhinosinusitis or foreign body (especially if unilateral)
- *Blood stained:* (with unilateral symptoms) tumors, a bleeding diathesis, or trauma

---

Box 6.7 Some causes of epistaxis

- Trauma from nose-picking, surgery, or infection
- Prolonged bleeding may be caused by hypertension, alcohol, anticoagulants, coagulation defects, and hereditary telangiectasia.
- Neoplasia and angiomas of the postnasal space and nose may present with epistaxis.

Sneezing

Sneezing is a very frequent accompaniment to viral upper respiratory tract infection and allergic rhinitis. It is commonly associated with rhinorrhea and itching of the nose and eyes.

Ask about exacerbating factors and explore the timeline carefully, looking for precipitants.

Disorders of smell

Patients may complain of a decreased sense of smell *(hyposmia)* or, more rarely, a total loss of smell *(anosmia)*. Ask about the exact timing of the hyposmia and any other associated nasal symptoms.

Anosmia is most commonly caused by nasal polyps but may be caused by head injury disrupting the olfactory fibers emerging through the cribiform plate. It may also complicate a viral upper respiratory tract infection (viral neuropathy).

Cacosmia is the hallucination of an unpleasant smell and may be caused by infection interfering with the olfactory structures.

Nasal deformity

Nasal deformity may occur as a result of a trauma causing pain ± swelling ± epistaxis ± displacement of nasal bones and septum.

Disruption of the bones and nasal septum may produce a "saddle" deformity. Other causes of a saddle nose include Wegener's granulomatosis, congenital syphilis, and long-term snorting of cocaine.

Rosacea (acne rosacea) can cause an enlarged, red, and bulbous rhinophyma. Widening of the nose is an early feature of acromegaly.

Nasal and facial pain

Facial pain is not normally due to local nasal causes. More frequently, it is related to infection within the sinuses, trigeminal neuralgia, dental infection, migraine, or mid-facial segment pain.

Symptoms of throat disorders

Oral pain
- The most common cause of pain in the oral cavity is dental caries and periodontal infection. Periodontal disease can cause pain with tooth-brushing and is associated with halitosis.
- Gum disease is a common cause of oral pain.
- In elderly patients, dentures may cause pain if improperly sized or if they produce an abnormal bite.
- Take a full pain history (📖 p. 34) and ask about other mouth and throat symptoms.

Throat pain
- A sore throat is an extremely common symptom. Clarify the full nature of the pain as discussed on 📖 p. 34. It is important to establish exactly where the pain is felt.
- Most acute sore throats are viral in origin and are associated with rhinorrhea and a productive cough. Consider infectious mononucleosis in teenagers.
- Acute tonsillitis is associated with systemic symptoms such as malaise, fever, and anorexia.
- Consider malignancy in adults with a chronically sore throat (see also Box 6.8).
- Ask about symptoms associated with cancer, such as dysphagia, dysphonia, weight loss, and a history of smoking or excessive alcohol.

▶ It is important to remember that oral and throat problems may be indicative of sexually transmitted infections. Tactfully ask about sexual encounters, if indicated. Such questioning is often difficult for new providers, but one can preface the question with a brief comment as to why such questions need to be asked.

▶ Throat pain often radiates to the ear because the pharynx and external auditory meatus are innervated by the vagus (X) nerve.

Lumps in the mouth
- *Lips* are a common site for localized malignancy, e.g., basal cell carcinoma (BCC), squamous cell carcinoma (SCC).
- *Tongue*: lumps here are nearly always neoplastic.
- *Oral cavity*: blockage of a minor salivary gland might give rise to a cystic lesion called a ranula and is usually sited in the floor of the mouth.

Box 6.8 Questions regarding chronic pharyngitis
- Ask about irritants such as tobacco smoke and alcohol.
- Consider chronic tonsillitis, postnasal drip from chronic sinusitis, acid reflux, and chronic noninfective laryngitis.

Most malignant lesions on the floor of the mouth present late: pain, dysphagia, and odynophagia (pain on swallowing) are common symptoms. The buccal lining is also another very common site for cancer.

Globus hystericus (globus pharyngeus)

This is the sensation of a lump in the throat (globus hystericus or globus syndrome). It is important to ask about symptoms of gastroesophageal reflux (GER) (📖 p. 206) or postnasal drip.

It is occasionally associated with a malignancy. Ask about dysphagia, odynophagia, hoarseness, and weight loss.

Lumps in the neck

Neck lumps are usually secondary to infection but a minority are due to malignant disease. The most common cause of neck swelling is lymph node enlargement. A comprehensive history and examination of the head and neck is important.

▶ In the adult, remember that metastatic neck disease may represent spread from structures below the clavicle, including lung, breast, stomach, pancreas, kidney, prostate, and uterus. If malignancy is suspected, the history and examination should include a search for symptoms and signs in other systems.

As well as the full standard history, ask especially about the following:

• Duration of the swelling
• Progression in size
• Associated pain or other symptoms in the upper aerodigestive tract
  • Odynophagia
  • Dysphagia
  • Dysphonia
• Systemic symptoms (weight loss, night sweats, malaise)
• Smoking and alcohol habits

Dysphonia

This is an alteration in the quality of the voice. The history should be aimed at identifying any of the several possible causes:

• *Inflammatory*: acute laryngitis, chronic laryngitis (chronic vocal abuse, alcohol, smoke inhalation)
• *Neurological*
  • *Central*: pseudobulbar palsy, cerebral palsy, multiple sclerosis, stroke, Guillain–Barré syndrome, head injury
  • *Peripheral*: lesions affecting cranial nerve X and recurrent laryngeal nerves (e.g., lung cancer, post-thyroidectomy, cardiothoracic and esophageal surgery), myasthenia gravis, motor neuron disease
• *Neoplastic*: laryngeal cancer, for example
• *Systemic*: rheumatoid arthritis, angiogenic edema, hypothyroidism
• *Psychogenic*: These are dysphonias in the absence of laryngeal disease and are mainly due to an underlying anxiety or depression (i.e., musculoskeletal tension disorders, conversion voice disorders). Like all other nonorganic disorders, you must rule out organic pathology.

Halitosis

This is offensive-smelling breath. It is commonly caused by poor dental hygiene or diet. Tonsillar infection, gingivitis, pharyngeal pouch, and chronic sinusitis with purulent postnasal drip can also cause bad breath.

Stridor

This is a noise from the upper airway (see also 📖 p. 187) and is caused by narrowing of the trachea or larynx. The main causes of stridor in adults are laryngeal cancer, laryngeal trauma, epiglottitis, and cancer of the trachea or main bronchus.

Examining the ear

Inspection and palpation
- Briefly inspect the external structures of the ear (Fig. 6.2), paying particular attention to the pinna, noting its shape, size, and any deformity.
- Carefully inspect for any skin changes suggestive of cancer.
- Don't forget to look behind the ears for any scars or a hearing aid.
- Gently pull on the pinna and push on the tragus and ask the patient if it is painful.
  - Pain indicates infection of the external auditory meatus
- Palpate the area in front of the tragus and ask if there is any pain.
  - Pain indicates temporomandibular joint disease.
- Look for any discharge.

Otoscopy
The otoscope allows you to examine the external auditory canal, the eardrum, and a few middle ear structures.

Otoscope
The otoscope consists of a light source, removable funnel-shaped speculum, and viewing window that often slightly magnifies the image. On many otoscopes, the viewing window can be slid aside for insertion of instruments (e.g., curettes and swabs) down the auditory canal (Fig. 6.3).

Technique
The following is the method for examining the patient's right ear. Examination of the left ear should be a mirror image of this.
- Explain the procedure to the patient and obtain verbal consent.
- Turn the light source on.
- Place a clean speculum on the end of the scope.
- Gently pull the pinna upward and backward with your left hand.
  - This straightens out the cartilaginous part of the canal, allowing easier passage of the scope.
- Holding the otoscope in your right hand, place the tip of the speculum in the opening of the external canal. Do this under direct vision *before* looking through the viewing window.
- Slowly advance the otoscope while looking through it.
  - It is often helpful to stabilize the otoscope by extending the little finger of the right hand and placing it on the patient's head.
- Inspect the skin of the auditory canal for signs of infection, wax, and foreign bodies.
  - If wax is causing obstruction, it may be necessary to perform ear lavage before continuing.
- Examine the tympanic membrane (Fig. 6.4).
- A healthy eardrum should appear grayish and translucent.
- Look for the light reflex. This is the reflection off the surface of the drum visible just below the malleus.
- Notice any white patches (tympanosclerosis) or perforation.
- A reddened, bulging drum is a sign of acute otitis media.
- A dull gray, yellow drum may indicate middle ear fluid.

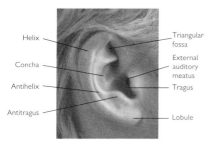

Fig. 6.2 The surface anatomy of the normal ear.

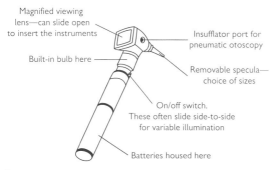

Fig. 6.3 A standard otoscope.

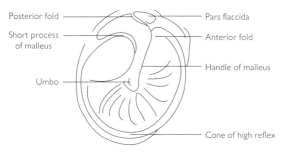

Fig. 6.4 The appearance of the normal eardrum on otoscopy.

A note on pneumatic otoscopy: Remember that this simple evaluation, when used by a reasonably skilled provider, may help avoid the necessity of sending the patient for a costly procedure. Simple procedures can be accurate and cost-effective.

Box 6.9 Testing auditory and vestibular function

See 📖 Chapter 10, Cranial Nerve VIII (📖 p. 287).

Examining the nose

External inspection
- Inspect the external surface and appearance of the nose, noting any disease or deformity.
- Stand behind the patient and look down over their head to detect any deviation.

Palpation
- Gently palpate the nasal bones and ask patient to alert you to any pain.
- If a visible deformity is present, palpate to determine if it is bony (hard and immobile) or cartilaginous (firm but compressible).
- Feel for facial swelling and tenderness.
  - Tenderness suggests underlying inflammation.

Nostril patency
Assess whether air moves through both nostrils effectively.
- Push on one nostril until it is occluded.
- Ask the patient to inhale through their nose.
- Then repeat on the opposite side.
Air should move equally well through each nostril; however, remember that nasal cycling may occur in a substantial portion of the population.

Internal examination
The postnasal space (nasopharynx) can be examined using fine-bore endoscopy. This is done by trained professionals; the student or nonspecialist should examine the anterior portion of the nose only.
- Ask the patient to tilt their head back.
- Push up slightly on the tip of the nose with the thumb (see Fig. 6.5).
  - You should now be able to see just inside the anterior vestibule.
- In adults, you can use a nasal speculum (see Fig. 6.6) to widen the nares to enable easier inspection.
- Pinch or release the speculum to the closed position, place the prongs just inside the nostril, and squeeze or release your grip gently, allowing the prongs to spread apart.
- Look at the following:
  - Color of the mucosa
  - Presence and color of any discharge
  - Septum (which should be in the midline)
  - Any obvious bleeding points, clots, crusting, or perforation
  - Middle and inferior turbinates along the lateral wall for evidence of polypoid growth, foreign bodies, and other soft tissue swelling

Testing olfaction
This is described in 📖 Chapter 10, Cranial Nerve I (📖 p. 263).

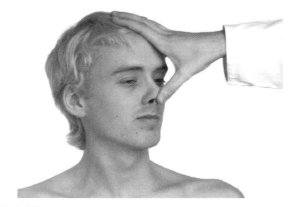

Fig. 6.5 Examination of the anterior vestibule: press nose upward with your thumb.

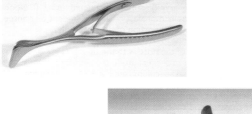

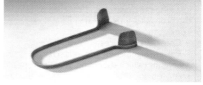

Fig. 6.6 A standard nasal speculum and Thudicum speculum.

Examining the nasal sinuses

The reader should revisit the anatomy of the sinuses and Fig. 6.1 on 📖 p. 121. The frontal and maxillary sinuses are the only two that can be examined, albeit indirectly.

Palpation
- Palpate and percuss the skin overlying the frontal and maxillary sinuses.
- Tap on the upper teeth (which sit in the floor of the maxillary sinus).
  - In both of the above, pain suggests inflammation (sinusitis).

Examining the mouth and throat

Ensure that the room is well lit. You should have an adjustable light-source. An otoscope or penlight should be adequate for nonspecialists.

Inspection

Face

Look at the patient's face for obvious skin disease, scars, lumps, signs of trauma, deformity, or facial asymmetry (including parotid enlargement).

Lips, teeth, gums

Inspect the lips at rest first.

- Ask the patient to open their mouth and take a look at the buccal mucosa, teeth, and gums.
- Note signs of dental decay or gingivitis.
- Ask the patient to evert the lips and look for any inflammation, discoloration, ulceration, nodules, or telangiectasia.

Tongue and floor of the mouth

Inspect the tongue inside and outside the mouth. Look for any obvious growths or abnormalities.

- Included in this should be an assessment of cranial nerve XII (📖 p. 293).
  - Ask the patient to touch the roof of the mouth with their tongue.
  - This allows you to look at the underside of the tongue and floor of the mouth.

Oropharynx

In order to look at the posterior oropharynx (Fig. 6.7), ask the patient to say "aaah" (which elevates the soft palate).

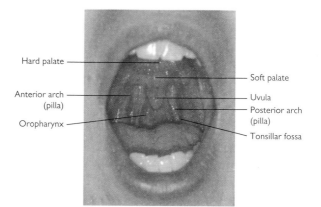

Hard palate —

Anterior arch (pilla) —

Oropharynx —

— Soft palate

— Uvula

— Posterior arch (pilla)

— Tonsillar fossa

Fig. 6.7 The normal appearance of the oral cavity.

- Use of a tongue depressor may provide a better view or it may just serve to gag the patient.

Uvula

The uvula should hang down from the roof of the mouth, in the midline. With an "aaah" the uvula rises up. Deviation to one side may be caused by cranial nerve IX palsy (see 📖 p. 289 for more detail), tumor, or infection.

Soft palate

Look for any cleft, structural abnormality, or asymmetry of movement and note any telangiectasia.

Tonsils

Inspect the tonsils, noting their size, color, and any discharge.
- The tonsils lie in an alcove between the posterior and anterior pillars (arches) on either side of the mouth.

Palpation

This is reserved for any abnormal or painful areas detected on initial inspection.
- Put on gloves and palpate the area of interest with *both* hands (one hand outside on patient's cheek or jaw and the other inside the mouth).
  - Note the characteristics of any lump (📖 p. 88).

The rest of the neck

Palpate the cervical and supraclavicular lymph nodes (📖 p. 58) and thyroid (📖 p. 104) and look for any additional masses (describe each as on 📖 p. 98).

Findings

- *Mucosal inflammation:* bacterial, fungal (candidiasis), and viral (e.g., herpes simplex) infections, or after radiotherapy treatment
- *Oral candidiasis:* radiotherapy, use of inhaled steroids, and immunodeficiency states (e.g., leukemia, lymphoma, HIV)
- *Gingivitis:* inflammation of the gums may occur in minor trauma (teeth brushing), vitamin and mineral deficiency, or lichen planus (see also Box 6.10).
- *Tonsillitis:* mucopus on the pharyngeal wall implies bacterial infection. Posterior pharyngeal wall vesicles may imply a viral origin. In teenagers think of infectious mononucleosis, particularly if the tonsils are covered with a white pseudomembranous exudate.

Box 6.10 Gum changes in systemic conditions

- Chronic lead poisoning: punctuate blue lesions
- Phenytoin treatment: firm and hypertrophied
- Scurvy: soft and hemorrhagic
- Cyanotic congenital heart disease: spongy and hemorrhagic

- Acute tonsillitis is often associated with systemic features of malaise, fever, anorexia, cervical lymphadenopathy, and candidiasis. Remember to consider HIV or other immune disorders in the presence of candidiasis!
- See Box 6.11 for causes of neck masses.

Box 6.11 Some causes of neck masses

Midline
- Lesions of the thyroid gland, thyroglossal cysts (lump moves when patient sticks out tongue), midline dermoids, submental lymph nodes, parathyroid gland enlargement (very rare)

Lateral
- Neoplasia (primary cancer, lymphoma, schwannoma, metastatic cancer), infection (mumps, glandular fever, TB, HIV), autoimmune (e.g. Sjogren's syndrome), normal variants (transverse process of C2, cervical rib, elongated styloid process), sarcoidosis, branchial cyst

Important presentations

Otitis externa

This is inflammation of the outer ear and is commonly caused by bacterial infection of the ear canal (e.g., *Streptococci, Staphylococci, Pseudomonas*) and fungi. Heat, humidity, swimming, and any irritants causing pruritis can all predispose a patient to otitis externa.

Otitis externa often occurs in patients with eczema, seborrheic dermatitis, or psoriasis due to scratching. Symptoms can vary from irritation to severe pain ± discharge.

Pressure on the tragus or movement of the auricle may cause pain.

Malignant otitis externa is a very aggressive form caused by a spreading osteomyelitis of the temporal bone (usually *Pseudomonas pyocaneus*). The infection may spread to involve the middle ear and lower cranial nerves. It is seen in immunocompromised patients and diabetics.

Furunculosis

This is an infection of hair follicles in the auditory canal. It presents with severe throbbing pain, exacerbated by jaw movement, with pyrexia and often precedes rupture of an abscess.

Otitis media and glue ear

This inflammation of the middle ear usually follows an upper respiratory tract infection.

In the early stages, the eardrum becomes retracted as the Eustachian tube is blocked, resulting in an inflammatory middle ear exudate. If there is infection, pus builds up, causing the middle ear pressure to rise. This is seen on otoscopy as bulging of the eardrum. The eardrum may eventually rupture if untreated.

Complications

These include inflammation in the mastoid air cells (mastoiditis), labyrinthitis, facial nerve palsy, extradural abscess, meningitis, lateral sinus thrombosis, and cerebellar and temporal lobe abscess.

Chronic suppurative otitis media

This is associated with a central persistent perforation of the pars tensa. The resulting otorrhea is usually mucoid and profuse in active infection.

Glue ear

Glue ear, or otitis media with effusion, is the most common cause of acquired conductive hearing loss in children (peaks at 3–6 years). There is a higher incidence in patients with cleft palate and Down syndrome. The etiology is usually Eustachian tube dysfunction with thinning of the drum.

Cholesteatoma

This is a destructive disease consisting of overgrowth of stratified squamous epithelial tissue in the middle ear and mastoid causing erosion of local structures and the introduction of infection.

When infected, there may be a foul-smelling aural discharge. Bone destruction and marked hearing loss can occur. Cholesteatoma may be complicated by meningitis, cerebral abscesses, and facial nerve palsy.

Menière's disease

This is also known as endolymphatic hydrops. There is distension of the membranous labyrinthine spaces; the exact cause is not known.

Symptoms include attacks of vertigo with prostration, nausea, vomiting, a fluctuating sensorineural hearing loss at the low frequencies, tinnitus, and aural fullness or pressure in the ear.

Attacks tend to occur in clusters with quiescent periods between. Each attack lasts only a few hours, and the patient usually has normal balance in between. Over years, hearing gradually deteriorates in the affected ear.

Vestibular neuronitis

This is typically associated with sudden vertigo, vomiting, and prostration. The symptoms are exacerbated by head movement. It often follows a viral illness in the young or a vascular lesion in the elderly. There is no deafness or tinnitus. The vertigo lasts for several days, but complete recovery of balance can take months or may never be achieved.

Otosclerosis

This is a localized disease of bone that affects the capsule of the inner ear. Vascular, spongy bone replaces normal bone around the oval window and may fix the footplate of the stapes.

Otoscopic examination is usually normal. There may be progressive conductive deafness manifesting after the second decade, possibly with tinnitus and, rarely, vertigo. Pregnancy and lactation aggravate the condition. There is often a strong family history. Both ears are affected in >50% of patients.

Benign positional vertigo

These are attacks of sudden-onset rotational vertigo provoked by lying down flat or turning over in bed. The condition is caused by crystalline debris in the posterior semicircular canal. It can follow an upper respiratory tract infection or head injury, but often there is no preceding illness.

The Dix-Hallpike maneuver (also referred to as Nylen-Barany maneuver) is diagnostic (see 📖 p. 288). If diagnosed, the person should undergo an Epley maneuver, which is often curative. This repositions the debris in the posterior semicircular canal into the utricle.

Labyrinthitis

This is a localized infection of the labyrinth apparatus and is difficult to distinguish clinically from vestibular neuronitis, unless there is hearing loss due to cochlear involvement.

Acoustic neuromas

These are benign, slowly growing tumors of the vestibular element of cranial nerve VIII. They usually present in middle age and occur more frequently in females. Bilateral neuromas occur in 5% of patients.

The early symptoms are unilateral or markedly asymmetric, progressive sensorineural hearing loss and tinnitus. Vertigo is rare, but patients with large tumors may have ataxia.

Presbycusis (senile deafness)

Presbycusis is a progressive loss of hair cells in the cochlea with age, resulting in a loss of acuity for high-frequency sounds. It becomes clinically noticeable from the age of 60–65 years, although the degree of loss and age of onset is variable.

Hearing is most affected in the presence of background noise.

Glomus jugulare tumor

This is a highly vascular tumor arising from glomus jugulare tissue lying in the bulb of the internal jugular vein or the mucosa of the middle ear.

It usually presents with a hearing loss or pulsatile tinnitus. Examination of the ear may show a deep red mass behind the ear drum. Occasionally, they are associated with other tumors, such as pheochromocytomas or carotid body tumors.

Allergic rhinitis

In allergic rhinitis, inhaled allergens are responsible for an antigen–antibody type I hypersensitivity reaction.

Common allergens in seasonal allergic rhinitis (hay fever) are pollen (including from grass) and flowering trees. In perennial allergic rhinitis, the principal allergens are animal dander,* dust mites,** and feathers. Rarely, digested allergens, such as wheat, eggs, milk, and nuts, are also involved.

The main symptoms include bouts of sneezing, a profuse rhinorrhea due to activity of glandular elements, postnasal drip, nasal itching, and nasal obstruction due to nasal vasodilatation and edema.

Nonallergic (vasomotor) rhinitis

This has all the clinical features of allergic rhinitis but the nose does not respond to an antigen–antibody type 1 reaction. The reactions tend to be to inhaled chemicals, such as deodorants, perfumes, or smoke, although alcohol and sunlight can provoke symptoms.

Allergies can coexist, and some people seem to have instability of the parasympathetic system in the nose, with excessive secretion of watery mucus and congestion (vasomotor rhinitis).

Nasal polyps

Nasal polyps are pale, grayish, pedunculated, edematous mucosal tissue that project into the nasal cavity. They most frequently arise from the ethmoid region and prolapse into the nose via the middle meatus and are nearly always bilateral.

In most cases, they are associated with nonallergic rhinitis and late-onset asthma. Other causes to consider include chronic paranasal infection, neoplasia (usually unilateral ± bleeding), cystic fibrosis, and bronchiectasis.

---

* The field of allergy research is rather interesting. Cat allergy, for example, is actually an allergy to one of the proteins in feline saliva—their fur is covered in it through licking.
** Actually an allergy to dust mite feces.

The main symptoms are watery anterior rhinorrhea, purulent postnasal drip, progressive nasal obstruction, anosmia, change in voice quality, and taste disturbance.

Septal perforation

Septal perforation may be idiopathic or caused by trauma (especially postoperative nasal surgery), infection (e.g., tuberculosis, syphilis), neoplasia (SCC, BCC, malignant granuloma), or inhaling cocaine and toxic gases.

The main clinical complaints include crusting, recurrent epistaxis, and a whistling respiration.

Tonsillitis

Acute tonsillitis is uncommon in adults in comparison to its frequency in children. The diagnosis is made from the appearance of the tonsils, which are enlarged with surface exudates. The patient is usually systemically ill with pyrexia, cervical lymphadenopathy, dysphagia, halitosis, and, in children, abdominal pain.

Complications include peritonsillar abscess (quinsy) and retropharyngeal abscess.

Laryngitis

This is frequently associated with an upper respiratory tract infection and is self-limiting. There may be associated secondary infection with *Staph.* and *Strep.* species. The patient typically complains of hoarseness, malaise, and fever. There may also be odynophagia, dysphagia, and throat pain.

Epiglottitis

🔴 This is a medical emergency. It is caused by group B *Haemophilus influenzae*. Epiglottitis is characterized by gross swelling of the epiglottis and is seen primarily in 3- to 7-year-olds, although adults may also be affected.

Clinical features include pyrexia, stridor, sore throat, and dysphagia. Remember the classic radiological feature, the "thumb sign."

Croup (laryngotracheobronchitis)

Most cases are viral (parainfluenza or respiratory syncytial virus). Croup occurs mainly between the ages of 6 months and 3 years.

Branchial cyst

These are an embryological remnant of the branchial complex during development of the neck. They are located in the anterior triangle just in front of the sternomastoid.

Presentation is typically at the age of 15–25 years.

Cardiovascular system

Applied anatomy and physiology

Cardiologists consider this system to be the most important one in the body. This system is fundamentally straightforward, and a good deal of information about its functioning can be gleaned from physical examination. The basic anatomy of the cardiovascular system should be familiar to readers. Following is a summary of some points that have particular implications for the clinical assessment.

The heart

The heart rotates counterclockwise during embryonic development, finally settling in such a way that the left ventricle lies almost entirely posteriorly and the right anteriorly—the whole seeming to hang in the chest, held by the aorta (*aorta* comes from the Greek "aorte," meaning "to suspend").

The myocardium is arranged in a complex spiral such that a contraction causes the heart to elongate and rotate slightly, hitting the anterior chest wall as it does—this can be felt as the apex beat.

All of this movement is lubricated by a double-lined cavity filled with a very small amount of fluid that the heart sits in—the pericardial sac.

Heart sounds

As the ventricles contract, the tricuspid and mitral valves close, heard as the first heart sound. As the ventricles relax, intraventricular pressure drops, and blood expelled into the great vessels begins to fall back, the aortic and pulmonary valves slam closed—this is heard as the second heart sound. The sounds are often described as sounding like *lub dub*.

As each heart sound is, in fact, *two* valves closing, any mistiming will cause a double, or "split," heart sound as one valve closes shortly after the other. A split second heart sound is normal in young adults and children. During inspiration, intrathoracic pressure drops, drawing blood into the chest, ↑ delivery to the right side of the heart, and ↓ delivery to the left as it pools in the pulmonary veins.

Consequently, the stroke volume will be greater on the right than on the left and the right ventricular contraction will take slightly longer. Thus, the pulmonary valve will close very slightly later than the aortic valve, producing the split second sound (*lub da-dub*). This is called "physiological splitting." Split heart sounds are considered on 📖 p. 168.

Jugular venous pulse (JVP)

There is no valve between the right heart and the large vessels supplying it. Thus, filling and contraction of the right atrium will cause a pressure wave to travel back through the vena cava. This can actually be seen in the neck at the internal jugular vein (IJV). See 📖 p. 161.

Arteries

As the ventricle expels blood into the arteries, it sends a pulse wave to the periphery that can be felt. This is *not* the actual flow of blood from the ventricle at that contraction but a pressure wave. The shape and feel of the wave can be altered by the force of expulsion, any obstacles (such as the aortic valve), and the state of the peripheral vasculature.

The arteries have their own intrinsic elasticity, allowing a baseline, or diastolic, pressure to be maintained between each pulse wave.

Veins

Blood flows at a much lower pressure in the veins.

Above the level of the heart, gravity does most of the work in returning the blood. Below, blood return is facilitated by contraction of muscles surrounding the deep veins, helped by numerous one-way valves to prevent backflow. Blood moves initially from the surface to the deep veins before moving upward, again mediated by one-way valves (if these valves become damaged, blood flows outward to the surface veins, causing them to swell and look tortuous—varicose veins).

Blood return is also aided by a negative pressure created by blood being pumped out of the right ventricle, and therefore drawn in through the right atrium at each beat.

Chest pain

This is the most common—and most important—cardiovascular symptom. Patients who mention it may be surprised to find themselves whisked away for an ECG before they can say anything more. It is, however, usually possible to determine the probable cause of the pain with a detailed history.

As for any other type of pain, the history must include the following:

- Nature (crushing, burning, aching, stabbing, etc.)
- Exact location
- Any radiation
- Severity (scored out of 10)
- Mode and rate of onset. What was the patient doing at the time?
- Change in the pain over time (and current score out of 10)
- Duration (if now resolved)
- Exacerbating factors (particularly, is it affected by respiration or movement?)
- Relieving factors (including the use of nitroglycerin)
- Associated symptoms (nausea, vomiting, sweating, belching, etc.)

Patients with a history of cardiac pain can also tell you whether the pain experienced is the same as or different from their usual angina.

Angina

Angina pectoris, or *angina*, is the pain caused by myocardial ischemia and the buildup of toxic products of respiration in the muscle. This is usually due to coronary artery disease but can also be caused by other cardiac diseases, such as aortic stenosis or hypertrophic cardiomyopathy.

Angina comes from the Latin for "choking," and this is often what the patient describes. As the brain cannot interpret pain from the heart per se, it is felt over the central part of the anterior chest and can radiate up to the jaw or shoulder, or down the arms or even to the umbilicus. This pattern is due to the common embryological origins of the heart and these parts of the body. Indeed, some patients may experience angina pain *only* in the arm, for example.

The "pain" of angina is usually an unfamiliar sensation; consequently, patients may be more comfortable with the term *discomfort*.

In true angina, you can expect the following features:

- Retrosternal
- Descriptions such as "crushing," "heaviness," or "like a tight band"
- Worse with physical or emotional exertion, with cold weather, and after eating
- Relieved by rest and nitrate spray, pill, or paste (within a couple of minutes)
- Not affected by respiration or movement
- Sometimes associated with breathlessness

In addition, patients classically clench their right fist and hold it to their chest when describing the pain.

In patients with known angina, a change in the nature of the symptom is important. Ask them how much exercise they can do before feeling the discomfort and whether this has changed.

Myocardial infarction (MI)

Patients will know this as a "heart attack." The pain is similar to that of angina but much more severe, persistent (despite nitroglycerin), and associated with nausea, sweating, and vomiting. Patients may also describe a feeling of impending doom or death—*angor animi*.

Pericarditis

The most common causes are viral or bacterial infection, MI, or uremia.
- Constant retrosternal soreness
- Worse on inspiration (pleuritic pain)
- Relieved slightly by sitting forward
- Not related to movement or exertion

Esophageal spasm

This is often mistaken for MI or angina.
- A severe, retrosternal burning pain
- Onset often after eating or drinking
- May be associated with dysphagia
- May have a history of dyspepsia
- May be relieved by nitroglycerin, as this is a smooth muscle relaxant (hence the confusion with angina). But nitroglycerin will take up to 20 minutes to relieve this pain, whereas angina is relieved within a few minutes.

Gastroesophageal reflux disease ("heartburn")

- Retrosternal, burning pain
- Relieved by antacids, onset after eating

Dissecting aortic aneurysm

This must be differentiated from MI as thrombolysis here may prove fatal.
- Severe, "tearing" pain
- Felt posteriorly—classically between the shoulder blades
- Persistent, most severe at onset
- Patient is usually hypertensive and marfanoid (see 📖 p. 68)

Pleuritic (respiratory) pain

This is covered in more detail in 📖 Chapter 8. It may be caused by a wide range of respiratory conditions, particularly pulmonary embolus (PE) and pneumothorax.
- Sharp pain, worse on inspiration and coughing
- Not central—may be localized to one side of the chest
- No radiation
- No relief with nitroglycerin
- Associated with breathlessness, cyanosis, etc.

Musculoskeletal pain

This pain may be caused by injury, fracture, or chondritis, among other etiologies. It is localized to a particular spot on the chest and worsens with movement and respiration. The area may be tender to palpation.

Tietze's syndrome is costochondritis (inflammation of the costal cartilages) at ribs 2, 3, and 4. It is associated with tender swelling over the costosternal joints.

Breathlessness and edema

Breathlessness and edema are presented together here, as usually they are linked pathophysiologically in the cardiovascular patient.

Excess tissue fluid caused by a failing heart will settle wherever gravity pulls it. In someone who is on their feet, it will settle in their ankles, causing swelling. If the patient is sitting in bed, the swelling will occur about their sacrum, and if the patient is lying down, fluid will collect in their lungs (pulmonary edema), causing breathlessness.

Dyspnea (breathlessness)

Dyspnea is an abnormal awareness of one's breathing and is described in detail in Chapter 8. Certain aspects of breathlessness should be asked of the cardiovascular patient in particular.

As with everything in clinical medicine, you must *quantify* the symptom, if you are able, in order to gauge its severity and as a baseline so that the effects of treatment or disease progression can be monitored. The New York Heart Association (NYHA) has devised a classification of breathlessness, shown in Box 7.1. In practice, it makes sense to measure the functional abilities of the patient. For example:

- How far can the patient walk on a level surface before they have to stop ("march tolerance")?
- What about stairs and hills—can they make it up a flight?
- Are they sure that they stop because of breathlessness or is it some other reason (arthritic knees, for example)?
- Has the patient had to curtail their normal activities in any way?

Orthopnea

This is shortness of breath when lying flat. Patients will not usually volunteer this as a symptom, so ask them about the following:

- How many pillows does the patient sleep with and has this changed?
  - Some patients may describe having to sleep sitting upright in a chair.
- If the patient sleeps with a number of pillows, ask why. Are they breathless when they lie down or is it for some other reason?

Paroxysmal nocturnal dyspnea (PND)

As the name suggests, PND constitutes episodes of breathlessness occurring at night—usually thought to be due to pulmonary edema. Again, patients won't usually volunteer this information and will often react with

---

Box 7.1 Framework for the cardiovascular examination

- I-none at rest, some on vigorous exercise
- II-none at rest, breathless on moderate exertion
- III-mild breathlessness at rest, worse on mild exertion
- IV-significant breathlessness at rest and worse on even slight exertion (the patient is often bed-bound)

Source: The Criteria Committee of the New York Heart Association (1994). *Nomenclature and Criteria for Diagnosis of Diseases of the Heart and Great Vessels.* 9th ed. Boston: Little, Brown & Co., pp. 253-256.

surprised pleasure when you ask them about it. Sufferers will experience waking in the night spluttering and coughing—they find they have to sit up or stand and many go to the window for "fresh air" in an attempt to regain their normal breathing.
• Do they wake up in the night coughing and trying to catch their breath?
• If so, describe in as much detail as you can, including how often and how badly the symptom is disturbing the patient's sleep cycle.

Cough

Pulmonary edema may cause a cough productive of frothy white sputum. This may be flecked with blood (pink) due to ruptured bronchial vessels.

Ankle edema

As already mentioned, in ambulatory patients, fluid will collect at the ankles and cause swelling. It is often surprising just how severe the swelling can get before people seek medical attention. Ask the following:
• How long has this been going on for?
• Is it worse at any particular time of day? (Typically, cardiac edema is worse toward evening and resolved somewhat overnight as the fluid redistributes itself.)
• Exactly how extensive is the swelling? Is it confined to the feet and ankles, or does it extend to the shin, knee, thigh, or even the buttocks, genitalia, and anterior abdominal wall?
• Is there any evidence of abdominal swelling and ascites? (📖 p. 239)

Palpitations

To have palpitations is to have an awareness of one's own heartbeat. This is one of the many situations in which the patient may have a very different idea of the word's meaning than yours. You should spend some time understanding exactly what they mean. Patients may be unfamiliar with the term altogether and instead describe the heart as "jumping," "skipping," or "missing a beat." Attempt to determine the following:

- When did the sensation start and stop?
- How long did it last?
- Did it come on suddenly or gradually?
- Did the patient lose consciousness? If so, for how long?
- Was the heartbeat felt as fast, slow, or some other pattern?
- Was it regular or irregular?
  - it is useful at this stage to ask the patient to tap out on their knee or a nearby table what they felt.
- What was the patient doing when the palpitations started?
- Is there any relationship to eating or drinking (particularly tea, coffee, wine, chocolate)?
- Could it have been precipitated or terminated by any medication?
- Has this ever happened before? If so, what were the circumstances?
- Are there any associated symptoms? (chest pain, shortness of breath, syncope, nausea, dizziness)
- Did the patient have to stop their activities or lie down?
- Was the patient able to stop the palpitations somehow? (Often, people discover they can terminate their palpitations with a vagal maneuver, such as a Valsalva maneuver, a cough, or swallow.)

Syncope

This is a faint or a blackout. You must determine whether there truly was a loss of consciousness and not simply the feeling that the patient was about to faint (presyncope). In particular, can the patient remember hitting the floor? If there really was a loss of consciousness, attempt to gain a collateral history from witnesses. Ask about the following:

- Was the onset gradual or sudden?
- How long was the loss of consciousness?
- What was the patient doing at the time? (standing, urinating, coughing)
- Were there any preceding or associated symptoms such as chest pain, palpitations, nausea, or sweating? (see Chest Pains, 📖 p. 148, and Palpitations, 📖 p. 152, this chapter)
- Was there any relationship to the use of medication? (Antihypertensives and use of nitroglycerin spray are common culprits.)
- When the patient came to, were there any other symptoms remaining?
- Was there any tongue-biting or urinary or fecal incontinence?
- Was there any motor activity during the unconscious episode?
- How long did it take for the patient to feel "back to normal"?

Other cardiovascular symptoms

Claudication

This comes from the Latin "claudicatio" meaning "to limp." These days, however, it is used to describe muscle pain that occurs during exercise as a sign of peripheral ischemia.

In true claudication, the patient describes the pain thus:
- Feels like a tight cramp in the muscle
- Usually occurs in the calf, thigh, buttock, and foot
- Appears *only* with exercise
- Disappears at rest
- May also be associated with numbness or pins-and-needles sensation on the skin of the foot (blood is diverted from the skin to the ischemic muscle).

As always, you should attempt to quantify wherever possible. In this case, determine the "claudication distance"—that is, how far the patient is able to walk before the pain starts. This will be useful in judging the severity of the disability and in monitoring the condition.

Rest pain

This pain, similar to claudication, comes on *at rest* and is usually continuous, a sign of severe ischemia. The patient may describe the following:
- Continuous, severe pain in the calf, thigh, buttock, or foot
- Aching in nature
- Lasts through the day and night
- Exacerbations of the pain may wake the patient from sleep.
- The patient may find slight relief by hanging the affected leg off the side of the bed.

Fatigue

Fatigue is a difficult symptom to determine, as you will find that most people claim to be more tired than normal if asked. However, this pathological fatigue is caused by ↓ cardiac output and ↓ blood supply to muscles and needs to be taken seriously. Again, quantify and determine the following:
- Is the patient able to do less than they were previously?
- Is any ↓ in activity due to fatigue or some other symptom (e.g., breathlessness)?
- What activities has the patient had to give up because of fatigue?
- What are they able to do before they become too tired?

The rest of the history

Cardiac risk factors

These are important aspects of the history that have an impact on the risk of cardiovascular disease. When documenting a history of a cardiovascular case, it is worth pulling these factors out of the usual order and documenting them, with details where appropriate, at the end of the presenting complaint (as below). They should *not* then be repeated again later in the write-up.

- *Age:* ↑ risk with age
- *Gender:* risk in males > females
- *Obesity:* How heavy is the patient? (Calculate their BMI—see 📖 p. 56.)
- *Smoking:* See 📖 p. 38 for further advice. Quantify in pack-years. Don't be fooled by the "ex-smoker" that gave up yesterday.
- *Hypertension:* Find out when it was diagnosed. How was it treated? Is it being monitored?
- *Hypercholesterolemia:* Increasingly, patients will know about this; some will even know their latest blood test results. When was it diagnosed? How is it being treated and monitored?
- *Diabetes:* what type? When was it diagnosed? How is it being treated and monitored? What are the usual glucose readings?
- *FH:* particularly first-degree relatives who have had cardiovascular events or diagnoses before the age of 60

Past medical history

Ask especially about the following:

- Angina—if the patient has nitroglycerin, ask how often they need to use it and whether this use has changed significantly recently.
- MI—when? How was it treated?
- Ischemic heart disease—how was the diagnosis made? Any angiograms? Any stent placements? What other investigations has the patient had?
- Cardiac surgery—bypass? How many arteries?
- Atrial fibrillation (AF) or other rhythm disturbance—what treatment? On warfarin?
- Rheumatic fever
- Endocarditis
- Thyroid disease

Drug history

Take particular note of cardiac medications and attempt to assess compliance and the patient's understanding of what the medication does. Remember, some recreational drug use can be a major cardiac stressor.

Social history

As in any other case, take note of the patient's employment—both how the disease has affected their ability to work and how any cardiac diagnosis may affect the patient's employability.

Also record the home arrangements—whether there are any caregivers present, aids or adaptations, stairs, and so on.

General inspection and hands

The full examination framework is shown in Box 7.2. While the order need not be strictly adhered to, the authors feel that this is the easiest routine, working from the hands and face to more intimate areas of the body.

Positioning

The patient should be seated, leaning back to 45°, supported by pillows, with their chest, arms, and ankles (if appropriate) exposed. Their head should be well supported, allowing relaxation of the muscles in the neck. Ensure that the room is warm and that there is enough privacy. In an exam condition, the patient should be undressed to their underwear with appropriate drapes and gown.

If you intend to measure that patient's blood pressure seated and standing (remember to have the patient stand for 3 minutes before measuring), it may be wise to do this at the beginning of the examination.

General inspection

As always, take a step back and take an objective look at the patient.
• Do they look ill? If so, in which way?
• Are they short of breath at rest?

Box 7.2 Framework for the cardiovascular examination

Following is an example framework for a thorough examination of the cardiovascular system—the information in this chapter is presented in a slightly different order for the purpose of clarity.

This is the authors' recommendation. Other methods exist and none are right or wrong, so long as nothing is missed.
• General inspection
• Hands
• Radial pulse
• Brachial pulse
• Blood pressure
• Face
• Eyes
• Tongue
• Carotid pulse
• Jugular venous pressure and pulse waveform
• Inspection of the precordium
• Palpation of the precordium
• Auscultation of the precordium
• Auscultation of the neck
• Dynamic maneuvers (if appropriate)
• Lung bases
• Abdomen
• Peripheral pulses (lower limbs)
• Edema assessment
• Peripheral veins

- Is there any cyanosis (see 📖 p. 191)?
- What is their nutritional state?
  - Are they overweight?
  - Are they cachectic (underweight with muscle wasting)?
- Do they have features of any genetic syndrome such as Turner, Down, or Marfan?

Hands

Take the patient's right hand in yours as if to greet them, look at it carefully, and compare with the other side. Look especially for the following:
- Temperature (may be cold in congestive cardiac failure)
- Sweat
- State of the nails
  - Blue discoloration if peripheral blood flow is poor
  - Splinter hemorrhages (small, streak-like bleeding in the nail bed) seen especially in bacterial endocarditis, but may also be a sign of rheumatoid arthritis, vasculitis, trauma, or sepsis from any source
- Finger clubbing (see 📖 p. 191). Cardiac causes include infective endocarditis and cyanotic congenital heart disease.
- Xanthomata—raised yellow lesions caused by a buildup of lipids beneath the skin. This is often seen on tendons at the wrist.
- Osler's nodes—rare manifestation of infective endocarditis (a late sign, and the disease is usually treated before this develops). There are red, tender nodules on the finger pulps or thenar eminence.
- Janeway lesions—nontender macular–papular erythematous lesions seen on palm or finger pulps as a rare feature of bacterial endocarditis

Peripheral pulses

All of the major pulses are described below but should be examined in the order described on the previous page. For each, you should attempt to detect the rate and rhythm of the pulsation. For the brachial and carotid pulsations in particular, you should also determine the volume and character (waveform) of the pulse.

Technique

Examination technique is described below and illustrated in Fig. 7.1.

It is good practice *not* to use your thumb to feel pulses, as you may mistake your own pulse (which can be felt weakly in the thumb) for the weak pulse of the patient, especially in the peripheral arteries.

Radial artery

Feeling for the waveform is not useful here as it is too far from the heart.

Use the first and second fingers to feel just lateral to the tendon of the flexor carpi radialis and medial to the radial styloid process at the wrist.

Brachial artery

Feel at the medial side of the antecubital fossa, just medial to the tendenous insertion of the biceps.

Carotid artery

This is the best place to assess the pulse volume and waveform.

Find the larynx, move a couple of centimeters laterally, and press backward medial to the sternomastoid muscle.

ⓘ Be sure not to compress both carotids at once, for fear of diminishing blood flow to the brain, particularly in the frail and elderly.

Femoral artery

This is another useful place for assessing the waveform unless there is disease or abnormality in the abdominal aorta.

The patient is usually stripped to their underwear by this point in the examination and should be lying on a bed or exam table with their legs outstretched. Ask them to lower their clothes a little more, exposing the groin area. The femoral pulsation can be felt midway between the pubic tubercle and the anterior superior iliac spine.

Popliteal artery

This lies deep in the popliteal fossa and is surrounded by strong tendons. It can be difficult to feel and usually requires more pressure than you expect. There are several techniques but we recommend the following:

With the patient lying flat and knees slightly flexed, press into the center of the popliteal fossa with tips of the fingers of the left hand and use the fingers of the right hand to add extra pressure to these.

Posterior tibial artery

Palpate at the ankle just posterior and inferior to the medial malleolus.

Dorsalis pedis

This runs lateral to the exterior hallucis longus tendon on the superior surface of the foot between the bases of the first and second metatarsals.

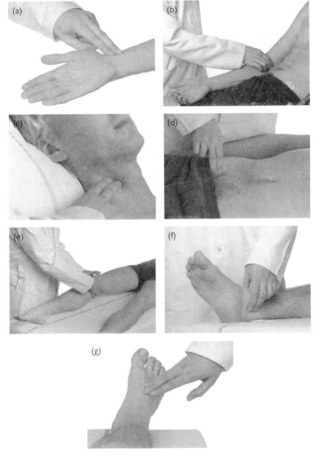

Fig. 7.1 Palpation of the peripheral pulses. a) The radial pulse. b) The brachial pulse. c) The carotid pulse. d) The femoral pulse. e) The popliteal pulse. f) The posterior tibial pulse. g) The dorsalis pedis pulse.

Pulse rate

This should be expressed in beats per minute (bpm). A rate <60 bpm is called *bradycardia* whereas *tachycardia* is a pulse >100 bpm. A normal healthy adult pulse rate should be ~60–100 bpm.

The most accurate method is to count the pulse for a full minute. In practice, count for a portion of this time and calculate the rate by multiplication. Commonly, people count for 15 seconds and multiply the number by 4.

Rhythm

You should feel the pulse for as long as it takes to be sure of the rhythm. In general, the pulse can be either regular or irregular but variations exist.

- *Regular:* a self-explanatory definition. Remember that the pulse rate may ↓ with inspiration and ↑ with expiration in the normal state.
- *Irregularly irregular:* a completely random pattern of pulsation synonymous with AF. The atria twitch and contract in an irregular fashion, sending electrical impulses to the ventricles (and, therefore, causing contraction and arterial pulsation) at random intervals.
- *Regularly irregular:* not quite the contradiction that it seems—a nonregular pulse can occur in some other regular pattern. For example, pulsus bigeminus will cause regular ectopic beats, resulting in alternating brief gaps and long gaps between pulses. In Wenckebach's phenomenon, you may feel increasing time between each pulse until one is "missed," and then the cycle repeats.
- *Regular with ectopics:* a very difficult thing to feel and be sure of without an ECG. A normal regular heart rate may be intermittently interrupted by a beat that is out of step, making the pulse feel almost irregularly irregular.

Character/waveform and volume

This is best assessed at the carotid artery. Feel for the speed at which the artery expands and collapses and for the force with which it does so. This takes some practice to master, and it may be useful to imagine a graph such as those shown in Fig. 7.2. Some examples follow:

- *Aortic stenosis:* a "slow rising" pulse, perhaps with a palpable shudder. This is sometimes called *anacrotic* or a *plateau* phase.
- *Aortic regurgitation:* a "collapsing" pulse that feels as though it suddenly hits your fingers and falls away just as quickly. Try feeling at the brachial artery and raising the arm above the patient's heart. This is sometimes referred to as a *waterhammer* pulse.
- *Pulsus bisferiens:* a waveform with two peaks, found where aortic stenosis and regurgitation coexist
- *Hypertrophic cardiomyopathy:* this pulse may feel normal at first but recedes quickly. It is often described as "jerky."
- *Pulsus alternans:* an alternating strong and weak pulsation, synonymous with a severely impaired left ventricle in a failing heart
- *Pulsus paradoxus:* pulse is weaker during inspiration (causes include cardiac tamponade, status asthmaticus, and constrictive pericarditis)

Other tests of arterial pulsation

These are not routinely performed unless the history and the rest of the examination have made the examiner suspicious of the specific pathologies that they represent.

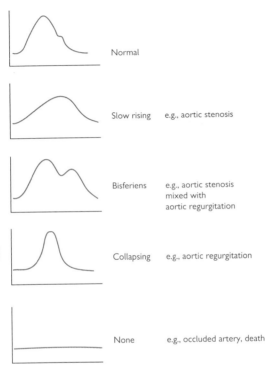

Fig. 7.2 Graphical representation of different arterial pulse waveforms and their causes.

Radioradial delay
Feel both radial pulses simultaneously. In the normal state, the pulses will occur together. Any delay in the pulsation reaching the radial artery on one side may point to pathology, such as an aneurysm at the aortic arch or subclavian artery stenosis.

Radiofemoral delay
Palpate the radial and femoral pulses on the same side simultaneously. They should occur together. Any delay in the pulsation reaching the femoral artery may point to aortic pathology, such as coarctation.

The face and neck

Face

Examine the patient's face at rest. It's a good idea to develop your own pattern for this. The authors recommend starting with an overview, moving to the eyes, mouth, then neck. The order is not important as long as all aspects are examined. Be sure to ask the patient to:

- Look up while you gently pull down one lower eyelid, exposing the conjunctiva.
- Open wide. Look inside their mouth.
- Stick out their tongue.

In the cardiovascular examination, look especially for the following:

- *Jaundice:* seen as a yellow discoloration of the sclera
- *Anemia:* seen as an unusually pale conjunctiva (experience is needed here)
- *Xanthelasma:* yellow, raised lesions found particularly around the eyes, indicative of high serum cholesterol
- *Corneal arcus:* a yellow ring seen overlying the iris. This is significant in patients <40 years but not in older persons.
- *Mitral facies:* rosy cheeks suggestive of mitral stenosis
- *Cyanosis:* seen as a bluish discoloration of the lips and tongue
- *High arched palate:* suggestive of diseases such as Marfan syndrome
- *Dental hygiene:* periodontal disease is a common source of organisms causing endocarditis.

Carotid pulse

At this point, the carotid pulse should be examined (📖 p. 157).

Jugular venous pressure

Theory

The jugular veins connect to the superior vena cava (SVC) and the right atrium without any intervening valves. Therefore, changes in pressure in the right atrium will transmit a pressure wave up these veins that can be seen in the neck. By measuring the height of the impulse, the pressure in the right side of the circulation can be expressed in centimeters.

Examination

It is often said that the JVP must only be measured in the internal jugular vein (IJV). This is not strictly the case. The external jugular vein (EJV) is easily seen as it makes a winding course down the neck (see Fig. 7.3). Its tortuous course means that impulses are not transmitted as readily or as reliably. It is for this reason that the IJV is used.

The center of the right atrium lies ~5 cm below the sternal angle, which is used as the reference point.

The normal JVP is ~8 cm of blood (therefore 3 cm above the sternal angle). With the patient tilted back to 45°, the upper border of the pulse is just hidden at the base of the neck. This, therefore, is used as the standard position for JVP measurement.

▶ Remember, it is the vertical distance from the sternal angle to the upper border of the pulsation that must be measured.

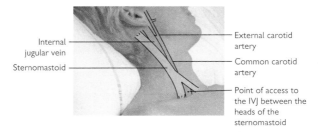

Fig. 7.3 The surface anatomy of the vasculature in the neck. Note that the IJV is partly hidden by the sternocleidomastoid at the base of the neck.

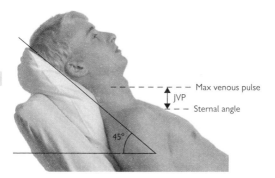

Fig. 7.4 Measuring the JVP. Measure the vertical distance from the top of the pulsation to the sternal angle and then add 5 cm to get the JVP.

▶ You must add 5 cm to the figure to give the true JVP (see Fig. 7.4).

• With the patient lying back at 45°, expose the neck.

• Ask the patient to turn their head away from you (their left) and ensure that the neck muscles are relaxed.

• Look for the JVP and measure the *vertical* distance from the top of the pulsation to the sternal angle.

ⓘ The result is often expressed along the lines of "3 cm above the sternal angle." Remember that that is a total JVP of 8 cm after adding the extra 5 cm that are not measured.

• Try to look upward, along the line of the sternomastoid. Don't get too close, and use oblique lighting to make the pulsation more obvious.

▶ It can sometimes be difficult to distinguish the JVP from the carotid pulse—see next section and Table 7.1 for some advice.

THE FACE AND NECK

Differentiating jugular and carotid pulsations

The rules for differentiating the jugular and carotid pulsations (Table 7.1) are guides only and not always true. For example, in severe tricuspid regurgitation, the jugular pulse is palpable and is not easily abolished by compression. If proving difficult, test the hepatojugular reflex.

Hepatojugular reflux
- Watch the neck pulsation.
- Exert pressure over the liver with the flat of your right hand.
  The JVP should rise by approximately 2 cm; the carotid pulse will not.

Character of jugular venous pulsation

This is rather difficult to detect without experience (see Box 7.3). The jugular pulsation has two main peaks (see Fig. 7.5). Establish the timing of the peaks in the cardiac cycle by palpating the carotid pulse at the same time. The key features are as follows:
- *a wave:* caused by atrial contraction; seen just *before* the carotid pulse
- *c point:* slight AV-ring bulge during ventricular contraction
- *x descent:* atrial relaxation
- *v wave:* tricuspid closure and atrial filling
- *y descent:* ventricular filling as tricuspid valve opens

Table 7.1 Characteristics of normal jugular and carotid pulsations

Jugular pulsation	Carotid pulsation
2 peaks (in sinus rhythm)	1 peak
Impalpable	Palpable
Obliterated by pressure	Hard to obliterate
Moves with respiration	Little movement with respiration

Box 7.3 A word about honesty in learning

Students often find the JVP hard to see while they are learning the various examination techniques. This reminds the authors of an important point.

In medicine, there is an almost overwhelming pressure to say "yes" when asked, "Can you see that?" by the teacher. One may be motivated by a fear of appearing stupid, taking too much of the teacher's time, or delaying the ward rounds further. If the real answer is "no," however, succumbing to this fear is useful to no one. The student fails to learn the correct technique or the correct identification of the sign, and the teacher fails to discover that their demonstration is inadequate. Misconceptions are born and passed on from person to person.

The authors thus urge students of medicine of all ages and at all stages to say "no, please show me again" when this is needed, and we will all be better for it.

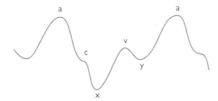

Fig. 7.5 Representation of the normal jugular venous pulsation.

Findings
- *Raised JVP:* right ventricular failure, tricuspid stenosis, tricuspid regurgitation, SVC obstruction, pulmonary embolus, fluid overload
- *Large a waves:* caused usually by a hypertrophied right atrium (pulmonary hypertension, pulmonary stenosis, tricuspid stenosis)
- *Absent a wave:* atrial fibrillation
- *"Cannon" a waves:* large, irregular waves caused by contraction of the atrium against a closed tricuspid valve; seen in complete heart block
- *Large v waves:* regurgitation of blood though an incompetent tricuspid valve
- *Sharp y descent:* characteristic of constrictive pericarditis
- *Sharp x descent:* characteristic of cardiac tamponade

Kussmaul's sign
The JVP will ↓ during inspiration in the normal state. The JVP will rise during inspiration (Kussmaul's sign) in the presence of pericardial constriction, right ventricular infarction, or, rarely, cardiac tamponade.

Examining the precordium

The *precordium* refers to that part of the chest overlying the heart. Inspection and palpation are discussed below. Auscultation is discussed in the next section (📖 p. 193).

Inspection

The patient should be lying at 45° with the chest exposed. Look for the following:

- Scars—sternal split is used to access the median structures and to perform coronary artery bypass graft (CABG) surgery. A left lateral thoracotomy may be evidence of previous closed mitral valvotomy, resection of coarctation, or ligation of a patent ductus arteriosus.
- Any abnormal chest shape or movements (📖 p. 193)
- Pacemaker or implantable defibrillator—usually implanted over the left pectoral region
- Any visible pulsations

Palpation

❶ Before starting the exam, explain what you are going to do and how you will do it, particularly to female patients. If possible, warm your hands.

General palpation

Place the flat of your right hand on the chest wall—to the left, then to the right of the sternum. Can you feel any pulsations?

- *Heave*—this is a sustained, thrusting pulsation usually felt at the left sternal edge indicating right ventricular enlargement.
- *Thrill*—this is a palpable murmur felt as a shudder beneath your hand. It is caused by severe valvular disease (if systolic: aortic stenosis, ventricular septal defect, or mitral regurgitation; diastolic: mitral stenosis)

Palpating the apex beat

This is the lowermost lateral point at which a definite pulsation can be felt. It is usually at the fifth intercostal space in the mid-clavicular line (Fig. 7.6).

Findings

- *Abnormal position of the apex beat:* usually more lateral than expected. This is caused by an enlarged heart or disease of the chest wall. With chronic lung disease, the apex may be more midline.
- *No apex beat felt:* usually caused by heavy padding with fat or internal padding with an overinflated emphysematous lung. It can sometimes be felt by asking the patient to lean forward or laterally.

Character of the apex beat

This can only be learned with experience, after having felt many normal impulses. Some common abnormalities are as follows:

- *Stronger, more forceful:* hyperdynamic circulation (e.g., sepsis, anemia)
- *Sustained:* impulse longer than expected (left ventricular hypertrophy, aortic stenosis, hypertrophic cardiomyopathy or hyperkinesia)
- *Double impulse:* (palpable atrial systole) characteristic of hyptertrophic cardiomyopathy

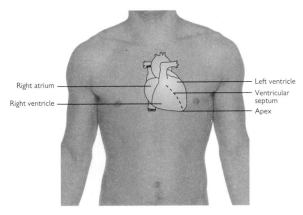

Fig. 7.6 Surface anatomy of the heart and most common location of the apex beat.

- *Tapping:* the description given to a palpable first heart sound in severe mitral stenosis
- *Diffuse:* a poorly localized beat caused by left ventricular aneurysm
- *Unpalpable:* emphysema, obesity, pericardial effusion, or death
- Beware of dextrocardia. If no beat is felt, check the right side.

Percussion

This is not useful and usually not included in the cardiovascular exam.

Auscultating the precordium

Technique

The bell of the stethoscope is used to detect lower-pitched sounds; the diaphragm, for higher-pitched sounds.

Auscultate at each of the four standard areas (Box 7.4; see Fig. 7.7).
These areas do not relate exactly to the anatomical position of the valves but are areas at which the sound of each valve can be best heard.

Different methods exist for this examination. A sensible approach would be to listen with the diaphragm at each area and then repeat, using the bell. You can then go back and concentrate on any abnormalities. You can then examine other areas looking for the features of certain murmurs and extra sounds as described on the following pages.

Practice is needed here; many hearts should be listened to in order to be familiar with the normal sounds. The physiology behind the heart sounds and physiological splitting were described on p. 146 and may be worth revisiting at this point.

If you are unsure which is the first and second heart sound—or where a murmur is occurring—you can palpate one carotid pulse while listening to the heart, enabling you to "feel" systole. The carotid pulsation occurs with S_1.

> **Box 7.4 The four areas for auscultation**
>
> - **Mitral**: fifth intercostal space in the mid-axillary line (the apex)
> - **Tricuspid**: fifth intercostal space at the left sternal edge
> - **Pulmonary**: second intercostal space at the left sternal edge
> - **Aortic**: second intercostal space at the right sternal edge

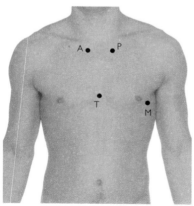

A = Aortic
P = Pulmonary
T = Tricuspid
M = Mitral

Fig. 7.7 The four standard areas for auscultation of the precordium and the valves that are best heard at each area.

ⓘ Remember to palpate only one carotid pulse at a time.

Findings—the heart sounds

First heart sound (S₁)

Mitral valve closure is the main component of S₁, and the volume depends on the force with which it closes.

- *Loud:* forceful closing (mitral stenosis, tricuspid stenosis, tachycardia)
- *Soft:* prolonged ventricular filling or delayed systole (left bundle branch block [LBBB], aortic stenosis, aortic regurgitation)
- *Variable:* variable ventricular filling (AF, complete heart block)

Second heart sound (S₂)

- *Soft:* ↓ mobility of aortic valve (aortic stenosis) or if leaflets fail to close properly (aortic regurgitation)
- *Loud:* aortic component loud in hypertension or congenital aortic stenosis (here the valve is narrowed but mobile). Pulmonary component loud in pulmonary hypertension

Splitting of S₂

See also Applied anatomy and Physiology, this chapter (📖 p. 146).

- *Exaggerated normal splitting:* caused by a delay in right ventricular emptying (right bundle branch block [RBBB], pulmonary stenosis, ventricular septal defect, or mitral regurgitation)
- *Fixed splitting:* no difference in the extent of splitting between inspiration and expiration. Usually due to atrial septal defect
- *Reversed splitting:* i.e., the pulmonary component of S₂ comes before the aortic component. Caused by a delay in left ventricular emptying (LBBB, aortic stenosis, aortic coarctation)

Third heart sound

This is a low-frequency (can just be heard with the bell) sound occurring just after S₂. It is described as a "triple" or "gallop" rhythm: *da-da-dum* or *ken-tuck-y*. It occurs at the end of rapid ventricular filling, early in diastole, and is caused by a shortening of the papillary muscles or by ventricular distension.

- *Physiological:* soft sound heard only at the apex, normal in children and fit adults up to age 30
- *Pathological:* indicates some impairment of left ventricular function or rapid ventricular filling (dilated cardiomyopathy, aortic regurgitation, mitral regurgitation, or constrictive pericarditis). May be associated with a high-pitched pericardial knock

Fourth heart sound

This is a late diastolic sound (just before S₁) caused by ↓ compliance or ↑ stiffness of the ventricular myocardium. It sounds like *da-lub dub* or *Ten-nes-see*. It coincides with abnormally forceful atrial contraction and raised end diastolic pressure in the left ventricle.

- Never physiological
- Causes are hypertrophic cardiomyopathy and systemic hypertension.

Findings—murmurs

These are "musical" humming sounds produced by the turbulent flow of blood. For each murmur heard, you should determine the following:

• Timing
• Site and radiation (where is it heard the loudest?)
• Loudness and pitch (see Box 7.5)
• Relationship to posture and respiration

The timing of the murmur is particularly essential in establishing the sound's origin. You must decide whether the noise occurs in systole or diastole (feel the patient's pulse at the carotid artery to be sure) and then when, within that period, it occurs.

Systolic murmurs

Pansystolic

This is a murmur that lasts for the whole of systole and tends to be due to backflow of blood from a ventricle to an atrium (tricuspid regurgitation, mitral regurgitation). A ventricular septal defect will also cause a pansystolic murmur.

Ejection systolic

These murmurs start quietly at the beginning of systole, quickly rise to a crescendo, and then decrescendo, creating a *whoosh* sound. They are caused by turbulent flow of blood out of a ventricle (pulmonary stenosis, aortic stenosis, hypertrophic cardiomyopathy). They are also found if flow is particularly fast (with fever, in healthy young adults).

Late systolic

There is an audible gap between S_1 and the start of the murmur, which then continues until S_2. Typically this is due to tricuspid or mitral regurgitation through a prolapsing valve.

Diastolic murmurs

• *Early:* usually due to backflow through incompetent aortic or pulmonary valves. It starts loudly at S_2 and decrescendos during

---

Box 7.5 Grading volume of a murmur

The experienced examiner should be able to give the murmur a grade according to its loudness:

• 1—very quiet (students may only hear it if they have already been told that it is there)
• 2—quiet but can be heard with a stethoscope wielded by an examiner with some experience
• 3—moderate; easily heard
• 4—loud, obvious murmur
• 5—very loud; heard over the whole of the precordium and may be accompanied by a palpable thrill
• 6—heard without the aid of a stethoscope

diastole. (You can produce a similar sound by whispering the letter *R* out loud).

- *Mid-diastolic:* begin later in diastole and may be brief or continue up to S_1. They are usually due to flow through a narrowed mitral or tricuspid valve. They are lower pitched than early diastolic murmurs.
- *Austin–Flint murmur:* audible vibration of the mitral valve during diastole as it is hit by flow of blood due to severe aortic regurgitation
- *Graham–Steele murmur:* pulmonary regurgitation secondary to pulmonary artery dilatation caused by ↑ pulmonary artery pressure in mitral stenosis

Continuous murmurs

These are murmurs heard throughout both systole and diastole. Common causes include a patent ductus arteriosus or an arteriovenous fistula.

Radiation

The murmur can sometimes be heard in areas where heart sounds are not normally auscultated—the murmur will tend to radiate in the direction of the blood flow that is causing the sound (see 📖 p. 171 for summary).

For example, murmur of aortic stenosis will radiate up to the carotids, whereas a mitral regurgitation murmur may be heard in the left axilla.

Position

Some murmurs will become louder if you position the patient in such a way that gravity aids the flow of blood creating the sound.
- Aortic regurgitation is heard louder if you ask the patient to sit up and lean forward; listen at the left sternal border.
- Mitral stenosis is louder if you ask the patient to lie on their left-hand side (listen with the bell at the apex).

Dynamic maneuvers

The following may help in identifying the origin of a murmur.
- *Respiration:* Right-sided murmurs (e.g., pulmonary stenosis) tend to be louder during inspiration and quieter during expiration (because of ↑ venous return—see 📖 p. 169). Ask the patient to breathe deeply while you listen. Left-sided murmurs are louder during expiration.
- *Valsalva maneuver:* This is forceful expiration against a closed glottis (consider straining over the toilet bowl). Replicate by asking the patient to blow into the end of a syringe, attempting to expel the plunger. This will ↓ cardiac output and cause most murmurs to soften. Murmurs of hypertrophic obstructive cardiomyopathy, mitral regurgitation, and mitral prolapse will get louder on release of Valsalva.

Findings—extra sounds

These are added sounds that are often associated with a specific murmur—see Table 7.2 (📖 p. 171).

Table 7.2 Selection of cardiac abnormalities and expected clinical findings (see also 📖 p. 175)

Abnormality	Primary site of murmur	Radiation	Timing	Added sounds*	Graphical Representation of the sounds
Aortic stenosis	Aortic area and apex	To carotid arteries	Ejection systolic	Ejection click (esp. bicuspid valve)	
Aortic regurgitation	Left sternal edge	Toward apex	Early diastolic	(Austin-Flint murmur 📖 p. 170)	
Mitral stenosis	Apex	Nil	Mid-diastolic	Opening snap	
Mitral regurgitation	Apex	Toward left axilla or base of left lung	Pansystolic	Mid-systolic click (if prolapsing)	
Tricuspid regurgitation	Lower left sternal edge	Lower right sternal edge, lung	Pansystolic		
Pulmonary stenosis	Upper left sternal edge	Left clavicular region	Ejection systolic		
Ventricular septal defect	Left sternal edge	whole of the precordium	Pansystolic		

*Note that added sounds, such as clicks and snaps, may only be present in certain patients and should not be expected when examining someone with a certain abnormality.

Opening snap

The mitral valve normally opens immediately after S_2. In mitral stenosis, sudden opening of the stiffened valve can cause an audible high-pitched snap. This may be followed by the murmur of mitral stenosis. If there is no opening snap, the valve may be rigid.

This is best heard over the left sternal border with the diaphragm of the stethoscope.

Ejection click

Similar to the opening snap of mitral stenosis, this is a high-pitched click heard early in systole, caused by the opening of a stiffened semilunar valve (aortic stenosis). It is associated with bicuspid aortic valves.

Ejection click is heard at the aortic or pulmonary areas and down the left sternal border.

Mid-systolic click

Usually caused by mitral valve prolapse, this is the sound of the valve leaflet flicking backward (prolapsing) midway through ventricular systole. It will be followed by the murmur of mitral regurgitation.

It is best heard at the mitral area.

Tumor plop

This is a very rare finding due to atrial myxoma. If there is a pedunculated tumor in the atrium, it may move and block the atrial outflow during atrial systole, causing an audible sound.

Pericardial rub

This is a scratching sound comparable to creaking leather that is heard with each heartbeat and caused by inflamed pericardial membranes rubbing against each other in pericarditis. It is louder as the patient is sitting up, leaning forward, and heard best in expiration.

Metallic valves

Patients who have had metallic valve replacement surgery will have an obviously audible mechanical "click" corresponding to the closing of that valve. These can often be heard without the aid of a stethoscope. Some valves have both opening and closing clicks.

If a patient's valve click is unusually soft, this may indicate dysfunction, e.g., thrombus or pannus.

All patients with prosthetic valves will have a flow murmur when the valve is open.

The rest of the body

The lung bases

Examination of the lungs should form part of a thorough cardiovascular examination (📕 Chapter 8). Look especially for crackles or sign of effusion.

The abdomen

See also 📕 Chapter 9. Look especially for the following:
- Hepatomegaly. Is the liver pulsatile (severe tricuspid regurgitation)?
- Splenomegaly
- Ascites
- Abdominal aortic aneurysm
- Renal bruits (renal artery stenosis)
- Enlarged kidneys

Peripheral edema

This is an abnormal ↑ in tissue fluid resulting in swelling—its causes are multiple but often due to heart failure. Edema is under gravitational control so will gather at the ankles if the patient is standing or walking, at the sacrum if sitting, and in the lungs if lying (orthopnea, 📕 p. 150).
- Make a note of any peripheral swelling, examining both the ankles and the sacrum.
- Note if the edema is "pitting" (are you able to make an impression in it with your finger?—best tested over the anterior of the tibia).
- Note how high the edema extends (ankles, leg, thighs, etc.).
- If the edema extends beyond the thighs, it is important to examine the external genitalia, particularly in men, where the swelling may cause outflow obstruction.

Varicose veins

Inspection

Varicosities appear as visible, dilated, tortuous, subcutaneous veins caused by the backflow of blood from the deep veins (usually a branch of the long saphenous vein).
- The patient should be examined in a standing position with the legs fully exposed.
- Note any stasis changes, such as surrounding edema, eczema, brown pigmentation, or ulcers.

Palpation
- Gently feel the varicose veins—hard veins may contain thrombus.
- Ask the patient to cough. If there is a palpable pulsation in the varicosity, there may be valvular incompetence at the long saphenous vein in the groin.

Percussion
- Apply the fingers of one hand to the upper part of the varicose vein.
- Gently flick the lower part of the vein with the other hand.
  - If there is a palpable wave sent up the vein, there are incompetent valves between those two points.

Trendelenburg test
- Ask the patient to lie down and raise their leg so as to drain the veins.
- Apply a tourniquet over the saphenous vein (upper half of thigh).
- Ask the patient to stand.
  - You can then determine the site of the incompetent perforating vein. Do the varicose veins fill above or below the tourniquet?
- Repeat the procedure until you are able to pinpoint the exact location of the incompetence and, by applying localized pressure, prevent the varicose veins from filling at all.

Important presenting patterns

Valvular disease (see also 📖 p. 171)

Mitral stenosis
- *Symptoms:* dyspnea, cough productive of frothy (pink?) sputum, palpitations (often associated with AF and resultant emboli)
- *Signs:* palmar erythema, malar flush, "tapping" apex beat, left parasternal heave, loud S_1, mid-diastolic murmur ± opening snap

Mitral regurgitation
- *Symptoms:* acute dyspnea and pulmonary congestion
- *Signs:* collapsing pulse, sustained apex beat displaced to the left, left parasternal heave, soft S_1, loud S_2 (pulmonary component), pansystolic murmur heard at the apex radiating to left axilla ± mid-systolic click, third heart sound

Aortic stenosis
- *Symptoms:* angina, syncope, dyspnea, sudden death
- *Signs:* Slow rising pulse, low blood pressure, narrow pulse pressure, sustained and powerful apex beat, ejection systolic murmur radiating to carotids, soft S_2, ± ejection click

Aortic regurgitation
- *Symptoms:* similar to aortic stenosis
- *Signs:* collapsing pulse, wide pulse pressure, sustained and displaced apex beat, soft S_2, early diastolic murmur at the left sternal edge (often described as "blowing" or decrescendo), ± ejection systolic murmur (↑ volume). You may also hear a "pistol shot" sound over the femoral artery with severe aortic regurgitation. See also Box 7.6.

Tricuspid stenosis
This usually occurs along with mitral or aortic valvular disease (e.g., in rheumatic fever) and is often the less serious of the patient's problems.
- *Signs:* auscultation similar to that of mitral stenosis, hepatomegaly, pulsatile liver, and venous congestion

---

Box 7.6 Some eponymous signs of aortic regurgitation

- Prominent carotid pulsation (Corrigan's sign)
- Head-nodding in time with the heartbeat (De Musset's sign)*
- Pulsation of the uvula in time with the heartbeat (Mueller's sign)
- Higher blood pressure in the legs than in the arms (Hill's sign)
- Nailbed capillary pulsation (Quincke's sign)

* Abraham Lincoln probably had Marfan syndrome, given his tall stature and long arms. In addition, a study of old photographs shows that he had De Musset's sign. During his lifetime cameras had longer shutter speeds, and President Lincoln's head-nodding caused his face to appear blurred in photographs, compared with the people sitting around him.

Tricuspid regurgitation
Signs include dilated neck veins, prominent v-wave in JVP that may, rarely, cause the earlobe to oscillate, pansystolic murmur louder on inspiration with a loud pulmonary component of S_2, left parasternal heave, pulsatile liver, peripheral and sacral edema, and ascites. You may also hear a third heart sound and evidence of AF.

Pulmonary stenosis
Signs include normal pulse with an ejection systolic murmur radiating to lung fields often with a palpable thrill over the pulmonary area. Other signs of right heart strain or failure can also occur.

Pulmonary regurgitation
This is usually a coincidental finding.
- *Signs:* loud S_2 that may be palpable, early diastolic murmur heard at the pulmonary area and high at the left sternal edge

Congenital heart disease
Ventricular septal defect (VSD)
- *Symptoms:* Children with VSD are often asymptomatic. If there is a large defect, the patient may suffer congestive cardiac failure with dyspnea and fatigue.
- *Signs:* There may be cyanosis and clubbing of fingers. Heart sounds usually appear normal, but if pulmonary hypertension develops, you may hear a loud pulmonary component of S_2 with a right-ventricular heave. A pansystolic murmur may also be heard at the left sternal edge, often accompanied by a palpable thrill. The signs may settle with time; the right heart pressure increases, causing less shunting and a softer murmur.

Atrial septal defect (ASD)
ASD is the most common congenital lesion and is often an asymptomatic finding discovered on investigating a murmur.
- *Symptoms of secundum defect:* asymptomatic if small. Symptoms include fatigue, dyspnea, palpitations (atrial arrythmias), recurrent pulmonary infections, and other symptoms of right heart failure. This defect is also associated with migraine and paradoxical emboli.
- *Symptoms of primum defect:* These include symptoms of heart failure in childhood with failure to thrive, chest infections, and poor development. In adults, there may be syncope (heart block) and symptoms suggestive of endocarditis.
- *Signs:* fixed splitting of S_2, ↑ flow over the normal pulmonary valve may give an ejection systolic murmur. There is also left parasternal heave with a normal or diffuse apical impulse. Particularly in ostium primum defects (endocardial cushion defects), you may hear the pansystolic murmur of mitral regurgitation or coexisting VSD (or both). Look also for signs of pulmonary hypertension.

Patent ductus arteriosus (PDA)
PDA is a persistent embryonic connection between the pulmonary artery and the aorta. Blood flows from the aorta into the pulmonary artery.

- *Symptoms:* often asymptomatic. Severe cases show dyspnea on exertion.
- *Signs:* collapsing pulse, heaving apex beat, "machinery" (continuous) murmur heard all over the precordium, S_2 not heard, systolic or diastolic thrill in the second intercostal space on the left

Coarctation of the aorta
This is a congenital narrowing of the aorta at or beyond the arch.
- *Symptoms:* usually asymptomatic. Symptoms may include headache, epistaxis, dizziness, and palpitations. Claudication, leg fatigue are also features. The coarctation may cause the heart to strain and give symptoms of congestive cardiac failure.
- *Signs:* ↑ blood pressure in the upper limbs, radiofemoral delay, ejection systolic murmur at the left sternal edge, sometimes palpable collateral arteries over the scapulae with interscapular bruits. Patients may also have underdeveloped lower limbs.
- Coarctation is often associated with aortic stenosis, aortic aneurysms, and bicuspid aortic valves. It is also seen in Turner syndrome.

Tetralogy of Fallot
This consists of pulmonary stenosis, VSD (infundibular), right ventricular hypertrophy, and an overriding aorta. (If associated with an ASD as well, this is Fallot's pentalogy.)
- *Symptoms:* syncope, squatting relieves breathlessness, growth retardation
- *Signs:* finger clubbing and central cyanosis with superadded paroxysms ("spells"). Murmurs of pulmonary stenosis or the VSD may be heard along with a systolic thrill and left parasternal heave.

Pericarditis
Causes include collagen diseases, infections such as TB, postinfarction, and idiopathic causes.
- *Symptoms of acute pericarditis:* constant retrosternal soreness, worse on inspiration (pleuritic), relieved slightly by sitting forward, not related to movement or exertion
- *If chronic, constrictive, may cause* Kussmaul's sign, impalpable apex beat, S_3, hepatomegaly, splenomegaly, ascities (pseudo-cirrhosis)

Pericardial effusion
- Pulsus paradoxus, ↑ JVP, impalpable apex beat, soft heart sounds, hepatomegaly, ascites, peripheral edema

Ischemic heart disease
See 📖 p. 148.

Congestive heart failure (CHF)
In simple terms, this refers to the inability of the heart to maintain an adequate cardiac output for perfusion of vital organs with variable severity. It is usually described in terms of "left" and "right" heart failure, but there is usually an element of both (biventricular).

Left ventricular failure
- *Symptoms* may include shortness of breath on exertion, orthopnea, paroxysmal nocturnal dyspnea, cough with pink frothy sputum, fatigue, weight loss, muscle wasting, and anorexia.
- *Signs:* The patient may appear tired, pale, sweaty, and clammy, and have tachycardic, thready pulse, low blood pressure, narrow pulse pressure, displaced apex beat (murmur of an underlying valvular abnormality?), third and fourth heart sounds, tachypnea, and crepitations at the lung bases.

Right ventricular failure
- *Symptoms:* as for LV failure, with peripheral edema and facial swelling
- *Signs:* many of those of LV failure. Also ↑ JVP, hepatomegaly, ascites, peripheral (sacral?) edema, pulsatile liver (if tricuspid regurgitation)

Hypertrophic cardiomyopathy
There may be a family history, although the vast majority of cases are sporadic, caused by new mutations.
- *Symptoms:* often none. If they are present, the patient may suffer from shortness of breath, angina, and syncope.
- *Signs:* sharp, rising (jerky) pulse, prominent JVP a-wave, double apex beat, late systolic murmur at left sternal border that ↑ with Valsalva maneuver

Peripheral vascular disease
- *Symptoms:* claudication, as on 🕮 p. 153.
- *Signs:* (see also Box 7.7) shiny, pale, cold limb, hair loss, absent peripheral pulse(s). If severe, ischemic ulceration and gangrene can occur.

Deep vein thrombosis (DVT)
DVT is often confused with cellulitis and a ruptured popliteal cyst.
- *Symptoms:* calf pain, swelling, and loss of use
- *Signs:* warm, tense, swollen limb, erythema, dilated superficial veins, cyanosis. There may be palpable thrombus in the deep veins. Often there is pain on palpating the calf.

Box 7.7 The acutely ischemic limb

Use the rule of Ps. The acutely ischemic limb will be
- **P**ainful (at first, then becoming)
- **P**ainless (numb)
- **P**ale
- **P**aralyzed
- **P**ulseless

The elderly patient

Geriatricians are equally interested in cardiovascular disease—with an aging population, the prevalence of cardiac, peripheral vascular, and stroke disease will rise. While age is one of many risk factors for vascular disease, older people are one of the biggest groups to benefit from primary and secondary risk factor reduction, so be comprehensive in all assessments. A careful history is of far more use than an inaccurate one and a list of physical findings.

History

Angina

Angina presents in a multitude of ways. Avoid labeling the symptoms as pain (which can irritate many patients); instead, listen to their complaints: "discomfort," "twinges," and "aches" are equally common presentations. Many older people have few symptoms and may present with sweating or breathlessness. Be astute and ask if these relate to exertion.

Orthopnea

Ask why patients sleep on extra pillows. Often this is due to other symptoms, such as arthritis. Do they sleep upright in a chair?

Breathlessness

This relates to a low-output state and not necessarily to pulmonary edema. Fatigue is a common presenting symptom and should not be overlooked.

Drug history

There is always a difficult balance of compliance, managing symptoms, achieving target doses, and avoiding side effects. Avoid rushing to optimize doses and upsetting a careful regimen. Ask about β-blocker eye drops, as they can be absorbed systemically and exert significant effects.

Lifestyle

Ask about smoking and seek opportunities to explore smoking cessation—it's never too late! Ask about alcohol use, as this may have a bearing on decisions around anticoagulation. Advice about healthy eating is often welcome; healthy eating is more palatable than more tablets.

Functional history

As ever, this is a key part of all histories. Targeted interventions, such as help with bathing to avoid overexertion (and symptoms), can have a significant impact.

Examination

General

Look for clues—e.g., the breathless patient returning from the bathroom, the nitroglycerin spray close at hand.

Auscultate and think

Think especially about valve lesions. It is important to assess how much a valvular problem could be contributing to a patient's symptoms and arrange for investigations to confirm this. Aortic valve replacement and CABG are often hugely successful in older people.

Edema
Be careful when palpating—contrary to popular teaching, pitting and non-pitting edema are painful! Could it be gravitational?

Peripheral pulses
These are often overlooked but are a vital part of the examination. Document them carefully, and look for skin changes and ulceration that might be causing significant problems but are not necessarily raised in the history.

Additional points

Alternative diagnoses
Respiratory illnesses often overlap and may mimic, e.g., pulmonary fibrosis and left ventricular failure. If things don't add up or there is little response to treatment, revisit your diagnosis.

Respiratory system

Applied anatomy and physiology

Anatomy

The respiratory tract extends from the nostrils to the alveoli and includes the pulmonary blood supply. Clinically, it is divided into the upper respiratory tract, which is the nose and pharynx, and the lower respiratory tract, which consists of the larynx and all distal structures.

Trachea, bronchi, and bronchioles

The trachea lies in the midline deep to the sternal notch and divides into the left and right main bronchi at the *carina*, level with the sternal angle.

There are about 25 further divisions before reaching the alveoli. The last 16 orders are termed *bronchioles* and differ from the bronchi by having no cartilage, fewer goblet cells, and progressively less muscular walls.

Lungs

The right lung has three lobes (upper, middle, and lower) whereas the left lung has two (upper and lower); see Fig. 8.1. Note the angle of the oblique fissure, dividing the upper and lower lobes such that examination of the anterior chest is mostly that of the upper (and middle) lobes; examination of the back is of the lower lobe.

The right middle lobe sits anterior, separated from the upper lobe by the horizontal fissure. The chest wall corresponding to this is between the right fourth and sixth ribs anterior and is easily missed. The same area on the left is the *lingula*, part of the left upper lobe, which reaches around the anterior side of the heart.

The slant of the diaphragm is such that the inferior border of the lungs is at the sixth rib anterior but extends down to the twelfth posterior.

Physiology

Lung function

Ventilation is under the influence of the respiratory center in the brain. This, in turn, can be influenced by higher voluntary centers and by chemoreceptors that respond to changes in blood gas partial pressures. In health, the most important ones are the brainstem chemoreceptors, stimulating breathing in response to rising blood CO_2.

The main muscle of breathing is the diaphragm, innervated by the phrenic nerve. Contraction causes a flattening of the central part and a slight elevation of the peripheral parts. This causes expansion of the chest cavity, and as the intrathoracic pressure drops, air is sucked into the lungs. The intercostal and scalene muscles maintain the chest wall stability. When a larger inspiration is needed, these "accessory" muscles, including the sternocleidomastoids, act to further expand the chest.

Expiration is largely passive, the air being expelled as the lungs recoil under their innate elasticity.

Aside from inadequate ventilation, ineffective lung functioning can result from inadequate perfusion of the ventilated areas. Also, impaired gas transfer across the alveoli may be a factor—either by a thickening of the wall (e.g., fibrosis), a loss of surface area (as in COPD), or fluid in the alveoli, such as edema, pus, or blood.

Defense

Mechanical defense against infection includes the narrow passages of the nose as well as the larynx, which separates the respiratory and gastrointestinal (GI) tracts. Cough receptors in the pharynx and lower airways initiate mechanisms resulting in a deep inspiration, followed by expiration against a closed glottis and a sudden glottal opening. This causes a rapid, forceful expulsion of air, which we know as a cough.

Most of the respiratory tract is lined with mucous secreted from goblet cells that catch small particles and microbes. This is continuously swept upward toward the larynx by beating cilia on the epithelium.

In the smaller airways and alveoli, macrophages and a variety of secreted defensive proteins act against microbes at a microscopic level.

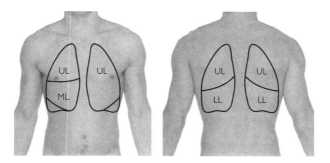

Fig. 8.1 Surface anatomy of the lungs. UL, upper lobe; ML, middle lobe; LL, lower lobe.

Dyspnea

Defining dyspnea

Shortness of breath (SOB), or *dyspnea*, is the sensation one has when using an abnormal amount of effort to breathe. Patients may describe "breathlessness," an inability to "get their breath," or being "short-winded."

"Tightness" is often described and may actually be the sensation of airway narrowing, as in asthma, or may be chest pain, as in cardiac disease. Tease out exactly what the patient means by this.

❶ Pleuritic chest pain is worse at the height of deep inspiration; patients may say they are "not able to get their breath." While their complaint is of breathlessness, their actual problem is pain on inspiration. Ask if they feel the need to breathe faster than normal or are unable to breathe deeply. If the latter, ask if that is due to pain or to some other sensation. If in doubt, ask the patient to take a deep breath and watch the results.

Onset and duration

How quickly did SOB come on? Pulmonary embolus, pneumothorax, and asthmatic attacks can come on suddenly. Pneumonia, heart failure, and anemia cause SOB that worsens over days or weeks. Smoking-related lung disease, by contrast, causes ↑ breathlessness over many years.

Slower onsets are poorly reported. The patient often reports the onset of a *worsening* of breathlessness. Ask when they were last able to run up the stairs, and the real duration of breathlessness becomes apparent.

Severity

Several classifications exist, but it is often more useful to quantify severity in terms of functional impairment. Ask, "How far can you walk before you have to stop? How many flights of stairs can you manage?" Restriction of hobbies such as gardening and dancing are also useful guides.

❶ Be sure that activities are restricted by SOB and not by arthritic hips or knees, chest pain, or some other ailment.

Exacerbating and relieving factors

What makes the breathlessness worse? Can it be reliably triggered by a particular activity or situation? Divide symptoms into SOB at rest and SOB on exertion and quantify as above. Remember to ask about position, e.g., orthopnea (📖 Chapter 7, p. 150).

Has the patient used inhalers? How frequently are they used? Did they help?

Associated symptoms

See the following pages for a full breakdown. Be aware of hyperventilation, in which the ↓ of blood CO_2 will cause paresthesia in the lips and fingers along with light-headedness and, in severe cases, tetany.

Cough and expectoration

Cough

Cough is a common but often overlooked symptom in respiratory disease usually caused by upper respiratory infection (URI) and/or smoking. Duration of cough is important, as well as character, exacerbating factors, and whether any sputum is produced.

Note that cough may be the only symptom of childhood asthma.

Chronic cough is that lasting >3 weeks and may be caused by asthma, carcinoma, interstitial disease and bronchiectasis, gastroesophageal reflux disease, and postnasal drip.

❶ Smokers will have a chronic cough, particularly in the mornings, so a history of a change in pattern is important.

The character of the cough often reveals the cause (Table 8.1).

Associated pain is common and the patient will be able to localize it to the upper respiratory tract (e.g., laryngitis; tracheitis is particularly painful) or the chest wall (i.e., pleurisy secondary to lobar pneumonia or collapse).

Remember nonpulmonary causes: postnasal drip (dry, tickly), gastroesophageal reflux (dry), pharyngeal pouch or tracheoesophageal fistula (worse after eating or lying down), and angiotensin-converting enzyme (ACE) inhibitors (dry).

Sputum

Sputum is excess respiratory secretions that are coughed up. Patients will usually understand the term *phlegm* or *mucous* better. Features to inquire about include the following: How often? How much? How difficult is it to cough up? Color? Consistency? Smell?

Table 8.1 Some characteristic coughs

Cause	Character
Laryngitis	Cough with a hoarse voice
Tracheitis	Dry and very painful
Pleurisy	Sharp pain (chest wall)
Postnasal drip	Tickly
Asthma	Chronic, paroxysmal, worse after exercise and at night
Esophageal reflux	Dry and nauseating. Often first thing in the morning.
Tracheo-esophageal fistula (rare)	Nauseating and worse after eating
Epiglottitis	Barking
Laryngeal nerve palsy	"Bovine" hollow, brassy
Left heart failure	Productive and worse on lying flat

Attempt to quantify sputum production in terms of well-known objects, such as teaspoons, etc. *Mucoid* sputum is white or clear in color but can be turned gray in cigarette smokers. Yellow or green sputum is termed *purulent* and usually indicates infection, although eosinophils in the sputum of asthmatics can also produce a green color. See Table 8.2.

Harder "plugs" of sputum from the airways are seen in asthmatic sputum. Miniature tree-like bronchial casts are produced in bronchopulmonary aspergillosis.

Hemoptysis

The coughing up of blood can vary from streaks or a pink hue (e.g., CHF) to massive, life-threatening bleeds. Establish the amount, color, frequency, and nature of any associated sputum. (Massive hemoptysis = >500 mL in 24 hours.) Hemoptysis is easily confused with blood originating in the nose, mouth, and GI tract (hematemesis). Ask about, and check for, bleeds in these areas.

Causes of hemoptysis include bronchitis, carcinoma, pulmonary embolus, and infarction, TB, cystic fibrosis, and lung abscesses. Infective causes will usually produce blood-stained sputum, not pure hemoptysis.

Be alert to other potential sites of bleeding (skin, GI tract, mouth) that could point to a coagulation disorder.

Table 8.2 Some characteristics of sputum

Nature of sputum	Causes
White/gray	Asthma Smoking
Green/yellow	Bronchitis Bronchiectasis
Green and offensive	Bronchiectasis Abscesses
Sticky, rusty	Lobar pneumonia
Frothy, pink	Congestive cardiac failure
Separates to 3 layers (mucoid, watery, rusty)	Severe bronchiectasis
Very sticky, often green	Asthma
Sticky, with "plugs"	Allergic aspergillosis (complication of asthma)

Other respiratory symptoms

Wheeze

This is a high-pitched, whistling, "musical" sound produced by narrowing of airways, large or small. It occurs with inspiration and expiration, but is usually louder and more prominent in the latter. If it is due to small-airway narrowing, as in asthma, it will be accompanied by a prolonged expiratory phase.

Causes include asthma, smoking-related lung disease, mucosal edema, airway obstruction, airway collapse, and pulmonary edema (cardiac asthma).

Stridor

Stridor has a harsh "crowing" inspiratory and expiratory sound with a constant pitch. It signals large-airway narrowing, usually at the larynx or trachea. It can precede complete airway obstruction so is treated as a medical emergency.

Hoarseness and dysphonia

This is described in 📖 Chapter 6 on p. 130.

Pain

Chest pain is explored fully in Chapter 7 (📖 p. 148). Pain arising from respiratory disease is usually pleuritic in nature and arises from the chest wall, parietal pleura, or mediastinum, as the lungs have no pain fibers. It is felt as a severe, sharp pain at the height of inspiration or on coughing. It is usually localized to a small area of chest wall. Note that patients will avoid deep breathing and may complain of breathlessness (see Dyspnea, this 📖 chapter, p. 185).

Pain resulting from lung parenchymal lesions may be dull and constant and is usually an ominous sign of spread into the chest wall.

The pain of tracheitis is a poorly localized, central soreness. Diaphragmatic pain may be felt at the ipsilateral shoulder tip, while pain from the costal parts of the diaphragm may be referred to the abdomen.

In general, muscular and costal lesions will be tender to touch over the corresponding chest wall and exacerbated by certain twisting movements, whereas pleurisy is not, although this is not always the case. Costochondritis is a common cause of pleuritic pain, of which Tietze's syndrome is a specific cause associated with pain and swelling of the superior costal cartilages.

Pain in a nerve-root distribution may be due to spinal lesions or herpes zoster virus (HZV).

The rest of the history

Other symptoms

Fever
Fever, particularly at night, may be a sign of infection such as TB, malignancy, or a connective tissue disorder.

Weight loss
This can be a symptom of carcinoma, chronic lung disease, or chronic infection. Attempt to quantify any loss (how much in how long?).

Peripheral edema
Edema manifesting as ankle swelling at the end of the day may be a sign of right heart failure secondary to chronic lung disease (cor pulmonale). If severe enough, patients may exhibit signs and symptoms of left heart failure (see 📖 Chapter 7, p. 177).

Obstructive sleep apnea
This is caused by upper-airway obstruction by the flaccid palatal muscles during REM sleep. This causes snoring and progressive hypoxia, which briefly wakes the patient from sleep, often accompanied by thrashing around, disturbing those sharing the bed. The bedtime partner will graphically tell this tale. The patient will describe early-morning headaches caused by CO_2 retention and daytime somnolence from sleep deprivation.

Past medical history
- Vaccination for respiratory illnesses, particularly bacillus Calmette-Guérin (BCG)
- Previous respiratory infections, especially TB before 1950, when operations could result in lifelong deformity
- X-ray abnormalities previously mentioned to the patient
- Childhood (a frequently coughing child may have had undiagnosed asthma)
- Previous intensive care unit (ICU) admissions or respirator dependency

Drug history
- What inhalers are used and how often? Check inhaler technique.
- Previous successful use of bronchodilators and steroids
- Oral steroid therapy predisposes to infection and TB especially.
- β-blockers may exacerbate obstructive lung diseases.
- ACE inhibitors cause a dry cough.
- If O_2 therapy—cylinders or concentrator? How many hours a day?
- Illicit drug use (Cocaine is associated with respiratory disease.)

Family history
- Asthma, eczema, and allergies
- Inherited conditions (e.g., cystic fibrosis [CF], A1-antitrypsin deficiency)
- Family contacts with TB

Smoking

Attempt to quantify the habit in pack-years: 1 pack-year is 20 cigarettes per day for 1 year (e.g., 40/day for 1 year = 2 pack-years; 10/day for 2 years = 1 pack-year).

❶ Beware of appearing judgmental.

Ask about previous smoking, as many patients will call themselves non-smokers if they gave up yesterday or even on the way to the hospital!

Remember to ask about passive smoking.

Alcohol

Alcohol abusers are at greater risk of chest infections, and bingeing may result in aspiration pneumonia.

Social history

Pets

Dogs and cats are a common source of allergens. Also ask about birds and caged animals. Ask about exposure beyond the home, at homes of close friends and relatives, and hobbies involving animal exposure.

Travel

Ask about travel (recent or previous) to areas where respiratory infections are endemic. Think particularly about TB. Remember that *Legionella* can be caught from water systems and air-conditioning even in developed countries.

Occupation

This factor is more important in chest medicine than in any other field. Be alert to exposure to asbestos, coal, cotton, nitrogen dioxide, metals such as tin, silver, iron oxide, and titanium, and hay, air conditioner systems, and so on.

Trace the patient's occupational history back, as there may be a lag of 20 or 30 years between exposure and resultant disease. Remember that exposure may not be obvious and that the patient may have been unaware of it at the time. Plumbers, builders, and electrical engineers may have been exposed to asbestos in the past.

Ask also about close personal contacts—partners may be significantly exposed by handling and washing clothing, for example (although this is relatively rare).

General appearance

Respiratory patients may be short of breath, and it may be easiest to examine them sitting at the edge of the bed instead of in the classic position of sitting back at 45°. Choose a position comfortable to you both. The patient should be undressed to the waist.

As ever, a surprising amount of information can be obtained by observing the patient before touching the patient.

Bedside clues
Look for evidence of the disease and its severity around the patient:
- Inhalers? Which ones?
- Any additional inhaler devices?
- Nebulizer?
- Is the patient receiving O_2 therapy? If so, how much and by what method (i.e., face mask, nasal cannula, etc.)?
- Sputum container? Sputum-laden tissues?
- Remember to inspect the sputum carefully and to record the findings.
- Any mobility aids nearby?
- Look for cigarettes, lighter, or matches at the bedside or in a pocket.

Respiration
Watch the patient from the foot of the bed. Or watch them approach your clinic room.
- Do they appear out of breath at rest?
- If so, do they appear in distress?
- Are they breathing through the mouth or the nose?
- Are they breathing through pursed lips? (↑ the expiratory pressure—an indication of smoking-related lung disease)
- If mobile, did they have to stop on the way to the room? How quickly did they recover?
- Count the respiratory rate. At rest, this should be <12/minute.
- Are the breaths of normal volume?
- Are they using the accessory respiratory muscles (e.g., sternomastoids)?
- Are they using their arms to splint their chest? (The classic position is sitting forward, hands on knees.)

Speech
- Is their speech limited by their breathlessness? If so, can they complete a full sentence? (an important indicator of severity in many conditions)
- Listen for hoarseness as well as the gurgling of excess secretions.
- A nasal voice may indicate neuromuscular weakness.

Cough and abnormal sounds
Watch and listen for coughing (see previous pages) as well as stridor and wheeze.

Hands, face, and neck

Temperature

- Cold fingers indicate peripheral vasoconstriction or heart failure.
- Warm hands with dilated veins are seen in CO_2 retention.

Staining

Fingers stained with tar appear yellow/brown where the cigarette is held (nicotine is colorless and does *not* stain). This indicates smoking but is not an accurate indicator of the number of cigarettes smoked.

Cyanosis

This is a bluish tinge to the skin, mucous membranes, and nails (see 📖 Chapter 3, p. 51), evident when >2.5g/dL of reduced hemoglobin is present (O_2 Saturation about 85%). It is easier to see in good, natural light.

Central cyanosis is seen in the tongue and oral membranes (severe lung disease, e.g., pneumonia, PE, COPD). Peripheral cyanosis is seen *only* in the fingers and toes and is caused by peripheral vascular disease and vasoconstriction.

Finger clubbing

There is ↑ curvature of the nails. Early clubbing is seen as a softening of the nail bed (nail can be rocked from side to side), but this is very difficult to detect. Progressive clubbing leads to a loss of the nail angle at the base and eventually to a gross longitudinal curvature and deformity.

Objectively check for clubbing by putting the patient's nails back to back as in Fig. 8.2. Clubbing leads to a loss of the diamond-shaped gap.

Important respiratory causes are carcinoma, asbestosis, fibrosing alveolitis, and chronic sepsis (bronchiectasis, abscess, empyema, CF).

Pulse

Check rate, rhythm, and character. A tachycardic bounding pulse = CO_2 retention.

Tremor

- *Fine tremor:* caused by use of β-agonist drugs (e.g., albuterol)
- *Flapping tremor (asterixis):* flapping when holding hands dorsiflexed with fingers abducted (Fig 8.3). This is identical to the flap of hepatic failure (see 📖 Chapter 9, p. 244) and is a late sign of CO_2 retention.

Blood pressure

Pulsus paradoxus (see 📖 Chapter 7, p. 159) is caused by pericardial effusion and severe asthma.

JVP

See 📖 Chapter 7, p. 161. JVP is raised in pulmonary vasoconstriction or pulmonary hypertension and right heart failure. It is markedly raised, without a pulsation, in SVC obstruction, with distended upper chest wall veins and facial and conjunctival edema (chemosis).

Nose

Examine inside and out, looking for polyps (asthma), deviated septum, and lupus pernio (red/purple nasal swelling of sarcoid granuloma).

Eyes

- *Conjunctiva:* evidence of anemia?
- *Horner's syndrome:* (⌸ Chapter 9, p. 274) caused by compression of the sympathetic chain in the chest cavity (tumor, sarcoidosis, fibrosis)
- *Iritis:* TB, sarcoidosis
- *Conjunctivitis:* TB, sarcoidosis
- *Retina:* Papilledema in CO_2 retention or cerebral metastases. Retinal tubercles in TB. Choroiditis in TB or syphilis

Lymph nodes

See ⌸ Chapter 3, p. 58, for a full description of examination technique. Feel especially the anterior and posterior triangles, the supraclavicular areas. Don't forget that the axillae receive lymph drainage from the chest wall and breasts.

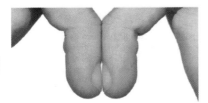

Fig. 8.2   Examining for clubbing. In the normal state, a diamond window will be seen between opposed nail beds, which is lost in finger clubbing.

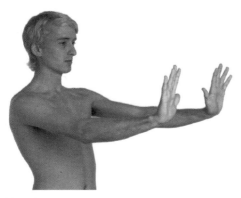

Fig. 8.3   Looking for a flapping tremor. Wrists are dorsiflexed and fingers abducted.

Inspection of the chest

Look at the shape and movement of the chest up close.

Surface markings

Check the whole chest for scars and lesions.

- **Scars** may indicate previous surgery. Look especially in the mid-axillary lines for evidence of past chest drains.
- **Radiotherapy** will often cause lasting local skin thickening and erythema.
- **Veins:** Look for unusually prominent surface vasculature.

Shape

- **Deformity:** Is there any asymmetry of shape? Remember to check the spine for scoliosis or kyphosis.
- **Surgery:** TB patients from the 1940s and 1950s may have had operations resulting in lasting and gross deformity (thoracoplasty).
- **Barrel chest:** a rounded thorax with ↑ anteroposterior (AP) diameter. Hyperinflation is a marker of smoking-related lung disease.
- **Pectus carinatum:** also called "pigeon chest." Sternum and costal cartilages are prominent and protrude from the chest. It is caused by ↑ respiratory effort when the bones are still malleable in childhood, from asthma or rickets.
- **Pectus excavatum:** also called "funnel chest." Sternum and costal cartilages appear depressed into the chest. This is a developmental defect, usually a normal variant with no significance to pathology.
- **Surgical (subcutaneous) emphysema:** Air in the soft tissues will appear as a diffuse swelling. It occurs especially in the neck; it may feel crackly to the touch.

Breathing pattern

Again, examine rate and depth of breathing.

- Fast, deep breaths are seen in anxiety states.
- Deep, sighing breaths are Kussmaul's respiration = systemic acidosis.
- Cheyne–Stokes breathing has an alternating pattern of deep, regular breathing with very slow, shallow breaths. It is due to failure of the normal respiratory regulation in response to blood CO_2 levels.
- Prolonged expiratory phase = marker of outflow limitation, a sign of smoking-related lung disease if coupled with pursed-lip breathing.

Movement

Observe chest wall movement during breathing at rest. Also, ask the patient to take a couple of deep breaths in and out, and watch closely.

- Look for asymmetry. ↓ Movement indicates lung disease on that side.
- ↓ Movement globally is seen in COPD, along with a "pump handle" movement of the ribs (hinged posteriorly only), compared with the normal "bucket handle" (hinged at the front and back).
- **Harrison's sulcus** is a depression of the lower ribs just above the costal margins and indicates severe childhood asthma.

Palpation

Mediastinal position

Trachea

The trachea should lie in the midline just beneath the sternal notch. The trachea will shift as the mediastinum is pulled or pushed laterally. This is a late sign and not easy to assess, unless the shift is marked.

There are several methods for checking the position, all of which are somewhat uncomfortable for the patient. The two most popular methods are as follows:

• Use a single finger to feel for the trachea; the distance between it and the sternomastoids on each side should be the same.
• Use two fingers and palpate the sulci on either side of the trachea at the same time. They should feel identical in size.

Apex beat or PMI (point of maximum impulse)

This is normally at the fifth intercostal space in the mid-clavicular line. It will shift with the mediastinum. However, it is very difficult to palpate in the presence of hyperexpanded lungs and may be shifted to the left if the heart is enlarged.

Chest expansion

This is an objective measure of chest movement, using your hands as a guide.

• Put both hands on the patient's posterior thorax, at a level just below the nipples, anchoring your fingers laterally at the sides.
• Extend your thumbs so that they touch at the spinous processes; don't press them against the chest.
• Ask the patient to take a deep breath. As they do this, watch your thumbs; they should move apart equally. Any ↓ in movement on one side should be visible.
• It is easy to move your thumbs yourself in the expected direction. Be aware of this and allow them to follow the movement of the chest.

🛈 This maneuver may also be done on the anterior chest, as illustrated in Fig. 8.4, but as one can see, personal comfort, breast size, and modesty may preclude a quality exam of a female. If chest expansion must be assessed on the anterior chest wall, it is important to explain what you are doing, as suddenly reaching for a female chest may be misconstrued!

Tactile vocal fremitus

This is the vibration felt on the chest as the patient speaks. Each part of the chest is tested, as for percussion.

• Place the medial edge of your hand horizontally against the chest.
• Ask the patient to say "99" or "1, 1, 1."
• You should feel the vibration against your hand.

This test is rather crude and often neglected by clinicians. The changes are identical to those for vocal resonance.

• ↑ Vibration in consolidation
• ↓ In pneumothorax, collapse, COPD and pleural effusion

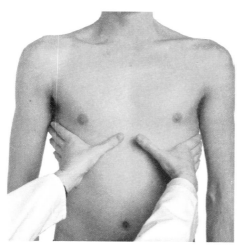

Fig. 8.4 Placement of the hands for testing chest expansion. Anchor with the fingers and leave the thumbs free-floating.

Percussion

Technique

This takes some practice to master fully, thus it can serve as an excellent indicator of how much time a student has spent performing the maneuver. The aim is to tap the chest by the standard method and listen to and feel for the resultant sound (see Figs. 8.5 and 8.6). For a *right-handed* provider:

- Place the left hand on the chest wall, fingers separated and lying between the ribs.
- Press the middle finger firmly against the chest.
- Using the middle finger of the right hand, strike the middle phalanx of the middle finger of the left hand (Fig. 8.5).
- The striking finger should be moved away again quickly, as keeping it pressed on the left hand may muffle the noise.
- The right middle finger should be kept in the flexed position, the striking movement coming from the wrist (much like playing the piano).

ⓘ Students quickly learn to keep the middle fingernail of their right hand well trimmed!

- Students should practice on themselves and each other. Learn the different sounds produced percussing over the lung and the more dense liver just below.
- In clinical practice, one should percuss each area of the lung, each time comparing right then left, as shown in Fig. 8.6.
- Don't forget the apices, which can be assessed by percussing directly onto the patient's clavicle (no left hand needed).
- If an area of dullness is heard (or felt), this should be percussed in more detail so as to map out the borders of the abnormality.

Findings

- Normal lung sounds *resonant*.
- *Dullness* = heard over areas of ↑ density (consolidation, collapse, alveolar fluid, pleural thickening, peripheral abscess, neoplasm)
- *Stony dullness* = the unique extreme dullness heard over a pleural effusion
- *Hyperresonant* = areas of ↓ density (emphysematous bullae or pneumothorax). COPD will create a globally hyperresonant chest.

▶There should be an area of dullness over the heart that may be diminished in hyperexpansion states (e.g., COPD or severe asthma).

▶The liver is manifested by an area of dullness below the level of the sixth rib anteriorly on the right. This may also be lost with hyperinflated lungs.

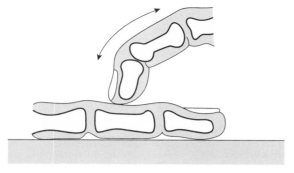

Fig. 8.5 Strike the middle phalanx of the middle finger of the left hand with the middle finger of the right hand.

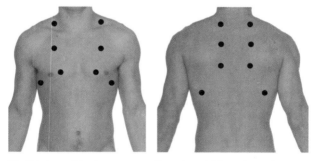

Fig. 8.6 Areas of the chest to percuss. Test right vs. left for each area, front and back.

Auscultation

Technique

The diaphragm should be used, except where better surface contact is needed in very thin or hairy patients.

- Ask the patient to take deep breaths in and out through the mouth.
- Listen to both inspiration and expiration.
- Listen over the same areas percussed, comparing left to right.
- If an abnormality is found, examine more carefully and define borders.
- Listen for the breath sounds and any added sounds, and note at which point in the respiratory cycle they occur.

ⓘ Many patients have difficulty performing correctly here. They may take one deep breath and hold it, may breath through the nose, or may take only one breath. Simple prompts ("keep going, in and out") will help. A brief demonstration will usually solve things if all else fails.

Findings

Breath sounds

- *Normal:* vesicular. Produced by airflow in the large airways and larynx and altered by passage through the small airways before reaching the stethoscope. Often described as rustling. This is heard especially well in inspiration and early expiration.
- *Reduced sound:* if local = effusion, tumor, pneumothorax, pneumonia, or lung collapse. If global = COPD or asthma (The "silent chest" is a sign of a life-threatening asthma attack.)
- *Bronchial breathing:* caused by ↑ density of matter in the peripheral lung, allowing sound from the larynx to the stethoscope unchanged, has a hollow, blowing quality, heard equally in inspiration and expiration, often with a brief pause between. (Think of a certain black-helmeted villain in a popular space movie series.) A similar sound can be heard by listening over the trachea in the neck. Bronchial breathing is heard over consolidation, lung abscess at the chest wall, and with dense fibrosis. It is also heard at the upper border of a pleural effusion.

Added sounds

- *Wheeze (rhonchi):* musical whistling sounds caused by narrowed airways. It is heard easier in expiration.
- Different-caliber airways = different-pitch note; thus asthma and COPD can cause a chorus of notes termed *polyphonic wheeze.*
  - *Monophonic wheeze* indicates that a single airway is narrowed, usually by a foreign body or carcinoma.
- ⓘ This is not a good marker of disease severity!
- *Crackles (crepitations, rales):* caused by air entering collapsed airways and alveoli producing an opening snap. They are heard in inspiration.
  - *Coarse* crackles are made by larger airways opening and sound like the snap and pop of a certain breakfast cereal. Causes include fluid or infection.

- *Fine* crackles occur later in inspiration. These sound like the tear of Velcro® and can also be reproduced by rolling hair at the temples between the thumb and forefinger. Causes include fluid, infection, or fibrosis (particularly at lung bases).

ⓘ Crackles are often a normal finding at the lung bases. If so, they will clear after asking the patient to cough.

- *Rub:* creaking sound likened to the bending of new leather or the creak of a footstep in fresh snow. This is heard at the height of inspiration and is caused by inflamed pleural surfaces rubbing against each other.
  - Causes include pneumonia and pulmonary embolism with infarction.

ⓘ Movement of the stethoscope on the chest wall sounds similar.

Vocal resonance

- Auscultatory equivalent of vocal fremitus
- Low-pitched sounds transmit well and create a vocal booming quality.
- Ask the patient to say "99" or 1, 1, 1" and listen over the same areas as before.
- The changes are the same as those for vocal fremitus.
- A marked ↑ resonance, such that a whisper can be clearly heard, is termed *whispered pectoriloquy.*

Important presenting patterns

Consolidation
- ↓ Air entry locally, secondary to infection
- ↓ Chest wall movement locally
- Dullness to percussion
- Bronchial breathing or ↑ breath sounds
- Coarse or fine crackles, localized
- ↑ Vocal resonance

Collapse
- Blockage of a major airway and collapse of the distal lung segment
- Mediastinal shift towards the abnormality
- ↓ Chest wall movement locally
- Dullness to percussion restricted to affected lobe
- ↓ Breath sounds
- ↓ Vocal resonance

Pleural effusion
- Collection of fluid between the two pleural layers, creating a sound barrier between the examiner and the patient's lung
- Mediastinal shift away from the lesion (with a large effusion)
- ↓ Chest wall movement locally
- Stony dull to percussion
- ↓ Breath sounds with bronchial breathing at the upper border
- ↓ Vocal resonance
- Sometimes a pleural rub just above

Pneumothorax
- Air in the pleural space
- Mediastinal shift away from the lesion (with a tension pneumothorax)
- ↓ Chest wall movement locally
- Hyperresonant to percussion
- ↓ Breath sounds
- ↓ Vocal resonance

Interstitial fibrosis
- No mediastinal shift. The trachea may move toward the fibrosis in upper-lobe disease.
- ↔ or ↓ chest wall movement
- ↔ percussion note
- ↔ breath sounds
- ↔ vocal resonance
- Fine crackles present

The elderly patient

Up to 60% of older people may suffer respiratory symptoms but less readily see their doctors about them. Lung function declines with age and exertional breathlessness rises, often with concurrent (nonrespiratory) illnesses. Careful, thoughtful assessment is therefore vital.

History

Clarify diagnosis

Not all disease in elders is COPD and many older people are lifelong non-smokers. Asthma and pulmonary fibrosis are often underdiagnosed.

Fatigue

Fatigue is often associated with chronic respiratory illnesses, and this may be more disabling to individuals than respiratory symptoms themselves.

Drug history

This should be comprehensive and dovetail with other medical problems. Anticholinergic drugs (e.g., atrovent) may precipitate glaucoma or worsen bladder and bowel symptoms, so be thorough. Ask about vaccinations—many people miss their annual flu vaccine because of hospitalization. Consider vaccination as appropriate.

Nutrition and mood

Undernutrition is common with chronic diseases and those in long-term care, affecting illnesses with higher resting metabolic rates (e.g., COPD). Depressed mood is similarly common and should be asked about.

Social history

Functional history is paramount and may reveal key interventions. A thorough occupational history is vital; many people do not know that they have worked or lived with someone exposed to, e.g., asbestos.

Examination

General

Poorly fitting clothes or dentures may point to weight loss (undernutrition, chronic disease, malignancy).

Hands

Arthritis and other deformities may make inhaler use difficult and point to related diagnoses (e.g., rheumatoid lung disease). Clubbing may not be present in later-onset pulmonary fibrosis.

Chest

Beware of basal crepitations, which are common in older age. Pick out discriminating signs—tachypnea, *position* of crackles, added sounds, etc.

Inhaler technique

This is a key examination. It may reveal why prior treatments were unsuccessful.

Diagnoses not to be missed

- *Asthma:* seen in up to 8% of individuals over 60 but underrecognized and undertreated. Spirometry is a key investigation.
- *Tuberculosis:* ↑ in the elderly, through reactivation, chronic illness, and undernutrition. TB presents nonspecifically, with cough, lethargy, and weight loss.

Abdomen

Applied anatomy

The abdomen includes the perineum, external and internal genitalia, and inguinal regions. These components are discussed in Chapters 12 and 14.

Boundaries

The abdomen is defined as the region lying between the thorax above and the pelvic cavity below. The anterior abdominal wall is bounded by the seventh to twelfth costal cartilages and the xiphoid process of the sternum superiorly and the inguinal ligaments and pelvic bones inferiorly.

The abdominal cavity is separated from the thoracic cavity by the diaphragm. There is no such delineation, however, between the abdomen and the pelvis; consequently, definitions vary.

Abdominal contents

The abdomen contains structures that form part of just about every body system.

The *digestive* organs of the esophagus, stomach, small intestine, large intestine, and the associated organs (liver, gallbladder, and biliary system, exocrine pancreas) all lie within the abdomen.

The *endocrine* portion of the pancreas, the adrenal glands, and gonads represent the endocrine system.

The *cardiovascular* system includes the abdominal aorta with its important branches to the liver, spleen, intestine, kidneys, and lower limbs.

The *immunological* system is represented by the spleen, the multiple lymph nodes surrounding the aorta and intestines, and the mucosa-associated lymphoid tissue (MALT) within the intestine itself.

The whole of the *urinary* system is present (kidneys, ureters, bladder, and urethra).

Much like the thorax, the abdomen is lined by a thin layer of membranous tissue: the *peritoneum*. This is a double lining—the *parietal peritoneum* covers the internal surface of the abdominal walls while the *visceral peritoneum* covers the organs. Between the two layers (the peritoneal cavity) is a small amount of fluid that acts as a lubricant enabling the abdominal contents to move against each other as the body changes position or, for example, as the gut contorts with peristalsis.

A select few organs lie behind the peritoneum on the posterior abdominal wall. They are the pancreas, a portion of the duodenum, the ascending and descending colon, and the kidneys.

Abdominal regions

The anterior abdominal wall is artificially divided into nine portions for descriptive purposes. Four imaginary lines can be drawn (see Fig. 9.1):
- 1horizontal line between the anterior superior iliac spines
- 1horizontal line between the lower border of the ribs
- 2vertical lines at the mid-clavicular point

To make life easier, the abdomen can also be divided into four quadrants by imagining one horizontal and one vertical line crossing at the umbilicus (see Fig. 9.2). Familiarize yourself with these along with the organs lying in each area.

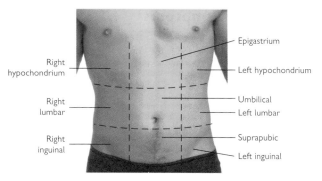

Fig. 9.1 The nine segments of the anterior abdominal wall.

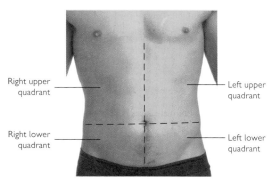

Fig. 9.2 The four quadrants of the anterior abdominal wall.

Esophageal symptoms

Dysphagia

This is difficulty swallowing and is the principal symptom of esophageal disease (see Box 9.1 for important causes). When a patient complains of dysphagia, you should attempt to establish the following:

- **Level of obstruction:** Where does the patient feel the food or liquid sticking? Patients can often point to a level on the chest, although the sensation usually correlates poorly with the actual level of obstruction.
- **Onset:** How quickly did the symptoms emerge? Obstruction caused by cancer, for example, may progress rapidly over a few months, whereas those with a benign peptic stricture may describe a very long history of GERD and progressive dysphagia.
- **Course:** Is it intermittent? Present for only the first few swallows (lower esophageal ring, spasm)? Progressive (cancer, stricture, achalasia)?
- **Solids/liquids:** Both solids and liquids being affected equally suggests a motor cause (achalasia, spasm). However, if solids are affected more than liquids, some physical obstruction is more likely (e.g., cancer).
- **Associated symptoms:** heartburn (leads to esophageal strictures), weight loss, wasting, fatigue (perhaps suggestive of cancer). Coughing and choking suggest pharyngeal dysphagia due to motor dysfunction (e.g., motor neuron disease causing bulbar or pseudobulbar palsy).

Odynophagia

This is pain on swallowing. It is usually an unpleasant substernal sensation *during* the swallow and suggestive of esophageal inflammation (infective esophagitis—candida, herpes, cytomegalovirus; peptic ulceration; caustic damage; esophageal perforation).

🔵 Remember to ask about potential causes during the drug history.

Heartburn and acid reflux

Also known as gastroesophageal reflux disease (GERD), this is caused by regurgitation of stomach contents into the esophagus due to an incompetent antireflux mechanism at the gastroesophageal junction (GEJ).

Typical features
- **Site:** midline, retrosternal
- **Radiation:** to the throat and occasionally the infrascapular regions
- **Nature:** burning
- **Aggravating factors:** worse after meals and when performing postures that raise the intra-abdominal pressure (bending, stooping, lying supine). Also worse during pregnancy
- **Associated symptoms:** often accompanied by acid or bitter taste (acid regurgitation) or sudden filling of the mouth with saliva* (waterbrash)

---

* The salivary glands can produce 10 mL of saliva/minute—the esophageo-salivary response.

Acid reflux may be worsened by certain foods (alcohol, caffeine, chocolate, fatty meals) and some drugs (calcium channel blockers, anticholinergics) that act to ↓ the GEJ sphincter pressure.

ⓘ Hiatal hernia is another important cause of reflux symptoms—be sure to inquire about this in the history.

Dyspepsia

This is commonly known as indigestion. It is very common and presents as a variety of symptoms:

- Upper abdominal discomfort
- Bloating
- Belching

Be on the alert for features suggestive of a serious pathology (anemia, weight loss, dysphagia, rectal blood loss, melena, and abdominal masses).

Box 9.1 Some causes of dysphagia

- *Oral:* painful mouth ulceration, oral, or throat infections
- *Neurological:* cerebrovascular event, bulbar and pseudobulbar palsies, myasthenia gravis
- *Dysmotility:* achalasia, systemic sclerosis, presbyesophagus
- *Mechanical:* pharyngeal pouch, esophageal cancer, peptic stricture, other benign strictures, extrinsic compression of the esophagus (e.g., large lung or thyroid tumor)

Nausea, vomiting, and vomitus

Nausea and vomiting

Nausea* is a feeling of sickness—the inclination to vomit. It usually occurs in waves and may be associated with retching or heaving. It can last from seconds to days depending on the cause.

Vomiting (emesis) usually follows nausea and autonomic symptoms, such as salivation. It is the forceful expulsion of the gastric contents by reflex contractions of thoracic and abdominal muscles. See Box 9.2 for causes.

The vomiting center is in the medulla and is composed of many efferent nuclei in serial communication with each other. When the entire circuit is activated by afferent stimuli, the complete set of actions required to cause vomiting is triggered.

Timing
You should be clear on exactly when the vomiting tends to occur, particularly its relation to meals—e.g., vomiting delayed for >1 hour after meals suggests gastroesophageal obstruction or gastroparesis. Early-morning vomiting is typical of pregnancy or raised intracranial pressure.

Nature of the vomitus
Although unpleasant, you should inquire about the exact nature of any vomited material and attempt to see a sample, if possible.

Blood (hematemesis)
Presence of blood indicates bleeding in the upper gastrointestinal tract (esophagus, stomach, duodenum). A history of bleeding must be explored in the context of other abdominal symptoms (Box 9.3). Ask especially about the following:

- Amount of blood and exact nature of it (see Box 9.4)
- Previous bleeding episodes, treatment and outcome (e.g., previous surgery?)
- Cigarette smoking
- Use of drugs such as aspirin, NSAIDs, and warfarin
- ❶ Remember to ask about weight loss, dysphagia, abdominal pain, and melena (consider the possibility of neoplastic disease).

Bile
Assess the presence or absence of bile. Remember that bile comes largely in two colors—the green pigment (biliverdin) often seen to color the vomitus in the absence of undigested food. The yellow pigment (bilirubin) appears as orange, often occurring in small lumps.**

Undigested food without bile suggests a lack of connection between the stomach and the small intestine (e.g., pyloric obstruction).

---

* *Nausea* comes from the Latin, meaning "sea-sickness," through the Greek *naus,* meaning "ship."
** This is the answer to the age-old question, why are there always carrots in vomit?. The orange globules are, in fact, dyed with bilirubin. We suggest saving that fact for your next dinner party.

Box 9.2 Important causes of vomiting

- *Acute:* GI tract infections (viral gastroenteritis, e.g., food poisoning, Norwalk, viral hepatitis), systemic bacterial infection, mechanical bowel obstruction, alcohol intoxication, acute upper GI bleed, urinary tract infection
- *Chronic:* pregnancy, uremia, drugs (narcotics, digitalis, aminophylline, cancer chemotherapy), gastroparesis (diabetes mellitus, scleroderma, drugs)
- *Other:* peptic ulcer disease, motor disorders (post-surgery or autonomic dysfunction), hepatobiliary disease, alcoholism, cancer
▶ Don't forget about central nervous system and vestibular problems.

Box 9.3 Causes of upper GI bleeding

- Peptic ulceration
- Erosive or ulcerative esophagitis
- Gastritis
- Varices (esophageal/gastric)
- Gastric and esophageal tumors
- Mallory–Weiss tear
- Dieulafoy's lesion
- Vascular anomalies (e.g., angiodysplasia, AV malformation)
- Hereditary hemorrhagic telangiectasia
- Connective tissue disorders
- Vasculitis
- Bleeding disorders

Box 9.4 Nature of hematemesis

- *Large volume of fresh, red* blood suggests active bleeding (coincident liver disease and/or heavy alcohol intake may suggest bleeding esophageal varices; abdominal pain and heartburn suggest a gastric or esophageal source such as a peptic ulceration or GERD).
- *Small streaks* at the end of prolonged retching may indicate minor esophageal trauma at the GEJ (Mallory–Weiss tear).
- *Coffee-grounds:* This term is used for blood that has been altered by exposure to stomach acid as the result of a bleeding site superior to the ligament of Trietz. It appears brown and in small lumps.

Abdominal pain

Like pain in any other region, abdominal pain may present in very different ways and has many different causes. You should establish the site, radiation, severity, character, frequency, duration, any exacerbating or relieving factors, and associated symptoms.

Site

Like most organs, those in the abdomen cannot be felt directly—the pain is referred to areas of the abdominal wall according to the organ's embryological origin (see Box 9.5 and Fig. 9.3).

- Ask the patient to point to the area affected. They often find this challenging and may indicate a wide area. In this case, ask them to use one finger and point to the area of maximum intensity: "Use one finger and point to where the pain is worst."

Box 9.5 Sites of abdominal pain and embryological origins

- *Epigastric:* foregut (stomach, duodenum, liver, pancreas, gallbladder)
- *Periumbilical:* midgut (small and large intestines including appendix)
- *Suprapubic:* hindgut (rectum and urogenital organs)

A very localized pain may originate from the parietal peritoneum. For example, appendicitis may begin as an umbilical pain (referred from the appendix) then move to the right iliac fossa as the inflammation spreads to the peritoneum overlying the appendix.

Radiation

Ask the patient if the pain is felt elsewhere or if they have any other pains (they may not associate the radiated pain with the abdominal pain).

Some examples include the following:

- Right scapula: gallbladder
- Shoulder tip: diaphragmatic irritation
- Mid-back: pancreas

Character

Ask the patient what *sort* of pain it is. Give some examples if they have trouble, but be careful not to lead the patient. A couple of examples include the following:

- *Colicky:* This is pain that comes and goes in waves and indicates obstruction of a hollow, muscular-walled organ (intestine, gallbladder, bile duct, ureter).
- *Burning:* This usually indicates an acid cause and is related to the stomach, duodenum, or lower end of the esophagus.

Aggravating and relieving factors

Ask the patient what appears to make the pain better or worse—or what they do to get rid of the pain if they suffer from it often.

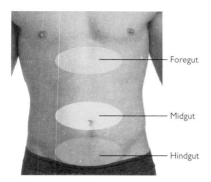

Foregut

Midgut

Hindgut

Fig. 9.3 Typical sites of pain according to origin.

Findings

Some characteristic pains:

- *Renal colic:* colicky pain at the renal angles ± loins, which are tender to touch, radiating to the groin, testicles, or labia. Typically, the patient writhes about, unable to find a position that relieves the pain.
- *Bladder pain:* a diffuse severe pain in the suprapubic region
- *Prostatic pain:* a dull ache that may be felt in the lower abdomen, rectum, perineum, or anterior thighs.
- *Urethral pain:* variable in presentation, ranging from a tickling discomfort to a severe sharp pain felt at the end of the urethra (tip of the penis in males) and exacerbated by micturition. It can be so severe that patients attempt to hold urine, causing yet more problems.
- *Small bowel obstruction:* colicky central pain associated with vomiting, abdominal distension ± constipation
- *Colonic pain:* as with small bowel obstruction but sometimes temporarily relieved by defecation or passing flatus
- *Bowel ischemia:* dull, severe, constant, right upper quadrant or central abdominal pain exacerbated by eating
- *Biliary pain:* severe, constant, right upper quadrant or epigastric pain that can last hours and is often worse after eating fatty foods.
- *Pancreatic pain:* epigastric, radiating to the back and partly relieved by sitting up and leaning forward
- *Peptic ulcer pain:* dull, burning pain in the epigastrium. Typically episodic at night, waking the patient from sleep. It is exacerbated by eating and sometimes relieved by consuming milk or antacids.

Bowel habit

Ask patients how often they move their bowels and if this has changed recently. Ask also about the other symptoms on these pages.

Constipation

This disorder can mean different things to different people. Normal bowel habit ranges from 3 times/day to once every 3 days.

Constipation is the passage of stool <3 times/week, or stools that are hard or difficult to pass. See Box 9.6 for causes.

A thorough history should include the following:

• Duration of constipation
• Stool size and consistency
• Straining, particularly at the end of evacuation
• Associated symptoms (nausea, vomiting, weight loss)
• Pain on defecation
• Rectal bleeding
• Intercurrent diarrhea
• Fluid and fiber intake
• Depression, lack of exercise
• Drug history (prescription and over-the-counter). Particularly ask about use of codeine, antidepressants, aluminum, and calcium antacids.
• Metabolic or endocrine diseases (thyroid disorders, hypercalcemia, diabetes, pheochromocytoma, Hirshsprung's disease)
• Neurological problems (autonomic neuropathy, spinal cord injury, multiple sclerosis)

Diarrhea

This is defined as an increase in stool volume (>200mL daily) and frequency(3/day). There is also a change in consistency to semiformed or liquid stool. See Box 9.7 for causes.

Establish the time course, since acute diarrhea is suggestive of infection. Ask especially about the following:

• Color, consistency, offensive smell, ease of flushing
• Duration
• Does the diarrhea disturb the patient's sleep?
• Is there any blood, mucus, or pus?
• Is there associated pain or colic?
• Is there urgency?
• Nausea, vomiting, weight loss?
• Any difference if the patient fasts?
    • No change in secretory diarrhea—e.g., *E. coli, Staph. aureus*
    • Disappears on fasting: *osmotic diarrhea*
• Foreign travel
• Recent antibiotics

Box 9.6 Some causes of constipation

- Low-fiber diet
- Physical immobility
- Functional bowel disease
- Drugs (e.g.,opiates, antidepressants, aluminumantacids).
- Metabolic and endocrine diseases (e.g.,hypothyroidism, hypercalcemia, hypokalemia, diabetes mellitus, porphyria, pheochromocytoma)
- Neurological disorders (e.g., autonomic neuropathy, spinal cord injury, multiple sclerosis)
- Colonic stricture
- Anorectal disease (e.g., anal fissure—causes pain to the extent that the patient may avoid defecating altogether)
- Habitual neglect
- Depression
- Dementia

Box 9.7 Some causes of diarrhea

- **Malabsorption:** may cause steatorrhea, a fatty, pale stool that is extremely odorous and difficult to flush. See Box 9.8 on 📖 p. 214.
- **↑Intestinal motility:** hyperthyroidism, irritable bowel syndrome (see below).
- **Exudative:** inflammation of the bowel causes small volume, frequent stools, often with blood or mucus (e.g., colonic carcinoma, Crohn's disease, ulcerative colitis)
- **Osmotic:** large volume of stool that disappears with fasting. Causes include lactose intolerance, gastric surgery.
- **Secretory:** high volume of stool that persists with fasting. No pus, blood or excessive fat. Causes include gastrointestinal infections, carcinoid syndrome, villous adenoma of the colon, Zollinger–Ellison syndrome, vasoactive intestinal polypeptide (VIP)-secreting tumor.

Rectal bleeding and melena

There are many causes of rectal blood loss (Box 9.9) but, as always, a detailed history will help. Determine the following:

- Amount
- ⓘ Small amounts can appear dramatic, coloring toilet water red.
- Nature of the blood (red, brown, black)
- Is it mixed within the stool or is it on the stool?
- Is it spattered over the bowl or with the stool, or only seen on the paper?
- Any associated features (Mucus may indicate inflammatory bowel disease or colonic cancer.)

Box 9.8 Fat malabsorption (steatorrhea)

This is a common feature of pancreatic insufficiency (e.g., due to chronic pancreatitis, cystic fibrosis). It is also caused by diseases such as celiac disease, inflammatory bowel disease, blind bowel loops, and short bowel syndrome.

You should be aware of these features and explore them all fully if one is mentioned by the patient:

• Pale stool
• Offensive smelling
• Poorly formed
• Difficult to flush (floats)

Melena

This is jet-black, tar-like, and pungent-smelling stool representing blood from the upper GI tract (or right side of the large bowel) that has been altered by passage through the gut.

The presence of melena is often asked about in hospitalized patients, but those who have smelled true melena rarely forget the experience!

Ask about iron supplementation or bismuth-containing compounds. These cause blackened stools but without the melena smell or consistency.

Mucus

This is a clear, viscoid secretion of the mucus membranes.* It contains mucus, epithelial cells, leukocytes, and various salts suspended in water.

The presence of mucus in or on stools may indicate the following:

• Inflammatory bowel disease
• Solitary rectal ulcer
• Small or large bowel fistula
• Colonic villous adenoma
• Irritable bowel syndrome

Flatus

Small amounts of gas frequently escape from the bowel via the mouth (eructation) and anus. A notable excess of this is a common feature of both functional and organic disorders of the gastrointestinal tract.

It is often associated with abdominal bloating and caused by the fermentation of certain foods by colonic flora.

Excessive flatus is a particular feature of the following

• Hiatal hernia
• Peptic ulceration
• Chronic gallbladder disease
• Air-swallowing (aerophagy)
• High-fiber diet

---

* Think "slime" or even "snot." Patients may find this easier to understand: "Have you noticed any slime-like mucus in your stools?"

Box 9.9 Causes of lower GI bleeding

- Hemorrhoids
- Anal fissure
- Diverticular disease
- Colonic carcinoma
- Colonic polyp
- Angiodysplasia
- Inflammatory bowel disease
- Ischemic colitis
- Meckel'sdiverticulum
- Small bowel disease (e.g., tumor, diverticulae, intussusception, Crohn's)
- Solitary rectal ulcer
- Hemobilia (bleeding into the biliary tree)

Jaundice and pruritus

Jaundice

Jaundice (icterus) is a yellow pigmentation of skin, sclera, and mucosa caused by excess bilirubin in the body fluids. It is usually considered a sign, as it is seen on examination. See also 📖 p. 51 and Box 9.10.

Ask about the following:
- Color of the urine (dark in cholestatic jaundice)
- Color and consistency of the stools (pale in cholestatic jaundice)
- Abdominal pain (e.g., caused by gallstones)

While the following factors should be included in any thorough history, you should make a special point of asking about them:
- Previous blood transfusions
- Past history of jaundice
- Drugs (e.g., antibiotics, NSAIDs, oral contraceptives, phenothiazines)
- IV drug use
- Tattoos and body piercing
- Foreign travel
- Sexual history
- Family history of liver disease
- Alcohol consumption
- Any personal contacts who also have jaundice

Pruritus

This is itching of the skin and may be either localized or generalized.

It has many causes—it is particularly associated with cholestatic liver disease (e.g., primary biliary cirrhosis, sclerosing cholangitis).

Box 9.10 Causes of jaundice

Prehepatic
- Hemolysis
- Gilbert's disease
- Dubin–Johnson syndrome
- Rotor syndrome

Hemodialysis
- Hepatocellular
- Cirrhosis
- Acute hepatitis (viral, alcoholic, autoimmune, drug induced)
- Liver tumors
- Cholestasis from drugs (e.g., chlorpromazine)

Posthepatic
Obstruction of biliary outflow due to the following:
- Luminal obstruction: gallstones
- Wall pathology: congenital bile duct abnormalities, primary biliary cirrhosis, trauma, tumor
- External compression: pancreatitis, lymphadenopathy, pancreatic tumor, ampulla of Vater tumor

Abdominal swelling

The five classic causes of abdominal swelling (the 5 F's) are shown in Box 9.11. To these you should also add *tumor*.

In decompensated cirrhosis, a combination of portal (sinusoidal) hypertension and Na and H_2O retention favors the transudation of fluid into the peritoneal cavity (ascites). The resultant swelling may be unsightly. It can also cause shortness of breath by putting pressure on the diaphragm from below, particularly when supine, and may be associated with pleural effusions.

See 📖 p. 672 for the causes and classification of ascites.

Box 9.11 Five causes of abdominal swelling—the 5 F's

- Fat
- Fluid
- Flatus
- Feces
- Fetus

Urinary and prostate symptoms

Urinary frequency
This is the passing of urine more often than is normal for the patient. Quantify this—how many times in a day—and also ask about the volume of urine passed each time (you are attempting to decide whether the patient is producing more urine than normal or simply feeling the urge to urinate more than normal).

Urgency
This is the sudden need to urinate, a feeling that the patient may not be able to make it to the toilet in time. Ask about the volume expelled.

Nocturia
This is urination during the night. Does the patient wake from sleep to urinate? How many times a night? How much urine is expelled each time?

Urinary incontinence
This is the loss of voluntary control of bladder emptying. Patients may be hesitant to talk about this, so try to avoid the phrase "wetting yourself." "You could ask about it immediately after asking about urgency" "Do you ever feel the desperate need to empty your bladder? Have you ever not made it in time?" Or ask about a "loss of control."

There are five main types of urinary incontinence:
- *True:* total lack of control of urinary excretion. This suggests a fistula between the urinary tract and the exterior or a neurological condition.
- *Giggle:* incontinence during bouts of laughter. This is common in young girls.
- *Stress:* leakage associated with a sudden ↑ in intra-abdominal pressure of any cause (e.g., coughing, laughing, sneezing)
- *Urge:* intense urge to urinate such that the patient is unable to get to the toilet in time. Causes include overactivity of the detrusor muscle, urinary infection, bladder stones and bladder cancer.
- *Dribbling or overflow:* continual loss of urine from a chronically distended bladder. Typically this occurs in elderly males with prostate disease.

Terminal dribbling
This is a male complaint and usually indicative of prostate disease. It is a dripping of urine from the urethra at the end of micturition, requiring an abnormally protracted shake of the penis and may cause embarrassing staining of clothing.

Hesitancy
This is difficulty in starting to micturate. The male patient describes standing and waiting for the urine to start flowing. Hesitancy is usually due to bladder outflow obstruction from prostatic disease or strictures.

Dysuria

Pain on micturition is usually described by the patient as "burning" or "stinging" and is felt at the urethral meatus. Ask whether it is throughout the passage of urine or only at the end (terminal dysuria).

Hematuria

This is the passage of blood in the urine. It is always an abnormal finding.
◐ Remember that microscopic hematuria will be undetectable to the patient, only showing on dip-testing.

Incomplete emptying

This is the sensation that there is more urine left to expel at the end of micturition. It suggests detrusor dysfunction or prostatic disease.

Intermittency

This is the disruption of urine flow in a stop–start manner. Causes include prostatic hypertrophy, bladder stones, and ureteroceles.

Oliguria and anuria

Oliguria is scanty or low-volume urination and is defined as the excretion of <300mL urine in 24 hours. Causes can be physiological (dehydration) or pathological (intrinsic renal disease, shock, or obstruction).

Anuria is the absence of urine formation. You should attempt to rule out urinary tract obstruction as a matter or urgency. Other causes include severe intrinsic renal dysfunction and shock.

Polyuria

This is excessive excretion of large volumes of urine and must be carefully differentiated from urinary frequency (the frequent passage of small amounts of urine).

Causes vary widely but include the ingestion of large volumes of water (including hysterical polydipsia), diabetes mellitus (the osmotic effect of glucose in the tubules results in more urine produced), failure of the action of antidiuretic hormone (ADH) at the renal tubule (as in diabetes insipidus) and defective renal concentrating ability (e.g., chronic renal failure).
◐ Remember also to ask the patient about the use of diuretic medication.

Appetite and weight

Loss of appetite and changes in weight are rather non-specific symptoms but should raise suspicion of a serious disease if either is severe, prolonged, or unexpected.

▶ Remember that weight loss has many causes outside of the abdomen and a thorough systems inquiry should be conducted.

Weight loss may not be noticed by patients if they don't regularly weigh themselves—ask about clothes becoming loose.

ⓘ Remember that the patient may have been intentionally losing weight, throwing you off track. Ask if the loss is expected.

▶ Ascites weighs 1kg/L and some patients with liver failure may have 10–20L of ascites, masking any dry-weight loss.

Ask the patient about their eating habit and average daily diet.

Try to determine the following:

• When the symptom was first noticed
• Quantify the problem. In the case of weight loss, determine exactly how and over what time period.
• Cause of the anorexia—does eating make the patient feel sick?
• Does eating cause pain (e.g., gastric ulcer, mesenteric angina, pancreatitis)?
• Any accompanying symptoms (abdominal pain, nausea, vomiting, fever)

Ask also about the following:

• Color and consistency of stools (e.g., steatorrhea?)
• Urinary symptoms (see 📖 p. 218)
• Recent change in temperature tolerance

In every case, you should calculate the patient's BMI as on 📖 p. 56.

The combination of weight loss with ↑ appetite may suggest malabsorption or a hypermetabolic state (e.g., thyrotoxicosis).

The rest of the history

Past medical history

Ask especially about the following:
- Previous surgical procedures, including peri- and postoperative complications and anesthetic complications
- Chronic bowel diseases (e.g., inflammatory bowel disease [IBD], including recent flareups and treatment to date)
- Possible associated conditions (e.g., diabetes with hemachromatosis)

Drug history

Think about drugs that can precipitate abdominal diseases and remember to ask about over-the-counter drugs. For example:
- *Hepatitis:* halothane, phenytoin, chlorothiazides, pyrazinamide, isoniazid, methyl dopa, HMG CoA reductase inhibitors (statins), sodium valproate, amiodarone, antibiotics, NSAIDs
- *Cholestasis:* chlorpromazine, sulfonamides, sulfonylureas, rifam-picin, nitrofurantoin, anabolic steroids, oral contraceptive pill
- *Fatty liver:* tetracycline, sodium valproate, amiodar-one
- *Acute liver necrosis:* acetaminophen
- Ask also about previous blood transfusions.

Smoking

Smokers are at ↑ risk of peptic ulceration, esophageal cancer, and colo-rectal cancer. Smoking may also have a detrimental outcome on the natural history of Crohn's disease. There is some evidence that smoking may protect against ulcerative colitis.

Alcohol

As always, a detailed history is required—see 📖 p. 37. If dependence is suspected, run through the CAGE questionnaire—see Box 9.12.

Box 9.12 CAGE questionnaire

A positive response to any of the four questions may indicate someone at risk of alcohol abuse. A positive answer to two or more questions makes the presence of alcohol dependence likely.

C   Have you ever felt that you should **C**ut down your drinking?
A   Have you ever got **A**ngry when someone suggested that you should cut down?
G   Do you ever feel **G**uilty about your drinking?
E   Do you ever need an **E**ye-opener in the morning to steady your nerves or get rid of a hangover?

Family history

Ask especially about a history of inflammatory bowel disease, celiac disease, peptic ulcer disease, hereditary liver diseases (e.g., Wilson's, hemochromatosis) bowel cancer, jaundice, anemia, splenectomy, and cholecystectomy.

Social history

- Risks of exposure to hepatotoxins and hepatitis through occupation
- Tattoos
- Illicit drug use (especially sharing needles)
- Social contacts with a similar disease (particularly relevant to jaundice)
- Recent foreign travel

Dietary history

- Amount of fruit, vegetables and fiber in the diet
- Evidence of lactose intolerance
- Change in symptoms related to eating certain food groups
- Sensitivities to wheat, fat, caffeine, gluten

Outline examination

As always, ensure adequate privacy. Ideally, the patient should be lying flat with the head propped on a single pillow, arms lying at the sides.

The abdomen should be exposed at least from the bottom of the sternum to the symphysis pubis—preferably the whole upper torso is uncovered. Do not expose the genitalia until needed.

The examination should follow an orderly routine. The authors' suggestion is shown in Box 9.13. It is standard practice to start with the hands and work proximally—this establishes a physical rapport before you examine more sensitive areas.

General inspection

Looking at the patient from the end of the bed, assess their general health and look for any obvious abnormalities described in 🕮 Chapter 3 before moving closer. Look especially for the following:

• High or low body mass
• The state of hydration
• Fever
• Distress
• Pain
• Muscle wasting
• Peripheral edema
• Jaundice
• Anemia

Box 9.13 Framework for abdominal examination

• General inspection
• Hands
• Arms
• Axillae
• Face
• Chest
• Inspection of abdomen
• Auscultation
• Palpation of abdomen
  • Light
  • Deep
  • Specific organs
  • Examination of hernial orifices
  • External genitalia
• Percussion (± examination for ascites)
• Digital examination of the anus, rectum ± prostate

Hand and upper limb

Take the patient's right hand in yours and examine carefully for the following signs.

Nails

See also Chapter 4.

- **Leukonychia:** whitening of the nail bed due to hypoalbuminemia (e.g., malnutrition, malabsorption, hepatic disease, nephrotic syndrome)
- **Koilonychia:** spooning of the nails, making a concave shape instead of the normal convexity. Causes include congenital and chronic iron deficiency
- **Muehrcke's lines:** transverse white lines. They are seen in hypoalbuminemic states, including severe liver cirrhosis.
- **Clubbing:** described on 📖 p. 191. abdominal causes are cirrhosis, inflammatory bowel disease, and celiac disease.
- **Blue lunulae:** a bluish discoloration of the normal lanulae seen in Wilson's disease

Palms

- **Palmar erythema:** "liver palms." This is a blotchy reddening of the palms of the hands, especially affecting the thenar and hypothenar eminences. It can also affect soles of the feet. It is associated with chronic liver disease, pregnancy, thyrotoxicosis, rheumatoid arthritis, polycythemia, and (rarely) chronic leukemia. It can also be a normal finding.
- **Dupuytren's contracture:** thickening and fibrous contraction of the palmar fascia. In early stages, palpable irregular thickening of the fascia is seen, especially that overlying the fourth and fifth metacarpals. This can progress to a fixed flexion deformity of the fingers starting at the fifth finger and working across to the third or second. Often bilateral, it may also affect the feet. It is seen especially with alcoholic liver disease but may also be seen in manual workers (or may be familial).
- **Anemia:** Pallor in the palmar creases suggests significant anemia.
- **Rash:** Remember syphilis in the differential.

Hepatic flap (asterixis)

This is identical to the flap seen in hypercapnic states (see 📖 p. 191).

Ask the patient to stretch out their hands in front of them with the hands dorsiflexed at the wrists and fingers out-stretched and separated (see Fig.9.4).

The patient should hold that position for at least 15 seconds. If flap is present, the patient's hands will move in jerky, irregular flexion and extension at the wrist and MCP joints. The flap is nearly always bilateral. It may be subtle and intermittent.

This is characteristic of encephalopathy due to liver failure.

If a sign of hepatic encephalopathy in a patient with previously compensated liver disease, it may have been precipitated by infection, diuretic medication, electrolyte imbalance, diarrhea or constipation, vomiting, centrally acting drugs, upper GI bleeding, abdominal paracentesis, or surgery.

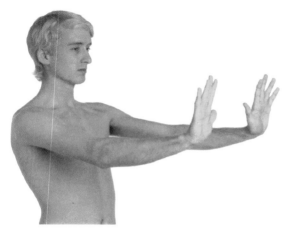

Fig. 9.4 Testing for hepatic flap. The patient should hold their arms outstretched with wrists dorsiflexed and fingers extended and abducted for at least 15 seconds.

Upper limb

Examine the arms for any signs of the following:

- *Bruising:* This may be a sign of the following:
  - Hepatocellular damage and the resulting coagulation disorder
  - Thrombocytopenia due to hypersplenism
  - Marrow suppression with alcohol
- *Petechiae:* pin-prick bleeds that do not blanch with pressure. Possibly a sign of thrombocytopenia
- *Muscle wasting:* seen as a decrease in muscle mass, possibly with overlying skin hanging loosely. A late manifestation of malnutrition and often seen in patients with chronic alcoholic liver disease
- *Scratch marks (excoriations):* suggests itch (pruritus) is present and may be the only visible feature of early cholestasis
- Be careful not to miss AV fistulae or hemodialysis catheters!

Axillae

Examine carefully for the following:

- Lymphadenopathy
- Acanthosis nigricans (a thickened, blackening of the skin. Velvety in appearance. May be associated with intra-abdominal malignancy)

Face and chest

Eyes

Ask the patient to look straight ahead while you look closely at their eyes, orbits, and surrounding skin. Then ask the patient to look up while you gently retract the lower lid with a finger, looking at the underlying sclera and conjunctiva. Look especially for the following:

- **Jaundice:** a yellow discoloration of the sclera. This is usually the first place that jaundice can be seen. This sign is particularly useful in patients with dark skin tones in whom jaundice would not otherwise be obvious.
- **Anemia:** pallor of the conjunctivae. You will need experience to spot this easily.
- **Kayser–Fleisher rings:** best seen with a slit lamp in an ophthalmology clinic. A greenish-yellow pigmented ring is just inside the cornea-scleral margin. It is due to copper deposition and seen in Wilson's disease.
- **Xanthelasma:** raised yellow lesions caused by a buildup of lipids beneath the skin. They are often seen encircling the eyes, especially at the nasal side of the orbit.

Mouth

Ask the patient to show you their teeth then open wide. Look carefully at the state of the teeth, the tongue, and the inner surface of the cheeks. You should also subtly attempt to smell the patient's breath.

Angular stomatitis

This is a reddening and inflammation at the corners of the mouth. It is a sign of thiamine, vitamin B_{12}, and iron deficiencies.

Circumoral pigmentation

Hyperpigmented areas surround the mouth. This is seen in Peutz–Jegher's syndrome.

Dentition

Note dentures or if there is evidence of tooth decay.

Telangiectasia

This is dilatation of the small vessels on the gums and buccal mucosa, seen in Osler–Weber–Rendu syndrome.

Gums

Look especially for ulcers (causes include celiac disease, inflammatory bowel disease, Behçet's disease and Reiter's syndrome) and hypertrophy (caused by pregnancy, phenytoin use, leukemia, scurvy [vitamin C deficiency],or inflammation [gingivitis]).

Breath

Smell especially for the following:
- *Fetor hepaticus:* a sweet-smelling breath
- *Ketosis:* sickly sweet pear-drop smelling breath
- *Uremia:* fishy smell

Tongue

Look especially for the following:

- *Glossitis:* smooth, erythematous swelling of the tongue. Causes include deficiencies of iron, vitamin B_{12}, and folate.
- *Macroglossia:* enlarged tongue. Causes include amyloidosis, hypothyroidism, acromegaly, Down syndrome, and neoplasia.
- *Leukoplakia:* a white-colored thickening of the tongue and oral mucus membranes. This is a premalignant condition caused by smoking, poor dental hygiene, alcohol, sepsis, and syphilis.
- *Geographical tongue:* painless red rings and lines on the surface of the tongue looking like a map. It can be caused by vitamin B_2 (riboflavin) deficiency or may be a normal variant.

Candidiasis

Also known as *thrush*, this is a fungal infection of the oral membranes seen as creamy, white curd-like patches that can be scraped off, revealing erythematous mucosa below. Causes include immunosuppression, antibiotic use, poor oral hygiene, iron deficiency, and diabetes.

Neck

Examine the cervical and supraclavicular lymph nodes as on 📖 p. 58.

Look especially for a supraclavicular node on the left-hand side, which, when enlarged, is called Virchow's node (Troisier's sign—suggestive of gastric malignancy).

Chest

Look at the anterior chest and look especially for the signs listed below.

Spider nevi

These are telangiectatic capillary lesions.

- A central red area with engorged capillaries spreading out from it in a spidery manner
- Caused by engorgement of capillaries from a central feeder vessel
- If the lesion is truly a spider nevus, it will be completely eliminated by pressure at the center from a penpoint or similar instrument and will fill outward when the pressure is released.
- Can range in size from those that are only just visible to up to 5 or 6mm in diameter
- Found in the distribution of the superior vena cava (see Fig. 9.5)
- A normal adult is allowed up to 5 spider nevi.
- Causes include chronic liver disease and estrogen excess.

Gynecomastia

This is the excessive development of male mammary glands due to ductal proliferation such that they resemble postpubertal female breasts.

- This is often embarrassing for the patient, so be sensitive in your approach.
- It is caused by alcoholic liver disease, congenital adrenal hyperplasia, and several commonly used drugs, including spironolactone, digoxin, and cimetidine.
- It can also be seen during puberty in the normal male.

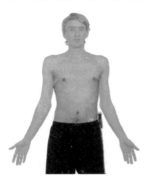

Fig. 9.5 Distribution of drainage to the superior vena cava and the area where one should look for spider nevi. The normal adult may have up to 5 such lesions.

Inspection of abdomen

With the abdomen exposed, you should make a careful and methodical inspection. Squat by the side of the bed or exam table so that the patient's abdomen is at your eye level when looking for waves or pulsations.

Note especially the features discussed on these pages.

Scars

These may be the result of trauma or previous surgery (Fig. 9.6). Recent scars will be pink and vascular. Old scars are white and may be indurated. Laproscopic surgery scars may be hidden in skin folds or the umbilicus.

Abdominal distension

Does the abdomen look swollen? Consider the 5 F's (Box 9.11 📖 p. 217) and note the state of the umbilicus (everted? deep?).

Focal swellings

Treat an abdominal swelling as you would do any other lump (📖 p. 88) and bear in mind the underlying anatomy and possible organ involvement.

Divarication of the recti

Particularly in the elderly and in patients who have had abdominal surgery, the twin rectus abdominis muscles may separate laterally on contraction, causing the underlying organs to bulge through the resultant midline gap.

Ask the patient to lift their head off the bed or to sit up slightly. Watch for the appearance of a longitudinal midline bulge.

Prominent vasculature

If veins are seen coursing over the abdomen, note their exact location. Attempt to map the direction of blood flow within them:

• Place two fingers at one end of the vein and apply occlusive pressure.
• Move one finger along the vein, emptying that section of blood in a milking action.
• Release the pressure from one finger and watch for the flow of blood back into the vein.

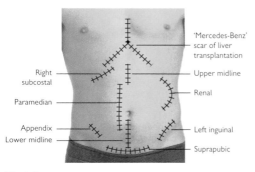

Fig. 9.6 Some common abdominal surgical scars.

- Repeat, emptying blood in the other direction.
- Given the venous valves, you should be able to determine the direction of blood flow in that vein.

Inferior flow of blood suggests superior vena cava (SVC) obstruction. Superior flow of blood suggests inferior vena cava (IVC) obstruction.

Flow radiating out from the umbilicus (caput medusae) indicates portal vein hypertension (porto-systemic shunting occurs through the umbilical veins which become engorged).

Obvious pulsations

Look across the abdomen for any pulsations. A pulsatile, expanding mass in the epigastrium may be an abdominal aortic aneurysm.

Peristaltic waves

These are usually only seen in thin, fit, young individuals. A very obvious bowel peristalsis is seen as rippling movements beneath the skin and may indicate intestinal obstruction.

Striae

Stretch marks are pink or white streaky lines caused by changes in the tension of the abdominal wall. These may be normal in rapidly growing pubescent teens. They are also seen in obesity, pregnancy (striae gravidarum), and ascites and following rapid weight loss or abdominal paracentesis.

Bear in mind that these will turn pink or purple in Cushing's syndrome, as will other scars (see 📖 p. 115).

Skin discoloration

There are two classical patterns of bruising or discoloration indicating the presence of retroperitoneal blood (seen especially in pancreatitis):

Cullen's sign: discoloration at the umbilicus and surrounding skin
Grey-Turner's sign: discoloration at the flanks

Stomas

Look for surgical stomas or fistulae, noting their exact location, nature of the stoma, and appearance of the exposed mucosa (if any). Remember that a stoma may be from the large bowel, small bowel, or renal tract. Look also at the contents of the stoma bag, noting any abnormalities such as diarrhea, pus, mucus, or blood.

- *Colostomy:* usually seen in the left iliac fossa and will be flush to the skin (bag may contain semisolid to formed stool)
- *Ileostomy:* usually in the right iliac fossa and formed as a spout of bowel mucosa extending from the abdominal wall to prevent the luminal contents from harming the abdominal wall (bag will contain semi-formed and liquid stool)
- *Urostomy:* often formed as an ileal conduit with ureters connected to a portion of small bowel and then to the abdominal wall. Usually in the right iliac fossa (bag will contain urine)
- *Nephrostomy:* drainage of urine from the kidney pelvis to the exterior. Usually a temporary measure following operative procedures to the renal tract or to decompress an obstructed system. Usually at the flank (bag will contain urine)

Auscultation

This is an important part of the abdominal examination that is easily missed. Listen before palpation or percussion of the abdomen.

Bowel sounds

These are low-pitched gurgling sounds produced by normal gut peristalsis. They are intermittent but will vary in timing depending on when the last meal was eaten. Practice listening to as many abdomens as possible to understand the normal range of sounds.

Listen with the diaphragm of the stethoscope just below the umbilicus.

- *Normal:* low-pitched gurgling, intermittent
- *High-pitched:* often called tinkling. These sounds are suggestive of partial or total bowel obstruction.
- *Borborygmus:* a loud, low-pitched gurgling that can even be heard without a stethoscope. (The sounds are called *borborygmi.*) These re typical of diarrheal states or abnormal peristalsis.
- *Absent sounds:* If no sounds are heard for 2 minutes, there may be a complete lack of peristalsis—i.e., a paralytic ileus or peritonitis.

Bruits

These are sounds produced by the turbulent flow of blood through a vessel—similar in sound to heart murmurs. Listen with the diaphragm of the stethoscope.

Bruits may occur in normal adults but raise the suspicion of pathological stenosis (narrowing) when heard throughout both systole and diastole. There are several areas you should listen at on the abdomen:

- Just above the umbilicus over the aorta (abdominal aortic aneurysm)
- Either side of midline just above the umbilicus (renal artery stenosis)
- At the epigastrium (mesenteric stenosis)
- Over the liver (AV malformations, acute alcoholic hepatitis, hepatocellular carcinoma)

Friction rubs

These are creaking sounds like that of a pleural rub (📖 p. 199) heard when inflamed peritoneal surfaces move against each other with respiration.

Listen over the liver and spleen in the right and left upper quadrants, respectively.

Causes include hepatocellular carcinoma, liver abscesses, recent percutaneous liver biopsy, liver or splenic infarction, and STI-associated perihepatitis (Fitz–Hugh–Curtis syndrome).

Venous hums

Rarely, it is possible to hear the hum of venous blood flow in the upper abdomen over a caput medusa (📖 p. 230) secondary to portosystemic shunting of blood.

Palpation

General approach

The patient should be positioned lying supine with the head supported by a single pillow and arms at their sides.

Each of the four quadrants (see 📖 p. 204) should be examined in turn with light and then by deep palpation before focusing on specific organs (📖 p. 233). The order in which they are examined doesn't matter—find a routine that suits you. Ask the patient if there is any area of tenderness, and remember to examine this part *last*.

Before you begin, ask the patient to let you know if you cause any discomfort. You should be able to examine the abdomen without looking at it closely. Instead, you should watch the patient's face for signs of pain.

Light palpation

For this use the fingertips and palmar aspects of the fingers.

● Lay your right hand on the patient's abdomen and gently press in by flexing at the metacarpophalangeal joints.

If there is pain on light palpation, attempt to determine whether the pain is worse when you press down or when you release the pressure (*rebound tenderness*).

If the abdominal muscles seem tense, determine whether it is localized or generalized. Ensure that the patient is relaxed—it may be helpful for the patient to bend their knees slightly, relaxing the abdominal muscles. An involuntary tension in the abdominal muscles, apparently protecting the underlying organs, is called *guarding*.

Deep palpation

● Once all four quadrants are lightly palpated, re-examine using more pressure. This should enable you to feel for any masses or structural abnormalities.

If a mass is felt, treat it as you would any other lump, describing its exact location, size, shape, surface, consistency, mobility, movement with respiration, and tenderness and whether or not it is palatial.

> **Box 9.14 Signs of peritonitis**
>
> ● Pain on light palpation
> ● Rebound tenderness
> ● Involuntary guarding
> ● Pain recurring with slight movement of the examining hand
> ● Absent bowel sounds (📖 p.231)

It is often possible to detect the putty-like consistency of stool in the sigmoid colon. You should treat this as you would any other lump, to be sure of its nature.

Palpating the abdominal organs

Liver

The normal liver extends from the fifth intercostal space on the right of the midline to the costal margin, hiding under the ribs so is often not normally palpable—don't worry if you can't feel one.

- Using the flat of the right hand, start palpation from the right iliac fossa.
- You should angle your hand such that the index finger is aligned with the costal margin (see Fig. 9.7).
- Exert gentle pressure and ask the patient to take a deep breath.
- With each inward breath, your fingers should drift slightly superiorly as the liver moves inferiorly with the diaphragm. Relax the pressure on your hand slightly at the height of inspiration.
- If the liver is just above the position of your hand, the lateral surface of your index finger will strike the liver edge and glide over it with a palpable step.
- If the liver is not felt, move your hand 1–2cm superiorly and feel again.
- Repeat the process, moving toward the ribs until the liver is felt.

If a liver edge is felt, you should note the following:
- How far below the costal margin it extends in finger-breadths or (preferably) centimeters and record the number carefully
- Nature of the liver edge (is the surface smooth or irregular?)
- Presence of tenderness
- Whether the liver is pulsatile

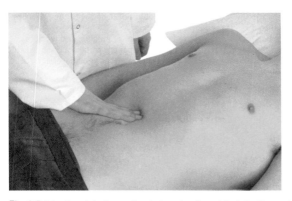

Fig. 9.7 Palpation of the liver—align the lateral surface of the index finger with the costal margin and palpate from the right iliac fossa to the ribs in a step-wise fashion.

Findings
- It is often possible to palpate the liver just below the costal margin at the height of inspiration in normal, healthy, thin people.
- An enlarged liver has many causes.
- A normal liver may be palpable in patients with COPD or asthma in whom the chest is hyperexpanded or in patients with a subdiaphragmatic collection.
- The liver may also be palpable in the presence of *Riedel's lobe*—a normal variant in which a projection of the liver arises from the inferior surface of the right lobe. It is more common in females and is commonly mistaken for a right kidney or enlarged gallbladder.

Gallbladder

The gallbladder lies at the right costal margin at the tip of the ninth rib, at the lateral border of the rectus abdominis. Normally it is only palpable when enlarged from biliary obstruction or acute cholecystitis (Box 9.15).
- Felt as a bulbous, focal, rounded mass that moves with inspiration
- Position the right hand perpendicular to the costal margin and palpate in a medial to lateral direction (see Fig. 9.8).

Spleen

The spleen is the largest lymphatic organ, which varies in size and shape between individuals—roughly the size of a clenched fist (12 × 7cm).

Normally, it is hidden beneath the left costal cartilages and is not palpable.

Enlargement of the spleen occurs in a downward direction, extending into the left upper quadrant (and even the left lower quadrant) across toward the right iliac fossa.
- It is palpated using a similar technique to that used to examine the liver (📖 p. 233).
- Your left hand should be used to support the left of the ribcage posterolaterally. Your right hand should be aligned with the fingertips parallel to the left costal margin (see Fig. 9.9).
- Start palpation just below the umbilicus in the midline and work toward the left costal margin, asking the patient to take a deep breath in and feeling for movement of the spleen under your fingers, much like palpating the liver.

Box 9.15 Important gallbladder signs

Murphy's sign
A sign of cholecystitis—pain on palpation over the gallbladder during deep inspiration. It is positive only if there is NO pain on the left at the same position.

Courvoisier's law
In the presence of jaundice, a palpable gallbladder is probably NOT caused by gallstones.

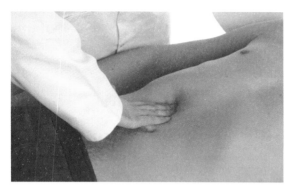

Fig. 9.8 Palpation of the gallbladder—the examining hand should be perpendicular to the costal margin at the tip of the ninth rib (where the lateral border of the rectus muscle meets the costal cartilages).

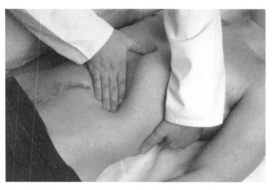

Fig. 9.9 Palpation of the spleen—align the fingertips of your right hand with the left costal border and start palpating just below the umbilicus, working toward the left upper quadrant.

- The inferior edge of the spleen may have a palpable notch centrally, which will help you differentiate it from any other abdominal mass.
- If a spleen is felt, measure the distance to the costal border in finger-breadths or (preferably) centimeters.
▶ A nonpalpable spleen may sometimes become palpable by reposition-ing the patient. Ask them to roll onto their right-hand side and repeat the examination as above.

Kidneys

The kidneys are retroperitoneal, lying on the posterior abdominal wall either side of the vertebral column between T12 and L3 vertebrae. They move slightly inferiorly with inspiration. The right kidney lies a little lower than the left (displaced by the liver).

Palpation is bimanual (both hands). You may be able to feel the lower pole of the right kidney in normal, thin people.

- Place your left hand behind the patient at the right loin.
- Place your right hand below the right costal margin at the lateral border of the rectus abdominis.
- Keeping the fingers of your right hand together, flex them at the metcarpophalangeal joints, pushing deep into the abdomen.
- Ask the patient to take a deep breath—you may be able to feel the rounded lower pole of the kidney between your hands, slipping away when the patient exhales.
- This technique of using one hand to move the kidney toward the other is called *renal ballottement.*
- Repeat the procedure for the left kidney, leaning over and placing your left hand behind the patient's left side (see Table 9.1 for comparison with enlarged spleen).

Findings

- **Unilateral palpable kidney:** hydronephrosis, polycystic kidney disease, renal cell carcinoma, acute renal vein thrombosis, renal abscess, acute pyelonephritis
- **Bilateral palpable kidneys:** bilateral hydronephrosis, bilateral renal cell carcinoma, polycystic kidney disease, nephrotic syndrome, amyloidosis, lymphoma, acromegaly

Table 9.1 Differentiating an enlarged spleen and an enlarged left kidney

Enlarged spleen	Enlarged kidney
Impossible to feel above	Can feel above the organ
Has a central notch on the leading edge	No notch, but you may feel the central hilar notch medially
Moves early on inspiration	Moves late on inspiration
Moves inferiomedially on inspiration	Moves inferiorly on inspiration
Not ballottable	Ballottable
Dullness to percussion	Resonant percussion note due to overlying bowel gas
May enlarge toward the umbilicus	Enlarges inferiorly lateral to the midline

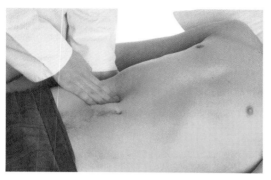

Fig. 9.10 Palpation of the right kidney.

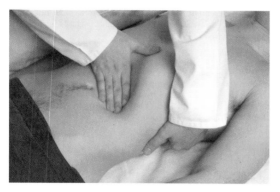

Fig. 9.11 Palpation of the left kidney.

Bladder

The urinary bladder is pyramid shaped and lies within the pelvic cavity. It is not palpable when empty.

As it fills, it expands superiorly and may even reach as high as the umbilicus or just beyond if very full.

It may be difficult to differentiate it from an enlarged uterus or ovarian cyst. The full bladder will be as follows:

- A palpable, rounded mass arising from behind the pubic symphysis
- Dull to percussion
- You will be unable to feel *below* it.
- Pressure on the full bladder will make the patient feel the need to urinate.

Aorta

The abdominal aorta may be palpated in the midline above the umbilicus, felt as a longitudinal pulsatile mass. It is particularly palpable in thin people. If it is felt:

- Position the fingers of each hand on either side of the outermost palpable margins.
- Measure the distance between your fingers. Normal diameter ≈2–3cm.
- Decide whether the mass you feel is pulsatile/expansile in itself (in which case your fingers will move outward) or whether the pulsation is transmitted through other tissue (in which case your fingers will move upward). See Fig. 9.12.

Inguinal lymph nodes

The inguinal chain of lymph nodes lies along the inguinal ligament between the pubic tubercle and the anterior superior iliac spine and should not be missed.

- Feel along this line for any lumps, treating each as you would any other lump (📖 p. 88).

Small, firm, mobile lymph nodes are common in healthy people and are often the result of minor sepsis or abrasions of the lower limbs.

▶ By this stage of the examination, you should have examined the nodes in the axillae, neck, supraclavicular areas, and inguinal regions.

Hernial orifices

Described on 📖 p. 243.

External genitalia

No thorough abdominal examination is complete without examining the genitalia, although in clinical practice, many leave this out, considering it inappropriate if you are not suspicious of any genitourinary pathology.

See 📖 Chapters 12 and 14.

(a)

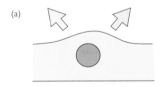

(b)

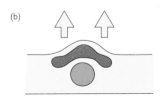

Fig. 9.12 Palpating a pulsatile mass. If the mass itself is expansile (a), your fingers will move outward. If the pulsatility is being transmitted through overlying tissues (b), your fingers will move upward.

Percussion

In the examination of the abdomen, percussion is useful for
• Determining the size and nature of enlarged organs or masses
• Detecting shifting dullness (below)
• Eliciting rebound tenderness (📖 p. 232)
Organs or masses will appear as dullness, whereas a bowel full of gas will seem abnormally resonant. Good technique comes with experience. Practice percussing your own liver. Percussion technique is described on 📖 p. 196.

Examining for ascites

If fluid is present in the peritoneal cavity (ascites), gravity will cause it to collect in the flanks when the patient is lying flat—this will give dullness to percussion laterally with central resonance as the bowel floats.

Ascites will produce a distended abdomen, often with an everted umbilicus. If you suspect the presence of ascites:
• Percuss centrally to laterally with the fingers spread and positioned longitudinally (see Fig. 9.13).
• Listen (and feel) for a definite change to a dull note.
There are then two specific tests to perform.

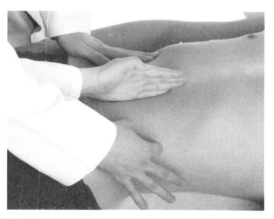

Fig. 9.13 Testing for a fluid thrill. Ask an assistant to place their hand centrally on the abdomen—this prevents transmission of the impulse through the abdominal wall.

*Shifting dullness**

- Percuss centrally → laterally until dullness is detected. This marks the air-fluid level in the abdomen.
- Keep your finger pressed there as you do the following:
- Ask the patient to roll onto the opposite side (i.e., if dullness is detected on the right, roll the patient to their left-hand side).
- Ask the patient to hold the new position for about half a minute.
- Repeat percussion, moving laterally to central over your mark.
- If the dullness truly was an air-fluid level, the fluid will now be moved by gravity away from the marked spot and the previously dull area will be resonant.

Fluid thrill

In this test, you are attempting to detect a wave transmitted across the peritoneal fluid. This is only really possible with massive ascites.

ⓘ You need an assistant for this test (you can ask the patient to help).

- Ask your assistant to place the ulnar edge of one of their hands in the midline of the abdomen (see Fig. 9.13).
- Place your left hand on one side of the abdomen, about level with the mid-clavicular line.
- With your right hand, flick the opposite side of the patient's abdomen.
- If a fluid thrill can be detected, you will feel the ripple from the flick transmitted as a tap to your left hand.

The assistant's hand is important—it prevents transmission of the impulse across the surface of the abdominal wall.

Liver

Percuss to map the upper and lower borders of the liver—note the length, in centimeters, at the mid-clavicular line.

Spleen

Percussion from the left costal margin toward the midaxillary line and the lower left ribs may reveal dullness suggestive of splenic enlargement that could not normally be palpated.

Kidneys

Percussion is useful in differentiating an enlarged kidney from an enlarged spleen or liver. The kidneys lie deep in the abdomen and are surrounded by perinephric fat, which makes them resonant to percussion. Splenomegaly or hepatomegaly will be dull.

Bladder

Dullness to percussion in the suprapubic region may be helpful in determining whether an ill-defined mass is an enlarged bladder (dull) or distended bowel (resonant).

---

* This is also the punchline to the medical student joke: "What's the definition of ward rounds?"

Rectal examination

This is an important part of the examination and should not be avoided simply because it is considered unpleasant. It is particularly important in patients with symptoms of rectal bleeding, tenesmus, change in bowel habit, and pruritus ani.
▶ Remember: If you don't put your finger in it, you may put your foot in it.

Before you begin

Explain to the patient what is involved and obtain verbal consent. Choose your words carefully, adjusting your wording to suit the patient. Favorite phrases include "hindend," "backside," and "bottom." Tell the patient that you need to examine their bottom with a finger. Warn that it 'probably won't hurt' but may feel cold and a little unusual.

Ask for another staff member to chaperone, to protect yourself against future claims of inappropriate treatment and to reassure the patient.*

As you proceed, explain each stage to the patient.

Equipment
- Chaperone
- Nonsterile gloves
- Tissues
- Lubricating jelly

Technique
- With informed verbal consent obtained, ensure adequate privacy.
- Uncover the patient from the waist to the knees.
- Ask the patient to lie in the left lateral position with their legs bent such that their knees are drawn up to their chest and their buttocks facing toward you—preferably projecting slightly over the edge of the bed or exam table.
- Ensure that there is a good light source, preferably a mobile lamp.
- Put on a pair of gloves.
- Separate the buttocks carefully by lifting the right buttock with your left hand.
- Inspect the perianal area and anus.
  - Look for rashes, excoriations, skin tags, ulcers, anal warts, fistulous openings, fissures, external hemorrhoids, abscesses, fecal soiling, blood, and mucus.
- Ask the patient to strain or bear down and watch for the projection of pink mucosa of a rectal prolapse.
- Lubricate the tip of your right index finger with the jelly.

* Accepted practice is that **all** providers have a chaperone when performing an intimate examination. In practice, male providers performing an examination on a female always have a chaperone present, while the need for a chaperone in other situations is judged individually at the time.

- Begin by placing the pulp of your right index finger against the anus in the midline and press in firmly but slowly.
  - Most anal sphincters will reflexively tighten when touched but will quickly relax with continued pressure.
- When the sphincter relaxes, gently advance the finger into the anal canal.
- Assess anal sphincter tone by asking the patient to tighten around your finger.
- Rotate the finger backward and forward, covering the full 360°, feeling for any thickening or irregularities.
- Push the finger further into the rectum.
- Examine all 360° by moving the finger in sweeping motions. Note:
  - Presence of thickening or irregularities of the rectal wall
  - Presence of palpable feces, and its consistency
  - Any points of tenderness
- Next, in the male, identify the prostate gland, which can be felt through the anterior rectal wall.
  - The normal prostate is smooth-surfaced, firm with a slightly rubbery texture, measuring 2–3cm diameter. It has two lobes with a palpable central sulcus.
- Gently withdraw your finger and inspect the glove for feces, blood, or mucus and note the color of the stool, if present. Test the stool for occult blood if a testing card is available.
- Tell the patient that the examination is over and wipe any feces or jelly from the gluteal cleft with the tissues. Some patients may prefer to do this themselves.
- Thank the patient and ask them to get dressed. You may need to help.

Findings

If any mass or abnormality is identified on the exterior or interior of the areas examined, its exact location should be noted. It is conventional to record as the position on a clock face, with 12 o'clock indicating the anterior side of the rectum at the perineum. Other features of the mass should be recorded as described on 📖 p. 88.

- *Benign prostatic hyperplasai (BPH):* The prostate is enlarged but the central sulcus is preserved, often exaggerated.
- *Prostate cancer:* The gland loses its rubbery consistency and may become hard. The lateral lobes may be irregular and nodular. There is often distortion or loss of the central sulcus. If the tumor is large and has spread locally, there may be thickening of the rectal mucosa either side of the gland, creating winging of the prostate.
- *Prostatitis:* The gland will be enlarged, boggy, and very tender.

▶ Hints

- If the patient experiences severe pain, with gentle pressure on the anal opening, consider anal fissure, ischiorectal abscess, anal ulcer, thrombosed hemorrhoid, or prostatitis.
- In this situation, you may have to apply local anesthetic gel to the anal margin before proceeding. If in doubt, ask a senior resident or attending physician.

Hernial orifices

A *hernia* is an abnormal protrusion of a structure, organ, or part of an organ out of the cavity in which it belongs. A hernia can usually be reduced—i.e., its contents returned to the original cavity either spontaneously or by manipulation.

Abdominal hernias are usually caused by portions of bowel protruding through weakened areas of the abdominal wall. In the abdomen, hernias usually occur at natural openings of the abdominal wall (e.g., inguinal canals, femoral canals, umbilicus, esophageal hiatus) or acquired weak spots such as surgical scars.

Most abdominal hernias have an expansile cough impulse—asking the patient to cough will increase the intra-abdominal pressure, causing a visible or palpable impulse.

Strangulation

Hernias that cannot be reduced (irreducible) may become fixed and swollen as their blood supply is occluded, causing ischemia and necrosis of the herniated organ. The hernias are painfully swollen with overlying erythema and may cause disruption of normal gut function (e.g., intestinal obstruction).

An approach to hernias

- Determine the characteristics as you would for any lump (📖 p. 88), including position, temperature, tenderness, shape, size, tension, and composition.
- Make note of the characteristics of the overlying skin.
- Palpate the hernia and feel for a cough impulse.
- Attempt reduction of the hernia.
- Percuss and auscultate the hernia (listening for bowel sounds or bruits).
- Always remember to examine the same site on the opposite side.

Inguinal hernias

Anatomy

The inguinal canal extends from the pubic tubercle to the anterior superior iliac spine. In the male, it carries the spermatic cord (vas deferens, blood vessels and nerves). In the female, it is much smaller and carries the round ligament of the uterus.

After testicular descent, the canal closes but the site is weakened.

The internal ring is an opening in the transversalis fascia lying at the mid-inguinal point, halfway between the anterior superior iliac spine and the pubic symphysis (about 1.5cm above the femoral pulse).

The external ring is an opening of the external oblique aponeurosis and is immediately above and medial to the pubic tubercle (see Fig. 9.14).

- **Direct inguinal hernia:** This is herniation at the site of the external ring.
- **Indirect inguinal hernia:** This is the most common site (85% of all hernias). Herniation is through the internal ring with bowel or omentum traveling down the inguinal canal and may protrude through the external ring into the scrotum. It is more likely to strangulate than direct inguinal hernias.

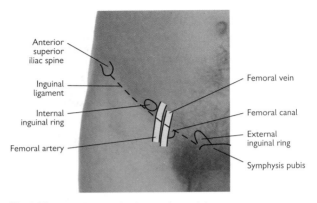

Fig. 9.14 Sites of the internal and external inguinal rings.

Examination
- The patient should be examined standing up and undressed from the waist down (some hernias may spontaneously reduce when supine).
- Palpate especially for tenderness and consistency of the lump.
  - Herniated omentum will appear rubbery, nonfluctuant, and dull to percussion.
  - Herniated gut will be fluctuant and resonant. You may be able to hear bowel sounds within the hernia.
- With two fingers on the mass, ask the patient to cough, and feel for an expansile cough impulse.
- Attempt to reduce the hernia by massaging it back toward its suspected site of origin.
  - For indirect hernias, you should use the flat of your hand, directing the hernia from below and guide it through the external ring, up the inguinal canal laterally toward the internal ring.
- Once reduced, the hernia should not reappear until you release the pressure.
- With the hernia reduced, try pressing over the site of the internal ring and asking the patient to cough. An indirect hernia will remain reduced, whereas a direct hernia will protrude once more (see Table 9.2).

Femoral hernias

Anatomy
The femoral canal is the small component of the femoral sheath medial to the femoral vessels and contains loose connective tissue, lymphatic vessels, and lymph nodes. It is bordered anteriorly by the inguinal ligament, the pectineal ligament posteriorly, the femoral vein laterally, and the lacunar ligament medially.

Table 9.2 Differentiation of inguinal hernias

Indirect inguinal hernia	Direct inguinal hernia
Can descend into the scrotum	Very rarely descends to the scrotum
Reduces upward, laterally, backward	Reduces upward and backward
Remains reduced with pressure at the internal ring	Not controlled by pressure over the internal ring
The causative defect is not palpable	Defect in the abdominal wall is palpable
Reappears at the internal ring and flows medially	Reappears in the same position as before reduction

Femoral hernias are protrusions of bowel or omentum through this space (see Box 9.16 for differential). They are more common in middle-aged and elderly women and can easily strangulate given the small, rigid opening they pass through.

Examination
- Examine with patient standing up and undressed from the waist down.
- Examine as you would any other hernia and attempt reduction.
- If present, a femoral hernia will appear as a lump just lateral and inferior to the pubic tubercle, about 2cm medial to the femoral pulse.

Other abdominal wall hernias
- *Umbilical/paraumbilical:* herniation through a defect near the umbilicus (considered congenital if identified in children)
- *Epigastric:* herniation through the linea alba above the umbilicus
- *Spigalean:* herniation through the linea semilunaris (lateral to the rectus sheath), usually below and lateral to the umbilicus; rare
- *Obturator:* herniation through the obturator canal, associated with increasing age and multiparity
- *Perineal:* herniation through the pelvic floor diaphragm; rare
- *Incisional:* herniation through the site of previous surgery. The bulge is usually seen underlying a surface surgical scar. There is increasing incidence with advanced age, but it can be caused by wound infection and associated fasciitis or muscle necrosis.

Box 9.16 **Differential diagnosis of femoral hernia**
- Inguinal hernia
- Very large lymph node
- Ectopic testicle
- Psoas bursa or abscess
- Lipoma

Important presenting patterns

Chronic liver disease

Any of the following features may be seen. With severe disease and decompensation, more will become apparent:

• Jaundice	• Purpura
• Palmar erythema	• Easy bruising
• Leuconychia	• Epistaxis
• Clubbing	• Menorrhagia
• Spider nevi	• Loss of libido
• Telangiectasia	• Hair loss
• Hepatomegaly	• Bilateral parotid swelling
• Ascites	• Encephalopathy
• Variceal bleeding—manifesting as hematemesis and/or melena.	

Men	Women
• Gynecomastia	• Breast atrophy
• Testicular atrophy	• Irregular menses
• Impotence	• Amenorrhea

Portal hypertension

Raised pressure in the hepatic portal vein is often secondary to liver disease or noncirrhotic causes such as portal vein thrombosis. Causes are portosystemic shunting and esophageal varices. Signs include
• Fetor hepaticus
• Splenomegaly
• Risk of gastrointestinal blood loss from varices (anemia, hematemesis, melena)
• Ascites
• Caput medusae

Alcoholic liver disease

This may cause all the features of chronic liver disease as described above. In addition, alcohol dependency or addiction is associated with the following:
• Tolerance
• Withdrawal symptoms
• Alcohol taken in larger amounts and for longer than intended
• Persistent desire to cut down

- Excessive time spent in activities related to alcohol intake
- Abandoning social, occupational or recreational activities
- Continued use despite an awareness of the adverse physiological and psychological effects of continued use

Fatty liver

Hepatic steatosis has many other causes, including drugs, pregnancy, and diabetes mellitus. Deposition of fat occurs as a result of preferential alcohol oxidation. It is reversible with abstinence but may proceed to cirrhosis with continued use. There are no specific clinical features.

Alcoholic hepatitis

This is hepatocellular inflammation with lymphocyte infiltration, steatosis, cholestasis, fibrosis, and necrosis. Clinical features include the following:
- Fever
- Jaundice
- Tender hepatomegaly
- May hear a bruit over the liver

Cirrhosis

This is severe hepatic fibrosis with micronodules. There is loss of hepatocytes, impaired synthetic function, and portal hypertension. Other causes of cirrhosis include chronic viral hepatitis (B or C), sclerosing cholangitis, Wilson's disease, hemachromotosis, α_1-antitrypsin deficiency, primary biliary cirrhosis, Budd–Chiari syndrome, and several drugs (e.g., amiodarone, methyldopa, and methotrexate). Clinical features can be any of those listed under Chronic Liver Disease, above.

Extrahepatic manifestations of alcoholic liver disease or alcoholism

• Obesity or malnutrition	• Osteoporosis
• Diarrhea	• Falls
• Gastric erosions	• Seizures
• Peptic ulcer disease	• Cognitive impairment (📖 p. 463)
• Pancreatitis	• Metabolic encephalopathy
• Varices	• Peripheral neuropathy
• Ascites	• Ataxic gait (📖 p. 321)
• Splenomegaly	• Wernicke's encephalopathy
• Hypertension	• Korsakoff's syndrome
• Loss of secondary sexual characteristics	• Cardiomyopathy
• Osteomalacia	• Arrhythmias (especially atrial fibrillation)

Hepatic encephalopathy

Shunting of blood away from the portal circulation, seen in chronic liver disease, allows potentially neurotoxic substances absorbed in the gut to bypass the liver where they would normally be removed.

Hepatic encephalopathy is graded as follows:

Grade 0   Normal mental state
Grade I   Altered mood or behavior ($\downarrow$ attention span, difficulty with numbers, and lack or awareness)
Grade II $\uparrow$ Drowsiness, slurred speech, mild to moderate confusion
Grade III Stupor but responsive to stimuli, significant confusion, restlessness
Grade IV   Coma

Malabsorption

Numerous disorders can cause malabsorption states. They can be grouped as pancreatic insufficiency, bile salt malabsorption, small bowel mucosa defects (celiac disease, tropical sprue, giardiasis, disaccharidase deficiency, Whipple's disease, short bowel syndrome), bacterial overgrowth, and specific delivery defects.

General symptoms and signs of malabsorption include the following:
- Muscle wasting
- Weight loss
- Pallor
- Diarrhea (watery)
- Steatorrhea: pale, fatty stools; offensive smelling and difficult to flush
- Glossitis
- Angular stomatitis (vitamin B_2, B_{12}, and folic acid deficiencies)
- Intraoral purpura and easy bruising (vitamin K deficiency)
- Follicular keratitis: hyperkeratotic white patches (vitamin A deficiency)

Acute pancreatitis

Symptoms
- Pain—central abdominal or epigastric, radiating through to the back. Sometimes relieved slightly by sitting forward.
- Vomiting

Signs
- Tachycardia
- Fever
- Jaundice (rarely)
- Peritonitis (bowel ileus, very tender abdomen, guarding)
- Retroperitoneal bleed: Cullen's or Grey–Turner's signs (📖 p. 230)

Chronic pancreatitis

In developed countries, the most common cause is chronic heavy alcohol intake. A small group of patients can inherit chronic pancreatitis through an autosomal dominant gene with incomplete penetrance.

Clinical features are usually due to pancreatic enzyme deficiencies and malabsorption and chronic pain. There may be acute exacerbations, presenting as acute pancreatitis. Loss of pancreatic endocrine function may cause diabetes.

Cholangitis

This is biliary sepsis. It is suggested by Charcot's triad:
- Right upper quadrant pain
- Fever
- Jaundice
  You may also be able to elicit Murphy's sign (📖 p. 234).

Celiac disease

This a common cause of malabsorption. It affects 1 in 133 (2 million) people in the United States. Incidence is much higher (up to 1/22) if a first-degree relative has the disease.[1] T-cell-mediated autoimmune disease of the small bowel mucosa is characterized by villous atrophy and ↑ intraepithelial lymphocytosis in response to ingestion of gluten.

Gluten is a high-molecular weight compound containing gliadins and peptides. It is found in a huge number of foods containing wheat, barley, and rye. Controversy exists over eating oats.

Clinical features are listed below.

Symptoms
- Tiredness
- Malaise
- Diarrhea or steatorrhea
- Abdominal discomfort and bloating
- Weight loss
- Anxiety
- Depression
- Peripheral paresthesia

Signs
- Muscle wasting
- Mouth ulceration
- Angular stomatitis
- Ankle edema (low serum albumin)
- Polyneuropathy
- Muscle weakness
- Tetany

Associated with
- Autoimmune thyroid disorders, chronic liver disease, fibrosing alveolitis, ulcerative colitis, insulin-dependent diabetes mellitus

Possible complications to be aware of
- Small bowel lymphoma (rare)
- Small bowel adenocarcinoma (rarer)
- Ulcerative jejunitis
- Splenic atrophy
- Anemia
- Osteomalacia
- Osteoporosis
- Secondary lactose intolerance

[1] http://digestive.niddk.nih.gov/ddiseases/pubs/celiac.

Inflammatory bowel disease: ulcerative colitis (UC)

This is a chronic relapsing disease of unknown etiology involving superficial inflammation of the colonic mucosa, starting from the rectum and working proximally without any breaks. The terminal ileum may be affected by backwash ileitis. Periods of remission may give no symptoms at all.

Symptoms
- Diarrhea (often with blood or mucus)
- Weight loss
- Fever
- Abdominal pain
- Proctitis may cause rectal bleeding, mucus, tenesmus, and constipation.

Complications to be aware of
- Toxic megacolon
- Iron deficiency anemia
- Increased risk of colorectal carcinoma
- Fistula formation (rare)

Inflammatory bowel disease: Crohn's disease

Like ulcerative colitis, this is a chronic inflammatory disease of the gastrointestinal tract but differs from UC in that lesions occur anywhere from the mouth to anus but especially at the terminal ileum and anorectum. Pathology involves deep ulceration, cobblestoning of the mucosa, fissuring and abscess formation with skip lesions, and non-caseating granulomas.

Symptoms
If disease is limited to the colon, symptoms may be identical to UC.
- Loose stools or diarrhea (usually not bloody)
- Anorexia
- Malaise
- Weight loss
- Abdominal pain (insidious, often in the right lower quadrant)
- Perianal pain
- Joint pains

Note on examination (these can occur in UC also)
- Aphthous mouth ulcers
- Uveitis
- Anemia
- Arthropathy

Active Crohn's disease
- Colicky pain often in the right iliac fossa
- May have diarrhea with blood and mucus
- Weight loss
- Borborygmus (📖 p. 231)
- May be a palpable inflammatory mass in the right iliac fossa
- Abdominal distension
- ± Bowel obstruction

Active Crohn's colitis
- Similar presentation to ulcerative colitis
- Perianal disease more likely to produce fissuring and fistula formation

Complications to be aware of
- Fistula formation (from the bowel to any other abdominal organ or the exterior)
- Small increased risk of colorectal carcinoma (especially in long-standing disease limited to the colon)
- Vitamin B$_{12}$ deficiency
- Iron deficiency
- Abscess formation
- Stricture formation
- Systemic infection

Extraintestinal features of inflammatory bowel disease
- Seronegative arthropathy of large or small joints (peripheral, non-deforming, particularly at the knees, ankles, and wrists)
- Sacroiliitis
- Anterior uvetitis
- Erythema nodosum
- Pyoderma gangrenosum
- Ureteric calculi
- Gallstones
- Sclerosing cholangitis
- Cholangiocarcinoma
- Nutritional deficiencies (Osteoporosis? Osteomalacia?)
- Bile salt malabsorption
- Osteoporosis secondary to long-term steroid use or malabsorption
- Systemic amyloidosis

Irritable bowel syndrome (IBS)—Rome III diagnostic criteria
Symptoms of abdominal discomfort or pain need to meet a frequency criterion (3 or more days a month for at least 3 months) in the preceding 6 months and has two out of three features:
- Relief or improvement with defecation
- Onset associated with a change in frequency of stool
- Onset associated with a change in form/appearance of stool

Other symptoms that support the diagnosis of IBS:
- Abnormal stool frequency (>3/day or <3/week)
- Abnormal stool form (lumpy/hard, loose/watery)
- Abnormal stool passage (straining, urgency, feeling of incomplete evacuation)
- Passage of mucus
- Bloating or feeling of abdominal distension

The elderly patient

Gastrointestinal disease presents as a huge spectrum in older patients, encompassing nutrition, oral care, and continence in addition to the range of presentations described in this chapter. While many older people suffer gastrointestinal symptoms, often due to underlying illnesses or the effect of medication, they may be embarrassed about discussing them. Thoughtful and holistic assessment is paramount, and simple interventions can pay dividends.

History
Oral care
This is an often overlooked but key part of any assessment. Dentures may be ill-fitting or lost, and dietary intake can suffer as a consequence. Hospitalized patients are particularly prone to losing their dentures.

Clarify symptoms and diagnoses
Does the patient really have an irritable bowel? (See below.) Many patients may describe themselves as having such diagnoses, but take the time to clarify what this means. Recent changes of bowel habit must always be viewed with a degree of alarm and causes considered.

Constipation
This can often lead to serious decline in patients. It is often easily remediable.

Weight and nutrition
Ask yourself why has the patient lost weight. The range of diagnoses is broad, but contemplate mood, dietary habits, and functional abilities in your assessments—it may be a matter of dislike of delivered frozen meals.

Drug history
Always consider the side effects of medication—analgesics and constipation, recent antibiotics, and diarrhea. Ask about over-the-counter drugs including NSAIDs (and topical drugs) and laxatives.

Continence
This is another key part of the assessment; try to discuss it sensitively and determine if there factors additional to any GI disturbance, including mobility, cognition and visual problems. This dovetails with the ever-important functional history.

Examination
General
Look out for signs of weight loss—wasting, poorly fitting clothes, etc. For inpatients, a completed weight chart and careful consideration may alleviate some of the problems of poor nutrition and acute illness.

Look in the mouth
A range of diagnoses is often apparent. Denture care should be assessed (poor cleaning associated with recurrent stomatitis), and other problems such as oral candida are obvious.

Observe

Look for other signs of systemic disease that might point to the cause of the gastrointestinal symptoms (e.g., multiple telangiectasia, valvular heart disease in GI bleeding).

Examine

Examine thoroughly for lymphadenopathy. Remember to examine hernial orifices—the cause of abdominal pain may be instantly obvious and correctable.

Rectal examination

This is vital—changes in bowel habit, continence, iron deficiency anemia, and bladder symptomatology all indicate that this should be performed.

Diagnoses not to be missed

Functional bowel disorders

These tend to be less common in older people, so always consider underlying organic problems. Endoscopic examinations are often well tolerated and have a good diagnostic yield.

Biliary sepsis

This is the third most common source of infection in older people (after chest and urine sepsis) and may lack many of the salient presenting features described previously in this chapter. Be alert to this possibility when considering differential diagnoses and choosing antibiotics.

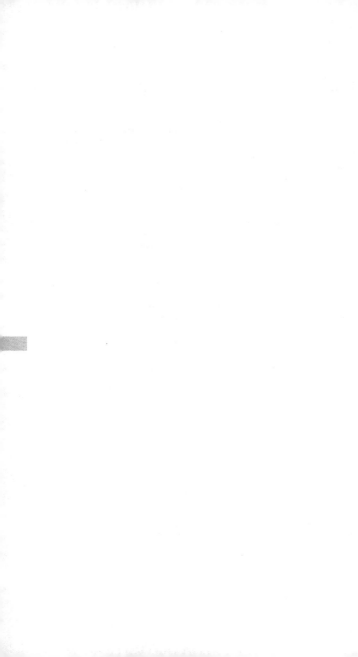

Nervous system

Presenting symptoms in neurology

The history is key in the examination of many neurological cases. If the patient cannot give a complete story (e.g., when describing a loss of consciousness or seizure), collateral histories should be gained from any witnesses to the event(s)—relatives, friends, the primary care provider, or even passers-by.

Approach to neurological symptoms

Symptoms can vary widely in neurology; the intricacies of a few are discussed below. For *all* symptoms, you should try to understand the following:

- Exact nature of the symptom
- Onset (Sudden? Slow—hours? Days? Weeks? Months?)
- Change over time (Progressive? Intermittent? Episodes of recovery?)
- Precipitating factors
- Exacerbating and relieving factors
- Previous episodes of the same symptom
- Previous investigations and treatment
- Associated symptoms
- Any other neurological symptoms

Dizziness

Narrow the exact meaning down without appearing aggressive or disbelieving. *Dizziness* is used by different people to describe rather different things:

- A sense of rotation = *vertigo*
- *Swimminess* or *light-headedness*—a nonspecific symptom that can be related to pathology in many different systems
- *Presyncope*—the unique feeling one gets just prior to fainting
- *Incoordination*—many will say they are dizzy when, in fact, they can't walk straight because of either ataxia or weakness.

Headache

This should be treated as any other type of pain. Establish character, severity, site, duration, time course, frequency, radiation, aggravating and relieving factors, and associated symptoms.

- Ask about facial and visual symptoms. (Some different types of headaches are described on □ p. 329.)

Numbness and weakness

These two words are often confused by patients, describing a leg as "numb" when it is *weak* with normal sensation. Also, patients may report numbness when, in fact, they are experiencing pins and needles (paresthesia)or pain.

Tremor

Here you should establish if the tremor occurs only at rest, only when attempting an action, or both. Is it worse at any particular time of the day? The severity can be established in terms of its functional consequence (can the patient hold a cup or bring food to their mouth?).

Again, establish exactly what is being described. A *tremor* is a shaking, regular or jerky involuntary movement.

Syncope

This is discussed in ▢ Chapter 7.

Falls and loss of consciousness (LOC)

An eyewitness account is vital. Establish also whether the patient actually lost consciousness. People often describe "blacking out" when in fact they simply fell to the ground (drop attacks have no LOC). An important question here is, "Can you remember hitting the ground?".

Ask about preceding symptoms and warning signs—they may point toward a different organ system (sweating or weakness could be a marker of hypoglycemia; palpitations may indicate a cardiac dysrhythmia).

Seizures

These are very difficult to assess, even for experienced history-takers! Establish early on if there was any impairment of consciousness, and seek collateral histories. Laypersons usually consider *seizure* = "fit" = tonic–clonic seizure. Doctors' understanding of *seizure* may be quite different. A surprising number of people also suffer *pseudoseizures*, which are nonorganic and have a psychological cause.

A few points to consider are as follows:
- Syncopal attacks can often cause a few tonic–clonic or myoclonic jerks, which may be mistaken for epilepsy.
- True tonic–clinic seizures may cause tongue-biting, urinary and fecal incontinence, or all of the above.
- People presenting with pseudoseizure can have true epilepsy *as well*, and vice versa.

Visual symptoms

Commonly, there is visual loss, double vision, or photophobia (pain when looking at bright lights). Here, establish exactly what is being experienced—"double vision" (diplopia) is often complained of when, in fact, the vision is blurred or sight is generally poor (amblyopia) or clouded.

The rest of the history

Ask if the patient is right- or left-handed (consider disability from loss of function; this may also be useful when thinking about cerebral lesions).

Direct questioning

In every patient, inquire about neurological symptoms other than the presenting complaint (headaches, fits, faints, blackouts, visual symptoms, pins and needles, tingling, numbness, weakness, incontinence, constipation, or urinary retention).

Past medical history

A birth history is important here, particularly in patients with epilepsy. Additional forms of neurological injury are often present at birth, for instance, in the case of brachial plexus injury during dystotic deliveries. Brain injury at birth has neurological consequences.

While a thorough history is required, inquire especially about the following:
- Hypertension—if so, what treatment?
- Diabetes mellitus—what type? What treatment?
- Thyroid disease
- Mental illness (e.g., depression)
- Meningitis or encephalitis
- Head or spinal injuries
- Epilepsy, convulsions, or seizures
- Cancer
- HIV/AIDS

Drug history

Ask especially about the following:
- Anticonvulsant therapy (current or previous)
- Oral contraceptive or other estrogen-based contraceptive preparation
- Corticosteroids
- Anticoagulants or antiplatelet agents

Family history

A thorough history, as always, is important. Ask about neurological diagnoses and evidence of missed diagnoses (seizures, blackouts, etc.).

Tobacco and alcohol

These are as important to ask about here as for any other system.

Social history

- Occupation: Neurological disease can have a significant impact on occupation, so ask about this at an early stage—some suggest right at the beginning of the history. Also ask about exposure to heavy metals or other neurotoxins.
- Is patient driving? Many neurological conditions have implications here.
- Ask about the home environment in detail (this will be very useful when considering handicaps and consequences of the diagnosis).
- Ask about support systems—family, friends, home help, day visits.

The outline examination

It is easy to get bogged down in some of the complexities of the neurological examination, but it is not something to be afraid of. Students should embrace it; practice often, as a competent neurological examination is a sure sign of someone who has spent plenty of time on honing their clinical skills. The following is a brief outline of how it should be approached:

- Inspection, mood, conscious level
- Speech and higher mental functions
- Cranial nerves (CN) II–XII
- Motor system
- Sensation
- Coordination
- Gait
- Any extra tests
- Other relevant examinations
  - Skull, spine, neck stiffness, eardrums, blood pressure, anterior chest, carotid arteries, breasts, abdomen, lymph nodes

General inspection and mental state

The neurological exam should start with any clues that can be gleaned from simply looking at and engaging with the patient.

- Is the patient accompanied by caregivers, and how does the patient interact with those people?
- Does the patient use any walking aids or other forms of support?
- Are there any abnormal movements? (📖 p. 315)
- Observe the gait as they approach the clinic room, if able (📖 p. 321).
- Is there any speech disturbance? (📖 p. 260)
- What is their mood like?
  - A detailed mood assessment (📖 p. 458) is not necessary here.
  - Ask the patient how they feel.
  - What is the state or their clothing, hair, skin, and nails?
  - Is there any restlessness, inappropriately high spirits, or pressure of speech?
  - Are they obviously depressed with disinterest?
  - Are they denying any disability?

Speech and language

Speech and language difficulties, especially expressive dysphasia, may be extremely distressing for the patient and their family. This topic must be approached with care, reassurance, and a calm seriousness in the face of possible bizarre and amusing answers to questions.

Examination

Speech and language problems may be evident from the start of the history and require no formal testing. You should briefly test the patient's language function by asking them to read or obey a simple written command (e.g., "close your eyes") and write a short sentence.

If apparently problematic, speech *can* be tested formally by asking the patient to respond to progressively harder questions, with answers ranging from yes/no, simple statements, to more complicated sentences, and finally by asking them to repeat complex phrases or tongue-twisters (see Dysarthria section).

Before jumping to conclusions, ensure that the patient is not deaf or that their hearing aid is working, and that they can understand English.

Dysarthria

This is a defect of articulation with language function intact (writing will be unaffected). There may be a cerebellar lesion, a lower motor neuron (LMN) lesion of the cranial nerves, an extrapyramidal lesion, or a problem with muscles in the mouth and jaws or their nerve supply.

- Listen for slurring and the rhythm of speech.
- Test function of different structures by asking the patient to repeat
  - "Yellow lion" or words with *D*, *L*, and *T* (tests *tongue* function).
  - "Peter Piper picked a pickle," or words with *P* and *B* (tests *lip* function).
- *Cerebellar lesions:* slow, slurred, low volume with equal emphasis on all syllables (scanning)
- *Facial weakness:* speech is slurred.
- *Extrapyramidal lesions:* monotonous, low volume, lacks normal rhythm

Dysphonia

This constitutes defective volume—huskiness. Dysphonia is usually from laryngeal disease, laryngeal nerve palsy, or, rarely, muscular disease, such as myasthenia gravis. It may also be "functional" (psychological).

Dysphasia

This is a defect of language, not just speech, so reading and writing may also be affected (some patients attempt to overcome speaking difficulties with a notepad and pen, only to be bitterly disappointed).

In very simple terms, the main language areas of the brain are illustrated in Fig. 10.1. Deficits can be understood in terms of lesions in one or more of these areas. There are four main types of dysphasia.

Global dysphasia

Both Broca's and Wernicke's areas are affected. The patient is unable to speak or understand speech at all.

Expressive dysphasia

This is also called *anterior*, *motor*, or *Broca's* dysphasia.

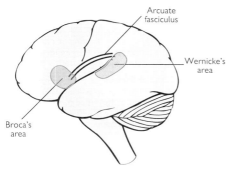

Fig. 10.1 Simple representation of the main language areas of the brain.

- Lesion in Broca's area (frontal lobe), involved in language production
- Understanding remains intact
- Unable to answer questions appropriately
- Speech is nonfluent, broken with abnormal word ordering
- Unable to repeat sentences
- Can be very distressing for patients. Ask, "Do you know what you want to say, but can't get it out?" and you'll be met with a grateful smile, nod, and handshake.

Receptive dysphasia

Also called *posterior*, *sensory*, or *Wernicke's* dysphasia.

- Lesion in Wernicke's area creates problems with understanding spoken or written language (dyslexia) and problems with word-finding
- Unable to understand commands or questions
- Speech is fluent with lots of meaningless grammatical elements.
- May contain meaningless words
- Unable to repeat sentences
- Patients are often unaware of their speech difficulty and will speak in a nonsensical way, often becoming frustrated with other people's lack of understanding.
- *Jargon dysphasia* describes a severe form of receptive dysphasia containing only meaningless words (neologisms) and sounds.
- *Paraphasia* is the supplementation of one word with another.

Conductive dysphasia

There is a lesion in the arcuate fasciculus and/or other connections between the two primary language areas.

- Patient can comprehend and respond appropriately
- Unable to repeat a sentence

Nominal dysphasia

- All language function is intact *except* for naming of objects.
- Caused by lesion in angular gyrus
- Patient may function with circumlocution (e.g., says "that thing that I write with" if unable to say "pen")

Cognitive function

Neurological diseases may affect function such that patients' appearance or communication skills are at odds with their social standing or educational level. Formal assessment of a person's mental state is thus important. This also allows for any future change to be noted and monitored.

Abbreviated mental test score (10 points)

This serves as a brief screening tool with a maximum score of 10 points. A more detailed, 30-point, score is shown in Box 15.11 (☐ p. 464).

Approach this gently—patients often dislike being tested without warning. Always explain the purpose of the questions, and ask permission to proceed.

Hints

When testing 5-minute recall:
- If thinking of an address for the patient to remember, be careful not to give out your own!
- Beware of repeating the test too often. Patients may well remember "42 West Street" from the last time it was asked.

Table 10.1 Abbreviated mental test score

1. Date of birth	"What is your date of birth?"
2. Age	"How old are you?"
3. Time	"What time is it?" • Correct to the nearest hour
4. Year	"What year is it now?" • Note that hospital patients often lose track of the day or month, not the year.
5. Place	"Where are we?" or "What is this place?" • Name of the hospital, clinic, or surgery ward
6. Head of state	"Who is the current president?" • A name is required. Such descriptions as "that man in all the trouble" won't do—even if it is potentially correct!
7. Current event	In recognition of the patient's age, culture, and education, it may be appropriate to ask the year of a noteworthy event, such as, "When was President Kennedy shot?" "When were aircraft crashed into the World Trade Center?"
8. 5-minute recall	Tell the patient an address (often "42 West Street" is used) and ask them to repeat it back to you to ensure they've heard it correctly. Ask them to remember it. Five minutes later, ask them to recall the address. • They must remember the address in full to score the point.
9. 20–1	"Count backward from 20 down to 1" • Patients sometimes need a prompt here: "Like this: 20, 19, 18, and so on."
10. Recognition	"What job do I do?" (doctor) and "What job does this man or woman do?" (nurse) • Both must be correct to score a point.

Cranial nerve I: olfactory

Applied anatomy

- *Sensory:* smell
- *Motor:* none

Fibers arise in the mucous membrane of the nose. Axons pass across the cribiform plate to the olfactory bulb. The olfactory tract runs backward below the frontal lobe and projects mainly in the uncus of the ipsilateral temporal lobe.

Note: Olfactory epithelium also contains free nerve endings of the first division of cranial nerve V.

Examination

This nerve is not routinely tested unless the patient complains of loss of sense of smell (anosmia) and exhibits other signs suggestive of a frontal or temporal lobe cause (e.g., tumor).

- *Casual:* Take a nearby odorous object (e.g., coffee or chocolate) and ask the patient if it smells normal.
- *Formal:* A series of identical bottles containing recognizable smells are used. The patient is asked to identify them. Commonly used agents include coffee, vanilla, camphor, and vinegar.

Test each nostril separately and determine if any loss of smell is uni- or bilateral.

Findings

- **Bilateral anosmia:** usually nasal, not neurological

Causes include upper respiratory tract infection, trauma, smoking, old age, and Parkinson's disease. Less commonly, there are tumors of the ethmoid bones or congenital ciliary dysmotility syndromes.

- **Unilateral anosmia:** mucous-blocked nostril, head trauma, subfrontal meningioma

Hints

Peppermint, ammonia, and menthol stimulate the free trigeminal endings so are not a good test of cranial nerve I.

Cranial nerve II: optic

Applied anatomy

With an understanding of anatomy of the optic nerves, defects in the visual field enable localization of a lesion within the brain.

The optic nerve begins at the retina (and is the only part of the central nervous system [CNS] that can be directly visualized). The nerve passes through the optic foramen and joins its fellow nerve from the other eye at the *optic chiasm* just above the pituitary fossa. Here, the fibers from the nasal half of the retina cross over. They continue in the optic tract to the lateral geniculate body. From there, they splay out such that those from the upper retina pass through the parietal lobe and the others through the temporal lobe.

Students easily get confused here and should focus on gaining full understanding of these processes at an early stage. Because of the refraction at the lens, images are represented on the retina upside down and back to front. Therefore, the *nasal* half of the retinal receives input from the *temporal* part of the visual field in each eye, while the temporal half of the retinal receives input from the nasal half of the eye.

Further back in the optic system, fibers from the nasal halves of the retinas cross, so, for example, the left side of the brain receives input from the right side of vision (the left temporal retina and the right nasal retina) and vice versa (see Fig. 10.2, p. 267).

Visual acuity

Sharpness or clarity of vision is formally tested using a Snellen's chart.
- In good light, the patient should stand 20 feet away from the chart.
- Each eye is tested in turn, and the patient is asked to read the chart.
- The number above each line indicates the distance at which a person with normal sight should be able to read it.
- Record the line reached—allow a maximum of two errors per line.
  - Indicate results as distance from chart/distance it should be read, e.g., 20/20.

If the patient can't see any of the letters, record whether they can
- Count fingers held in front of their face (CF)
- See hand movements (wave your hand)
- Perceive light
  - Record as CF, HM, PL, or NPL (not perceive light).

Color vision

- Not tested routinely and not considered in this book
- Tested using Ishihara plates

Visual fields

The area that each eye can see without moving can be mapped out. They are not circular—eyebrows and the nose obstruct superiorly and nasally, whereas there is no obstruction laterally.

Sitting opposite the patient, the examiner's left visual field (for example) should be an exact mirror image of the patient's right visual field. In this way, the patient's fields can be tested against the examiner's.

Gross defects and visual neglect (inattention)

Sit opposite the patient, ~1 m apart, at eye level Test first for gross defects and visual neglect, with both eyes open.

- Raise your arms up and out to the sides so that one hand is in the upper right quadrant of your vision and one in the upper left.
- Ask the patient to look directly at you ("look at my nose").
- Move one index finger and ask the patient, while looking straight at you, to point to the hand that is moving.
- Test with the right, left, and then both hands.
- Test the lower quadrants in the same way.
- If visual neglect is present, the patient will be able to see each hand moving individually but report seeing only one hand when both are moving (compare with sensory inattention, 📖 p. 312).

Testing each eye

In the same position as above, ask the patient to cover their right eye while you cover your left, and look directly at one another.

- If you were now to trace the outer borders of your vision in the air half-way between yourself and the patient, it should be almost identical to the area seen by the patient.

Test each quadrant individually:

- Stretch your arm out and up so that your hand is just outside your field of vision, an equal distance between you and the patient.
- Slowly bring your hand into the center (perhaps wiggling one finger) and ask the patient to say "yes" as soon as they can see it.
- You should both be able to see your hand at the same time.
- Test upper right and left, lower right and left individually, bringing your hand in from each corner of vision at a time.
- Ensure that the patient remains looking directly at you (many will attempt to turn and look at the hand if not prompted correctly).
- Map out any areas of visual loss in detail, finding borders. Test if any visual loss extends across the midline horizontally or vertically.
- Test each eye in turn (you both may require a short break between eyes, as this requires considerable concentration).

Repeat the above procedure with a red-headed pin or similar small red object to map out areas of visual loss in more detail.

- Ask the patient to say "yes" when they see the pin *as red.*
- Start by mapping out the blind spot, which should be ~15° lateral from the center at the midline (this tests both your technique and the patient's reliability as a witness before proceeding).

Decide if any defect is of a quadrant, half the visual field or another shape and in which eye, or both. Record by drawing the defect in two circles representing the patient's visual fields, as shown in Fig. 10.2 📖 p. 267.

If the patient is unable to cooperate

Like much of the neurological examination, gross defects can be seen without the patient's cooperation (confused or drowsy). Test for response to "menace" by bringing your hand in sharply from the side, stopping just short of hitting the patient in the eye. If your hand can be seen, the patient will blink. Test vision on the left and the right.

Some common visual field defects

Compare the defects below with the corresponding number on Fig. 10.2 showing the position of the lesion and a representation of the fields, as it should be recorded in the patient's notes.

- *Tunnel vision:* a confusing term. A constricted visual field, giving the impression of looking down a pipe or tunnel, may be caused by glaucoma, retinal damage or papilledema. Tubular vision is often functional.
- *Enlarged blind spot:* caused by papilledema
- *Unilateral field loss:* (1) blindness in one eye caused by devastating damage to the eye, its blood supply, or optic nerve.
- *Central scotoma:* a hole in the visual field (macular degeneration, vascular lesion or, if bilateral, toxins). If bilateral, this may indicate a very small defect in the corresponding area of the occipital cortex (multiple sclerosis).
- *Bitemporal hemianopia:* (2) the nasal half of both retinas and, therefore, the temporal half of each visual field is lost (damage to the center of the optic chiasm, such as a pituitary tumor, craniopharyngioma, suprasellar meningioma).
- *Binasal hemianopia:* the nasal half of each visual field is lost (very rare)
- *Homonymous hemianopia:* (3) may be left or right. Commonly seen in stroke patients. The right or left side of vision in both eyes is lost (e.g., the nasal field in the right eye and the temporal field in the left eye). If the central part of vision (corresponding to the macula) is spared, the lesion is likely in the optic radiation; without macula sparring, the lesion is in the optic tract.
- *Homonymous quadrantanopia:* corresponding quarters of the vision are lost in each eye (e.g., the upper temporal field in the right and the upper nasal field in the left)
  - Upper quadrantanopias (4) suggest a lesion in the temporal lobe.
  - Lower quadrantanopias (5) suggest a lesion in the parietal lobe.

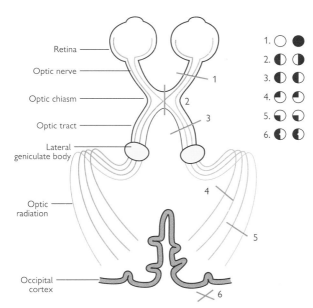

Fig. 10.2 Representation of the visual tracts from the retina to the occipital cortex showing main structures and expected visual field loss according to the site of the lesion.

Cranial nerve II: ophthalmoscopy

Direct ophthalmoscopic examination of the fundus is a vital part of any neurological examination but is often avoided, as it is considered difficult.

It can provide the observer with vital information about the condition of the optic nerve head. The exam takes practice, but the experienced observer can gain views of the fundus, macular region, and retinal vascular arcades. It is worth practicing at every opportunity. The direct ophthalmoscope gives a greatly magnified view of the fundus; gaining a view of the peripheral retina beyond the equator requires examination with a slit lamp or indirect ophthalmoscope, not covered in this book.

For a complete ophthalmoscopic examination, it is often worth dilating the pupil by instilling a few drops of a mydriatic medication (1% cyclopentolate) into the inferior conjunctival sac. With a little practice, one often finds that this is not necessary for a routine examination.

❶ If you plan to dilate the pupil, ask the patient if they have any history of angle-closure glaucoma or episodes of seeing haloes around lights at nighttime. If you suspect this, or the anterior chamber of the eye appears shallow, it is best to err on the side of caution—dilating the pupil could occlude the drainage angle and precipitate an acute attack.

Examination

- Performed in a dimly lit room with the patient sitting or lying down
- Ask the patient to focus on a distant object and keep their eyes still (this relaxes accommodation as much as possible).
- Look through the ophthalmoscope 30 cm away from the patient and bring light in nasally from the temporal field to land on the pupil.
  - The pupil will appear red, and opacities in the visual axis will appear as black dots or lines.
  - By cycling through the different lenses of the ophthalmoscope, you should be able to gain an impression of where these opacities lie. Possible locations are the cornea, aqueous, lens (and its anterior and posterior capsules), and vitreous.
- Dial up a hypermetropic (plus) lens on the ophthalmoscope to focus on the corneal surface and move in as close as possible to the patient's eye—by gradually ↓ the power of the lens, you can examine the cornea, iris, and lens. (Formal examination of these structures is best done with the slit lamp, although a great deal of information can be gained with the direct ophthalmoscope.)
- Continue to ↓ the power of the lens until you can sharply focus on the retinal vessels. It is often best to pick up one of the vascular arcades in the periphery and track them in toward the optic disc. This allows the peripheral quadrants to be examined before viewing the optic disc. Take time to look at the vessels carefully, particularly where the arteries cross the veins.
- Ask the patient to look directly into the light of the ophthalmoscope so you can gain a view of the macular region.

The normal fundus

Optic disc

- The healthy disc is a pale pink/yellow color and round or slightly oval (Fig. 10.3).
- The margins between the disc and the surrounding retina should be crisp and well defined. Occasionally, a surrounding ring is present, which may be slightly lighter or darker in color.
- At the center of the disc is the physiological cup. It appears paler in color than the rest of the disc.

Macular region

- Located temporally from the optic disc
- This is the region with the maximum concentration of cones.
- At the center of the macula is the *fovea*—a tiny pit devoid of blood vessels and responsible for fine resolution.
- Disease involving the macula and fovea can cause devastating visual loss.

Retinal vessels

- The central retinal artery and vein enter and leave the globe in the center of the optic disc.
- Veins appear larger and darker in color than the arteries.
- Spontaneous venous pulsations are seen in many normal eyes.
- Arterial pulsations should not be visible in normal eyes.

Hint

View the macula by directing light on the most sensitive part of the eye. This can often be unpleasant for the patient and will lead to more marked miosis and a restricted view.

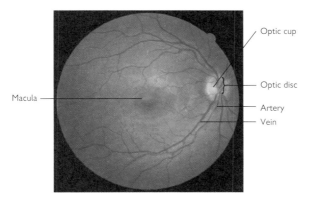

Fig. 10.3 The normal appearance of the fundus of the right eye.

Abnormal findings on fundoscopy

Optic disc swelling

Appearance

- The optic disc is raised, swollen, and enlarged.
- The disc often appears darker in color.
- The margins of the disc are blurred and become indistinct from the adjacent retina.
- Retinal vessels can be seen arching down from the raised disc toward the peripheral retina.
- In severe cases, retinal hemorrhage may be seen around the disc.

The term *papilledema* is often incorrectly used to describe optic disc swelling. *Papilledema* is swelling of the optic disc due to raised intracranial pressure (ICP) (Fig. 10.4).

Causes

- Space-occupying lesions, including intracranial malignancy, subdural hematoma, and cerebral abscess
- Subarachnoid hemorrhage (often associated with vitreous hemorrhage)
- Chronic meningitis
- Idiopathic intracranial hypertension (IIH)
- Malignant hypertension
- Ischemic optic neuropathy

Optic disc cupping

Appearance

- The physiological cup is indented with respect to the rest of the disc.
- Retinal vessels kink sharply as they emerge over the rim of the cup (Fig. 10.5).
- Hemorrhages may be present.

Causes

- Most commonly one of the various types of glaucoma

Optic atrophy

Appearance

- Pale optic disc due to loss of nerve fibers in the optic nerve head (Fig. 10.6)

Causes

- Ischemic optic neuropathy
- Optic neuritis
- Trauma
- Optic nerve compression

Retinal hemorrhages

Appearance

The appearance of a hemorrhage depends on its location within the various layers of the retina. Deep hemorrhages appear as dots from the close packing of cells in this region. More superficial hemorrhages in the nerve fiber layer appear as more widespread blotches.

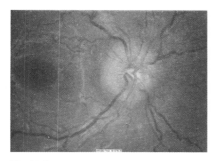

Fig. 10.4 Severe papilledema. Note how the disc margins are blurred and that there is a lack of normal cupping at the disc.

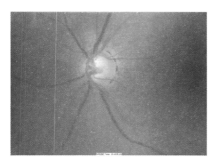

Fig. 10.5 Optic disc cupping, in this case secondary to glaucoma. Note how the vessels seem to disappear over the edge of the disc as if falling down a hole.

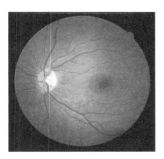

Fig. 10.6 Optic atrophy. The optic disc is pale and well demarcated.

Causes

Many pathological processes:
- Diabetes mellitus
- Hypertension
- Subarachnoid hemorrhage
- Blood dyscrasias
- Systemic vasculitis
- Valsalva related
- Trauma
- Bacterial endocarditis (known specifically as Roth spots)

Central or branch retinal artery occlusion

Appearance
- Large areas of ischemic white retina associated with sudden catastrophic visual loss
- Calcific, cholesterol, or fibrin-platelet emboli can often be seen occluding the retinal artery or branch.

Causes
- Either embolic or thrombotic (remember giant cell arteritis)

Central or branch retinal vein occlusion

Appearance
- Large, widespread flame-shaped hemorrhages classically giving the fundus a stormy-sunset appearance. It is associated with gradual-onset painless, blurred vision and visual loss.
- Optic disc swelling may be present.

Causes
- Blood dyscrasias
- Diabetes mellitus
- Glaucoma

Foster–Kennedy syndrome

Appearance
- Unilateral optic atrophy
- Contralateral papilledema
- Central scotoma
- Anosmia (variable)
- Systemic symptoms such as headache, dizziness, vertigo, and vomiting

Causes
- Meningioma of optic nerve, olfactory groove or sphenoid wing
- Frontal lobe tumor

Pupils

Applied anatomy

The pupil is the aperture at the center of the iris. Variation in pupil size is brought about by two muscles in the iris under the control of the autonomic nervous system:

- *Sphincter pupillae muscle:* found in the iris at margin of the pupil and innervated by parasympathetic fibers. It constricts the pupil (miosis).
- *Dilator pupillae muscle:* radially arranged smooth muscle. Innervated by sympathetic nervous system. It dilates the pupil (mydriasis).

The pupillary light response

The pupillary light response has afferent and efferent limbs that can be affected separately in a number of pathologies. The afferent fibers leave the eye in the optic nerve and separate in the midbrain to synapse with the third nerve nuclei. Efferent pathway fibers then travel to synapse in the ciliary ganglion before innervating the sphincter pupillae.

Examination

Inspect both pupils in good light—is there a discrepancy in size (anisocoria) or shape? (This is present in 25% of the normal population and does not necessarily indicate pathology. It may be secondary to previous ocular inflammatory disease, trauma, or surgery.) If anisocoria is present, one must determine which of the pupils is the correct size.

- A pathologically constricted pupil is more obvious in dim light as the normal pupil dilates.
- A pathologically large pupil will be more apparent in bright illumination when the normal pupil will constrict.

Test pupil responses to direct and consensual light. This is best done in a dimly lit room. Ask the patient to look into the distance to ensure the eye is relaxed and dis-accommodated. Shine a light upward from just inferior to the lower lid to avoid dazzling the patient.

- Constriction of the pupils should be seen almost instantaneously in response to illumination in both the illuminated eye (direct) and nonilluminated eye (consensual). Repeat for both eyes.

The afferent limb of the pupillary light pathway is assessed using the Marcus–Gunn swinging light test, to look for a relative afferent pupil defect (RAPD). If present, do the following:

- Shine light in the normal eye and both pupils constrict. (The consensual response in the affected eye is intact.)
- Swing light to the affected eye and both pupils dilate. (Afferent drive to cause constriction of the pupils from the affected eye is reduced compared to that of the unaffected eye.)
- Swing light back to the normal eye and both pupils constrict.
- Finally, check the near reflex (the efferent limb of the pupil reflex). Ask the patient to focus on a distant object and then look immediately to your index finger held ~30 cm in front of their face.

The normal response will be for the pupils to constrict in response to convergence and accommodation.

Findings: some pupil abnormalities

Argyll–Robertson pupil

Midbrain lesions caused by neurosyphilis target the more dorsally located fibers that subserve the light response. The ventrally located fibers responsible for accommodation are spared.

- *Appearance:* a small, irregular pupil that accommodates but does not react to light
- *Causes:* neurosyphilis and diabetes mellitus

Holmes–Adie pupil

There is denervation of the iris and ciliary body due to ciliary ganglionitis (although some would dispute this). Associated loss of tendon reflexes is seen in some patients and is termed *Holmes–Adie syndrome*.

Appearance

- Unilateral dilated pupil—accommodates (and relaxes) very slowly and shows absent or depressed light reflex. It is supersensitive to 0.1% pilocarpine (muscarinic agonist causing constriction).

Causes

- Usually idiopathic and predominates in young adult females ($♀:♂ ≈$ 2:1). It may also follow iridoplegia or ocular trauma.

Horner's syndrome

This involves interruption of the sympathetic nerve supply to the iris.

Appearance

- Unilateral miotic pupil with partial ptosis (due to paralysis of Muller's muscle—a small smooth muscle in the upper lid). Movement of the upper lid should be intact as the levator muscle is supplied by the oculomotor nerve. There is also a variable interruption of sudomotor innervation to the ipsilateral side of the face.
- Sweating is absent if the lesion occurs proximal to the carotid plexus, after which the sudomotor fibers separate.

Causes

The protracted course of the sympathetic pathway makes it vulnerable to disruption at many different points.

- Congenital—often associated with an alteration in iris pigment (heterochromia); injury or surgery to the neck (avulsion of C8 and T1 nerve roots results in Klumpke's paralysis); multiple sclerosis; cavernous sinus disease; neoplasia involving the mediastinum, cervical cord or apex of the lung; infarction—secondary to occlusion of the basilar or posterior inferior cerebellar artery; thoracic aortic aneurysm; syringomyelia or syringobulbia

Box 10.1 More on the RAPD

At rest, the patient's pupils are equal and of normal size. RAPD is *relative* because the response seen when light is shone on the affected pupil is less than that seen when light is shone in the normal pupil, and *afferent* because it demonstrates a problem in the afferent limb of the light response in the affected eye. The response indicates unilateral or asymmetrical optic nerve disease or extensive retinal pathology. An RAPD will not be seen in patients with corneal or lens opacities.

Cranial nerves III, IV, and VI

The third (oculomotor), fourth (trochlear), and sixth (abducens) nerves are considered together, as their primary function is to provide motor innervation to the extrinsic muscles of the eye. Connections exist with the horizontal gaze center in the pons and the vertical gaze center in the midbrain.

Applied anatomy: CN III

- *Motor:* levator palpebrae superioris, superior rectus, medial rectus, inferior rectus, inferior oblique (all the extrinsic muscles of the eye except the lateral rectus and superior oblique)
- *Autonomic:* parasympathetic supply to the constrictor (sphincter) pupillae of the iris and ciliary muscles

The main oculomotor nucleus lies anterior to the aqueduct of the midbrain. The Edinger–Westphal nucleus (accessory parasympathetic nucleus) lies posterior to the oculomotor nucleus. Fibers pass anteriorly, through the cavernous sinus and enter the orbit through the superior orbital fissure.

Applied anatomy: CN IV

- *Motor:* superior oblique

The nucleus lies just inferior to that of the oculomotor nerve and has connections with the cerebral hemispheres, visual cortex, and nerves III, VI, and VIII. Its fibers pass posteriorly and immediately cross one another. They then travel through the cavernous sinus, entering the orbit through the superior orbital fissure.

Applied anatomy: CN VI

- *Motor:* lateral rectus

The nucleus lies beneath the fourth ventricle. It connects with the nuclei of the III and IV cranial nerves through the medial longitudinal fasciculus (MLF). It emerges from the pons and travels through the cavernous sinus to enter the orbit through the superior orbital fissure.

Examination

The patient should be sitting facing you with their eyes straight ahead. Ensure that visual acuity has already been assessed and recorded.

- Inspect the position of the lids.
  - Is there ptosis (drooping of the lid)?
  - Are the epicanthic folds prominent? (This may cause pseudosquint.)
- Look at the position of the eyes in neutral gaze.
  - An asymmetrical position suggests strabismus (squint); this should be assessed with the cover test (see Box 10.2, 📖 p. 277).
- Ask the patient to follow your index finger in vertical, horizontal, and oblique planes, avoiding extremes of gaze. Draw a large imaginary *H* directly in front of the patient.
  - Is nystagmus present (rapid to-and-fro movements of the eyes)?
  - Ask the patient if they see double at any stage (diplopia).
- The patient's eyes should be able to follow the moving target smoothly. This is termed *pursuit*. (It is often slowed or interrupted with saccades in Huntington's chorea and Parkinson's disease.)

- Now hold up your index finger on one side of their head and your thumb on the other—in their temporal visual fields. Ask the patient to look quickly between the finger and thumb. This tests saccadic eye movements—they should be accurate, smooth, and rapid.
- Ask the patient to look from a distant object to a near object—the eyes should converge smoothly and equally in association with accommodation and pupil constriction. This is called *convergence*.

Hints

Patients will often attempt to turn their head to look at your moving finger. This can be overcome in two ways:
- Fully explain the examination before beginning. Often, an instruction, such as, "Please follow the tip of my finger with your eyes but keep your head still," works wonders.
- If the patient continues to turn their head, you can stabilize it by gently placing your free hand on their forehead.

Abnormal findings

Ptosis (drooping of the lid)

Causes include the following:
- Weakness of the levator muscle in myasthenia gravis
- Third-nerve palsy
- Disruption of insertion of the levator muscle into the tarsal plate of the lid, through either surgery or trauma

Strabismus or squint

This is an abnormality of coordinated eye movements. In divergent squint, one eye is directed toward the target, the other is turned laterally. In convergent squint, the other eye is turned medially.

Squint is broadly categorized into two forms:
- *Nonparalytic:* seen in childhood. Both eyes have full range of movement but only one eye is directed toward the target of fixation.
- *Paralytic:* Movement of one or more of the extraocular muscles is decreased because of disease of the muscle, a nerve palsy, or a physical obstruction to movement in a particular direction (e.g., tethering, trauma, or neoplasm).

Box 10.2 Cover–uncover test

This test is used for further analysis of nonparalytic squint.
- The patient should be sitting in front of you.
- Present a fixation target in front of them (the top of your pen, for example).
- Ask them to cover their right eye.
- Closely observe the uncovered left eye—one of three responses is possible:
  - The eye doesn't move—normal
  - The eye moves nasally to fixate—divergent squint present
  - The eye moves temporally to fixate—convergent squint present
- Now repeat the test, covering the left eye.

Pick up a subtle squint by holding a pen light about 10 inches away from the center of the patient's face. The reflection of light should be from the same position on the cornea in both eyes. If this is not the case, the fixating eye will have the central reflection.

ⓘ A more sophisticated assessment of squint is made in eye clinics, using a syntophore.

Further assessment of a squint should always involve a detailed examination of the cornea, lens, vitreous, and retina, to exclude opacities and abnormalities.

Nystagmus

For oscillating movements of the eyes, there are several subclassifications based on clinical appearance and lesion location. Watch the movements carefully. Are the to-and-fro phases of the movements the same speed in both directions, or is one more rapid than the other?

Vestibular

This is a type of jerk nystagmus (to-and-fro movements are of different velocities). It is caused by disease in the labyrinth or its central connections. The fast phase is away from the side of the lesion. There are often horizontal and rotary components. It is usually only present in the acute phase of labyrinthine disease.

Pendular nystagmus

The velocity of the movements is the same in both directions. This is often a congenital condition associated with ↓ visual acuity. It is also seen in cerebrovascular disease and multiple sclerosis.

Patients with acquired nystagmus will often complain of continual movement of their visual environment (oscillopsia), which is not the case with congenital nystagmus.

Optokinetic nystagmus

This is a normal response of the eye when trying to follow a moving object (e.g., when looking from the window of a train). It is formally assessed using a rotating drum painted with vertical black and white lines.

Movements are controlled by the cerebral hemisphere, toward which the drum is rotating, causing pursuit movement in the direction of rotation followed by saccadic movement back in the opposite direction. Defective optokinetic nystagmus is seen in lesions of the deep parietal lobe, when drum rotation is toward the affected cerebral hemisphere.

Upbeat nystagmus

The fast phase is upward. Causes include brainstem disease, intoxication with alcohol, and a number of other drugs, including phenytoin.

Downbeat nystagmus

The fast phase is downward. This is seen in toxic states and demyelinating disease. There is also herniation of cerebellar tissue through the foramen magnum, as seen in Chiari malformation.

Gaze-evoked nystagmus
The fast phase is toward the direction of action of the affected muscle. This is usually seen in dysfunction of extraocular muscles secondary to intrinsic weakness or nerve palsy.

Hint
When assessing nystagmus, try to avoid the extremes of lateral gaze (i.e., not >30°). This will elicit *end-point nystagmus*—a physiological response not to be confused with a pathological process.

Palsies of cranial nerves III, IV, and VI

CN III: oculomotor

Appearance

The pupil is dilated and responds to neither light nor accommodation. All of the extraocular muscles are paralyzed except for the lateral rectus and the superior oblique. The unopposed action of these causes the eye to look down and out. Paralysis of the levator muscle causes complete ptosis.

Causes

These include diabetes mellitus (pupil sparing), lesions involving the superior orbital fissure, cavernous sinus disease, aneurysm of the posterior communicating artery, and Weber's syndrome (associated contralateral hemiplegia).

CN IV: trochlear

Appearance

Paralysis of the superior oblique causes the eye to elevate when adducting. The patient will complain of diplopia and have difficulty looking downward and inward on the affected side. The patient may try to compensate for this by tilting their head away from the side of the lesion (ocular torticollis).

Causes

Trauma, surgery, diabetes mellitus, atherosclerosis, or neoplasia may be involved.

CN VI: abducens

Appearance

Paralysis of the lateral rectus muscle means the eye cannot be abducted from the midline and the unopposed action of the medial rectus leaves the eye deviated nasally at rest. The patient will complain of diplopia in horizontal gaze. Lesions in the sixth nerve nucleus also involve the lateral gaze center and lead to a gaze paresis.

Causes

These include diabetes mellitus, atherosclerosis, multiple sclerosis, neoplastic lesions, raised ICP leading to compression of the nerve on the edge of the petrous temporal bone (a false localizing sign), trauma, and surgery.

Combined nerve palsies

Given the close proximity of nerves III, IV, and VI at points along their courses, lesions at specific anatomical locations can lead to combined nerve palsies.

Cavernous sinus

All three nerves involved in oculomotor control, along with sympathetic fibers to the iris and the ophthalmic and maxillary divisions of the trigeminal nerve, pass through here.

Common lesions include caroticocavernous fistula; expanding pituitary tumor; cavernous sinus thrombosis, associated with proptosis and injection of conjunctival vessels (chemosis); and an aneurysm.

Orbit
A complex range of ophthalmoplegias can result from any compressive lesion located within the orbit. Proptosis may be present with variable optic nerve involvement. Many lesions may directly impinge on the extraocular muscles as well as the innervating nerves.

Superior orbital fissure
The superior orbital fissure transmits all the nerves supplying the extraocular muscles along with the ophthalmic division of the trigeminal nerve. Inflammation or a lesion at the superior orbital fissure leads to *Tolosa–Hunt syndrome*, a complex unilateral ophthalmoplegia associated with anesthesia over the forehead and ocular pain.

Some other eye movement disorders
Internuclear ophthalmoplegia
This is interruption of the MLF, connecting the nuclei of cranial nerves III and VI on opposite sides.

Voluntary gaze toward one side is initiated by the opposite cerebral hemisphere. Descending fibers then decussate to the horizontal gaze center in the pons and parapontine reticular formation where further impulses are transmitted directly to the sixth nerve nucleus, causing abduction of the ipsilateral eye.

Conjugate adduction of the contralateral eye is brought about by impulses transmitted via the medial longitudinal fasciculus to the third nerve nucleus, thus maintaining binocular single vision.

Appearance
- Impaired adduction in the ipsilateral eye in unilateral lesions. Nystagmus is often seen in the abducting eye.
- Bilateral lesions often cause vertical nystagmus and impaired vertical pursuit.
- Convergence remains intact.
- The patient will complain of horizontal diplopia due to impaired adduction on the affected side, not to nystagmus in the abducting eye.

Common causes
- Cerebrovascular disease, multiple sclerosis

Lesions of the parapontine reticular formation (PPRF)
The PPRF is responsible for conjugate eye movements in horizontal gaze.

Appearance
- Failure of horizontal eye movements toward the side of the lesion—a horizontal gaze paresis
- An ipsilateral internuclear ophthalmoplegia if the lesion extends to involve the MLF
- Preservation of vertical gaze
- Contralateral deviation of the eyes in the acute phase

Causes
- Vascular disease, demyelinating disease, neoplasia

Parinaud's syndrome

Lesions occurring in the dorsal midbrain involve the vertical gaze center, hence this syndrome is also known as dorsal midbrain syndrome.

Appearance
- Impaired upward gaze in both eyes, resulting in convergence, retraction of the globe into the orbit, and nystagmus
- Light-near dissociation of the pupils—the near reflex is intact but response to light is poor.

Causes
- Demyelinating disease, vascular disease affecting the dorsal midbrain, enlarged third ventricle

Cranial nerve V: trigeminal

Applied anatomy

Sensory
- Facial sensation in three branches—ophthalmic (V1), maxillary (V2), and mandibular (V3). Distribution is shown in Fig. 10.7.

Motor
- Muscles of mastication

Nerve originates in the pons, travels to trigeminal ganglion at the petrous temporal bone, and splits. V_1 passes through the cavernous sinus with CN III and exits via the superior orbital fissure; V_2 leaves via the infraorbital foramen (also supplies the palate and nasopharynx); V_3 exits via the foramen ovale with the motor portion.

Examination

Inspection
Inspect the patient's face—wasting of the temporalis will show as hollowing above the zygomatic arch.

Testing motor function
- Ask the patient to clench their teeth. Feel both sides for the bulge of the masseter and temporalis.
- Ask the patient to open their mouth wide—the jaw will deviate toward the side of a V lesion.
- Again ask them to open their mouth, but provide resistance by holding their jaw closed with one of your hands.

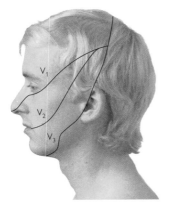

Fig. 10.7 Distribution of the sensory branches of the trigeminal nerve. V_1 = ophthalmic, V_2 = maxillary, V_3 = mandibular. Note that V_1 extends to the vertex and includes the cornea and V_3 does *not* include the angle of the jaw.

Testing sensory function
- Assess light touch for each branch and ask patient to say "yes" if felt.
  - Choose three spots to test on each side to make the examination easy to remember—forehead, cheek, and mid-way along jaw.
- For each branch, compare left to right. Ignore minor differences (it's difficult to press with exactly the same force each time).
- Test pin-prick sensation at the same spots, using a sterile pin.
- Temperature sensation is not routinely tested—consider this only if abnormalities in light touch or pin-prick are found. Use specimen tubes or other small containers full of hot or cold water.

Findings
- Wasting of muscles: long-term V palsy, motor neuron disease (MND), myotonic dystrophy
- Loss of all sensory modalities: V ganglion lesion (e.g., herpes zoster)
- Loss of light touch only—with loss of sensation on ipsilateral side of the body: contralateral parietal lobe (sensory cortex) lesion.
- Loss of light touch in V only: lesion at sensory root pons
- Loss of pin-prick only—along with contralateral side of body: ipsilateral brainstem lesion
- Loss of sensation in muzzle distribution (nose, lips, anterior cheeks): damage to the lower part of the spinal sensory nucleus (syringomyelia, demyelination)

Reflexes
Jaw jerk
ⓘ Explain to the patient what you will do; this could appear threatening!
- Ask the patient to let their mouth hang loosely open.
- Place your finger horizontally across their chin and tap your finger with a patella hammer.
- Feel and watch jaw movement.
  - There should be a slight closure of the jaw, but this varies widely in normal people. A brisk and definite closure may indicate an upper motor neuron (UMN) lesion above the level of the pons (e.g., pseudobulbar palsy).

Corneal reflex
Afferent = V_1, efferent = VII.
- Ask the patient to look up and away from you.
- Gently touch the cornea with a wisp of cotton wool. Bring this in from the side so it cannot be seen approaching.
- Watch both eyes. A blink is a normal response.
  - No response = ipsilateral V_1 palsy
  - Lack of blink on one side only = VII palsy
- Watch out for contact lenses, as they will give a reduced sensation. Ask the patient to remove them first.

Hints
- Note the sensory distribution. The angle of the jaw is not supplied by V_3 but by the great auricular nerve (C2, C3).
- When testing the corneal reflex, touch the cornea (overlies the iris), not the conjunctiva (overlies the sclera).

Cranial nerve VII: facial

Applied anatomy

- **Sensory:** external auditory meatus, tympanic membrane, small portion of skin behind the ear. Special sensation: taste anterior 2/3 of tongue
- **Motor:** muscles of facial expression, stapedius
- **Autonomic:** parasympathetic supply to lacrimal glands

The nucleus lies in the pons, the nerve leaves at the cerebellopontine angle with CN VIII. The nerve gives off a branch to the stapedius at the geniculate ganglion, while most of the nerve leaves the skull via the stylomastoid foramen and travels through the parotid gland.

Examination

Muscles of facial expression

Test both the left and right sides at the same time. Some patients have difficulty understanding the instructions—the authors recommend a quick demonstration following each command, allowing the patient to mirror you (e.g., "puff out your cheeks like this"). This exam can be quite embarrassing; the examiner making equally strange faces can lighten the mood and aid in the patient's cooperation and enthusiasm.

- Look at the patient's face at rest. Look for asymmetry in the nasolabial folds, angles of the mouth, and forehead wrinkles.
- Ask the patient to raise their eyebrows ("look up!"). Watch the forehead wrinkle.
- Attempt to press their eyebrows down and note any weakness.
- Ask patient to close their eyes tightly. Watch, then test against resistance with your finger and thumb, saying, "Don't let me pull them apart."
- Ask the patient to blow out their cheeks. Watch for air escaping on one side.
- Ask the patient to bare their teeth (e.g., "show me your teeth!"). Look for asymmetry.
- Ask the patient to purse their lips and to whistle for you. Look for asymmetry. The patient will always smile after whistling (see below).

Whistle-smile sign

Failure to smile when asked to whistle (whistle-smile negative) is usually due to emotional paresis of the facial muscles and is synonymous with Parkinsonism.

External auditory meatus

This should be examined briefly if only CN VII is examined—it can be done as part of CN VIII if examining all the cranial nerves.

Taste

This is rarely tested outside specialist clinics.

- Each side is tested separately, using cotton buds dipped in the solution of choice applied to each side of the tongue. Be sure to swill the mouth with distilled water between each taste sensation.
- Test sweet, salty, bitter (quinine), and sour (vinegar).

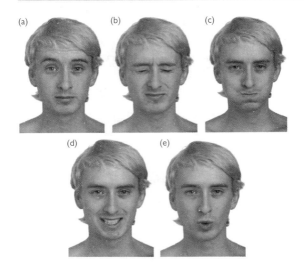

Fig. 10.8 Testing the muscles of facial expression as described on 📖 p. 285. (a) Eyebrows; (b) eyelids; (c) puffing out the cheeks; (d) baring teeth; (e) whistle.

Findings

- *Upper motor nerve lesion* will cause loss of facial movement on the ipsilateral side but with preservation of forehead wrinkling—both sides of the forehead receive bilateral nervous supply (unilateral = cerebrovascular accident [CVA], etc.; bilateral = pseudobulbar palsy, motor neuron disease).
- *Lower motor nerve lesion* will cause loss of all movement on the ipsilateral side of the face (unilateral = demyelination, tumors, Bell's palsy, pontine lesions, cerebellopontine angle lesions; bilateral = sarcoid, Guillain–Barré syndrome [GBS], myasthenia gravis).
- *Bell's palsy:* idiopathic unilateral LMN VII paresis
- *Ramsay–Hunt syndrome:* unilateral paresis caused by herpes at the geniculate ganglion (look for herpes rash on the external ear)

Hints

- *Bell's phenomenon* is the upward movement of the eyeballs when the eye closes. This occurs in the normal state but can be clearly seen if the eyelids fail to close because of VII palsy.
- VII palsy does *not* cause eyelid ptosis.
- Long-standing VII palsy can cause fibrous contraction of the muscles on the affected side, resulting in a more pronounced nasolabial fold (the reverse of the expected findings).
- Bilateral VII palsy will cause a sagging, expressionless face and is often missed.

Cranial nerve VIII: vestibulocochlear

Applied anatomy
- **Sensory:** hearing (cochlear), balance and equilibrium (vestibular)
- **Motor:** none

The eighth nerve comprises two parts.

The *cochlear branch* originates in the organ of Corti in the ear and passes through the internal auditory meatus to its nucleus in the pons. Fibers pass to the superior gyrus of the temporal lobes.

The *vestibular branch* arises in the utricle and semicircular canals, joins the auditory fibers in the facial canal, enters the brainstem at the cerebellopontine angle, and ends in the pons and cerebellum.

Examination
Inquire first about symptoms—hearing loss or changes, or balance problems. Peripheral vestibular lesions cause ataxia during paroxysms of vertigo but not at other times.

Begin by inspecting each ear as described in 📖 Chapter 6 (p. 132).

Hearing
Test each ear separately. Cover one by pressing on the tragus or create white noise by rubbing your fingers together at the external auditory meatus.

Simple test of hearing
- Whisper a number into one ear and ask the patient to repeat it.
- Repeat with the other ear.
- Be careful to whisper at the same volume in each ear (the end of expiration is best) and at the same distance (about 24 inches).

Rinne's test
- Tap a 512 Hz* tuning fork and hold adjacent to the ear (air conduction, Fig. 10.9a).
- Then apply the base of the tuning fork to the mastoid process (bone conduction)—see Fig. 10.9b.
- Ask the patient which position sounds louder.
  - Normal = air conduction > bone conduction = "Rinne's positive"
  - In neural (or perceptive) deafness, Rinne's test will remain positive.
  - In conductive deafness, the findings are reversed (bone > air).

Weber's test
- Tap a 512 Hz tuning fork and hold the base against the vertex or forehead at the midline (see Fig. 10.9c).
- Ask the patient if it sounds louder on one side.
  - In neural deafness, the tone is heard better in the intact ear.
  - In conductive deafness, the tone is heard better in the affected ear.

* This is the C above middle C for those musically inclined.

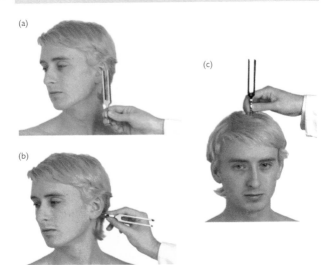

Fig. 10.9 (a) Testing air conduction. (b) Testing bone conduction. (c) Position of the tuning fork for Weber's test.

Vestibular function

Turning test

- Ask the patient to stand facing you, with arms outstretched.
- Ask them to march on the spot, then close their eyes (continue marching).
- Watch!
  - The patient will gradually turn toward the side of the lesion; sometimes they will turn right round 180°.

Hallpike's maneuver

This is a test for benign positional vertigo (BPV). Do **not** test those with known neck problems or possible posterior circulation impairment.

- Explain to the patient what will happen.
- Sit the patient facing away from the edge of the bed such that when they lie back, their head will not be supported (over the edge).
- Turn their head to one side and ask them to look in that direction.
- Lay them back quickly, supporting their head so that it lies about 30° below the horizontal.
- Watch for nystagmus (the affected ear will be lowermost).
- Repeat with the head turned in the other direction.
  - No nystagmus = normal
  - Nystagmus, with a slight delay (10 seconds) and fatigable (can't be repeated successfully for 10–15 minutes) = BPV
  - Nystagmus, no delay and no fatiguing = central vestibular syndrome

Cranial nerves IX and X

The ninth (glossopharyngeal) and tenth (vagus) nerves are considered together as they have similar functions and work together to control the pharynx, larynx, and swallowing.

Applied anatomy: IX

- *Sensory:* pharynx, middle ear. Special sensation: taste on posterior 1/3 of tongue
- *Motor:* stylopharyngeous
- *Autonomic:* parotid gland

This nerve originates in the medulla, passes through the jugular foramen.

Applied anatomy: X

- *Sensory:* tympanic membrane, external auditory canal, and external ear. Also proprioception from thorax and abdomen
- *Motor:* palate, pharynx, and larynx
- *Autonomic:* carotid baroreceptors

This nerve originates in the medulla and pons, leaves the skull via the jugular foramen.

Examination

Pharynx

- Ask the patient to open their mouth. Inspect the uvula (use a tongue depressor if necessary). Is it central or deviated to one side? If to one side, which side?
- Ask the patient to say "aah." Watch the uvula. It should move upward centrally. Does it deviate to one side?

Gag reflex

This is unpleasant for the patient and should only be tested if a IX or X nerve lesion is suspected (afferent signal = IX, efferent = X).

- With the patient's mouth open wide, gently touch the posterior pharyngeal wall on one side with a tongue depressor or other sterile stick.
- Watch the uvula (it should lift up).
- Repeat on the opposite side.
- Ask the patient if they felt the two touches and if there was any difference in sensation.

Larynx

- Ask the patient to cough. Normal character? Gradual onset or sudden?
- Listen to the patient's speech. Note volume and quality and whether it appears to fatigue (gets quieter as time goes on).

Test swallow

- At each stage, watch the swallow action. Are there two phases or one smooth movement? Delay between fluid leaving the mouth (oral phase) and pharynx and larynx reacting (pharyngeal phase)? Is there any coughing or choking? Any "wet" voice?
- Terminate the test at the first sign of the patient aspirating.

- Offer the patient a teaspoon of water to swallow. Repeat × 3.
- Offer the patient a sip of water. Repeat × 3.
- Offer the patient the glass for a mouthful of water. Repeat × 3.

Findings

Uvula

- Moves to one side = X lesion on the *opposite* side
- No movement = muscle paresis
- Moves with "aah" but not gag and ↓ pharyngeal sensation = IX palsy

Cough

- Gradual onset of a deliberate cough = vocal cord palsy
- "Wet," bubbly voice and cough (before the swallow test) = pharyngeal and vocal cord palsy (X palsy)
- Poor swallow and aspiration = combined IX and X or lone X lesion

Cranial nerve XI: accessory

Applied anatomy

- *Sensory:* none
- *Motor:* sternocleidomastoids and upper part of trapezii

The accessory nerve is composed of cranial and spinal parts. The cranial accessory nerve arises from the nucleus ambiguus in the medulla. The spinal accessory nerve extends from the lateral part of the spinal cord down to C5 as a series of rootlets. These join together and ascend adjacent to the spinal cord, passing through the foramen magnum to join with the cranial portion of the accessory nerve. It leaves the skull via the jugular foramen.

The cranial portion joins with the vagus nerve (X). The spinal portion innervates the sternocleidomastoids and the upper fibers of the trapezii.

▶ Note that each cerebral hemisphere controls the ipsilateral sternocleidomastoid and the contralateral trapezius.

Examination

The cranial portion of the accessory nerve cannot be tested separately.

- Inspect the sternocleidomastoids. Look for wasting, fasciculation, hypertrophy, and any abnormal head position.
- Ask the patient to shrug their shoulders, and observe.
- Ask the patient to shrug again, using your hands on their shoulders to provide resistance.
- Ask the patient to turn their head to each side, first without and then with resistance (use your hand on their cheek).

Findings

Isolated accessory nerve lesions are very rare. CN XI lesions usually present as part of a wider weakness or neurological syndrome.

- *Bilateral weakness:* with wasting caused by muscular problems or motor neuron disease
- *Unilateral weakness (trapezius and sternomastoid same side)* suggests a peripheral neurological lesion.
- *Unilateral weakness (trapezius and sternomastoid of opposite sides),* usually with hemiplegia, suggests a UMN lesion ipsilateral to the weak sternomastoid.

Hints

- Remember that the action of the sternocleidomastoid is to turn the head to the *opposite* side (e.g., poor head turning to the *left* indicates a weak *right* sternocleidomastoid).
- When providing resistance to head turning, be sure to press against the patient's cheek (see Fig. 10.10). Lateral pressure to the jaw can cause pain and injury, particularly in older and frail patients.

(a)

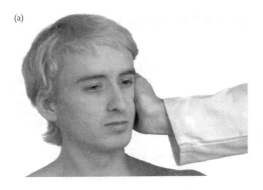

(b)

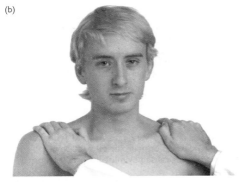

Fig. 10.10 (a) Using resistance against lateral head-turning. Be careful not to apply pressure to the patient's jaw. (b) Testing the trapezius against resistance.

Cranial nerve XII: hypoglossal

Applied anatomy
- *Sensory:* none
- *Motor:* muscles of the tongue

The nucleus lies on the floor of CN IV ventricle. Fibers pass ventrally, leaving the brainstem lateral to the pyramidal tracts. The nerve leaves the skull via the hypoglossal foramen.

Examination
- Ask the patient to open wide and inspect the tongue on the floor of the mouth. Look for size and evidence of fasciculation.
- Ask the patient to protrude the tongue. Look for deviation or abnormal movements.
- Ask the patient to move the tongue in and out repeatedly, then from side to side.
- To test for subtle weakness, place your finger on the patient's cheek and ask them to push against it from the inside, using their tongue.

Findings
- A LMN neuron lesion will cause fasciculation on the affected side and a deviation toward the affected side on protrusion. There will also be a weakness on pressing the tongue away from the affected side.
- A unilateral UMN lesion will rarely cause any clinically obvious signs.
- A bilateral UMN lesion will give a small, globally weak tongue with reduced movements.
- A bilateral LMN lesion (e.g., motor neuron disease) will also produce a small, weak tongue.
- Rapid in-and-out movement on protrusion (trombone tremor) can be caused by cerebellar disease, extrapyramidal syndromes, and essential tremor.

Hint
Rippling movements may be seen if the tongue is held protruded for long periods. This is normal and should not be mistaken for fasciculations.

Motor: applied anatomy

The motor system is complex. A detailed description is beyond the scope of this book; what follows is a brief overview.

Cortex

The primary motor area is the precentral gyrus of the cerebrum. It is here, along with adjacent cerebral areas, that initiation of voluntary movement occurs. Muscle groups are represented by areas of the cortex from medial to lateral, as shown in Fig. 10.11. The size of the area dedicated to muscle corresponds to the precision of movement (= the number of motor units that are involved).

Pyramidal (direct) pathways

These are concerned with precise, voluntary movements of the face, vocal cords, hands, and feet. The simplest pathways consist of two neurons. The upper motor neuron (UMN) originates in the cerebral cortex then passes down through the internal capsule, brainstem, and spinal cord where it synapses with a lower motor neuron (LMN). This, in turn, leaves the cord to synapse with the skeletal muscle fibers.

There are three pyramidal tracts:
- *Lateral corticospinal*: control of precise movement in the hands and feet and represents 90% of the UMN axons. These cross over (decussate) in the medulla oblongata before continuing to descend so that nerves from the right side of the brain control muscles on the left of the body and vice versa.

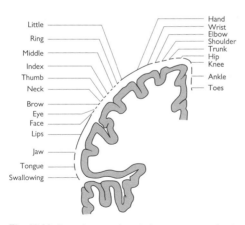

Fig. 10.11 Coronal section through the motor cortex showing the representation of different muscle groups. Note the larger areas given to those muscles performing precise movements—hands, face, and lips.

- *Anterior corticospinal:* control of the neck and trunk and holds 10% of the UMN axons. These do not cross in the medulla but descend in the anterior white columns of the spinal cord. They decussate at several spinal levels and exit at the cervical and upper thoracic segments.
- *Corticobulbar:* voluntary muscles of the eyes, face, tongue, neck, and speech. They terminate at nuclei in the pons and medulla, some crossed, others not. They control cranial nerves III, IV, V, VI, VII, IX, X, XI, and XII.

Extrapyramidal (indirect) pathways

These constiute all of the other descending pathways. They are complex circuits involving the cortex, limbic system, basal ganglia, cerebellum, and cranial nerve nuclei. There are five major tracts controlling precise movements of the hands and feet, movement of the head and eyes in response to visual stimuli, muscle tone, and truncal stability and balance.

Basal ganglia and nuclei are complex circuits concerned with the production of automatic movement and planning movement sequences. They also appear to inhibit intrinsically excitable circuits.

Cerebellum

This is involved in learning and performing skilled, automatic movements (e.g., running, playing the piano) and in posture and balance. It monitors intention, receives signals for actual movements, compares the difference, and makes corrective adjustments.

Box 10.3 A word about functional weakness

Large parts of the neurological examination rely on cooperation of the patient. Occasionally, patients can give the appearance of neurological disability that does not exist, for any number of psychiatric or psychosocial reasons. The examination here is very difficult even for very experienced practitioners. Consider a functional component to the problem if you see the following:
- Abnormal distribution of weakness
- Normal reflexes and tone despite weakness
- Movements are variable and power erratic.
- Variation is seen on repeat testing.

Be careful! Don't jump to conclusions. Do not assume symptoms are functional if they are unusual. All patients should be given the benefit of the doubt. Functional weakness is a diagnosis largely of exclusion.

Motor: inspection and tone

Inspection

As for any other system, the examination begins when you first set eyes on the patient and continues through the history-taking.

- Any walking aids or abnormal gait (see 📖 p. 321)?
- Shake hands—abnormalities of movement? Strength? Relaxation?
- Any abnormal movements when sitting?
- Any obvious weaknesses (e.g., hemiplegia)?
- Does the patient have good sitting balance?

Inspection can be formalized at the examination stage of the encounter. The patient should be seated or lying comfortably with as much of their body exposed as possible. Look at all muscle groups for the following:

- Abnormal positioning, due to weakness or contractures
- Wasting
- Fasciculation (irregular contractions of small areas of muscle)

Make a point of inspecting the shoulder girdle, small muscles of the hand, quadriceps, anterior compartment of the lower leg, and ankle. Look at the foot for contractures or abnormalities of shape.

Tone

The aim is to test resting tone in the limbs. This takes practice; the feel of normal, ↓ or ↑ tone can be taught only through experience.

❶The assessment can be difficult, as it relies on the patient being relaxed; telling the patient to relax usually has the opposite effect! They can be distracted by a counting task or told to relax the limb "as if you're asleep." Distracting the patient with light conversation is a generally successful ploy. You should also repeat the following maneuvers at different speeds and intervals to catch the patient at an unguarded moment.

Arms

- Take the patient's hand in yours (as if shaking it) and hold their elbow with your other hand (see Fig. 10.12a). From this position, you can
  - Pronate and supinate the patient's forearm.
  - Roll the patient's wrist through 360°.
  - Flex and extend the patient's elbow.

Legs

- *Hip:* With the patient lying flat, legs straight, hold onto the patient's knee and roll it from side to side (see Fig. 10.12b).
- *Knee:* With the patient in the same position, put your hand behind the patient's knee and raise it quickly (Fig. 10.12c). Watch the heel—it should lift from the bed or exam table slightly if tone is normal.
- *Ankle:* Holding the foot and the lower leg, flex and dorsiflex the ankle (Fig. 10.12d).

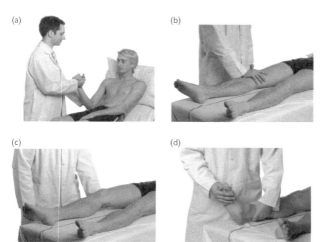

Fig. 10.12 Testing tone. (a) Testing the upper limb. (b) Testing tone at the hip. (c) Testing tone at the knee. (d) Testing tone at the ankle.

Findings

Normal tone
- Slight resistance in movement (feel through experience)

↓ Tone
- Flaccid due to LMN or cerebellar lesions or myopathies

↑ Tone
- *Spasticity (clasp-knife rigidity):* The limb appears stiff. With increased pressure, there is a sudden give and the limb moves. This is seen in UMN lesions.
- *Rigidity (lead pipe):* The limb is equally stiff through all movements.
- *Rigidity (cogwheel):* an extrapyramidal sign, caused by tremor superimposed on a rigid limb. The limb moves in a stop–go halting fashion.
- *Gegenhalten:* (paratonia) seen in bilateral frontal lobe damage and catatonic states. Tone ↑ with ↑ pressure from the examiner—the patient *appears* to be resisting movement.
- *Myotonia:* a slow relaxation after action. When asked to make a fist, the patient is unable the release it quickly and will be slow to let go of a handshake (e.g., myotonic dystrophy).
- *Dystonia:* The limb or head has an abnormal posture that looks uncomfortable.

Motor: upper limb power

As for the muscles of the face, the examiner should demonstrate each movement, mirroring the patient (see Fig. 10.13).

This also allows each action that the patient makes to be opposed by the same (or similar) muscle groups in the examiner—test their fingers against your fingers, and so on. Each muscle group should be graded from 0 to 5 according to the system shown in Box 10.4.

Examination of the upper limbs also allows both sides to be tested at once, providing direct comparison between left and right (see Fig.10.13).
🛈 Be careful not to hurt frail, elderly patients or those with osteoarthritis (OA), rheumatoid arthritis (RA), or other rheumatological disease.

Shoulder

- *Abduction* (C5): Ask the patient to abduct their arms with elbows bent. Ask them to hold still as you attempt to push their arms down.
- *Adduction* (C6, C7): The patient should hold their arms tightly to their sides with elbows bent. You attempt to push their arms out.

Elbow

- *Flexion* (C5, C6): The patient holds their elbows bent and supinated in front of them. Hold the patient at the elbow and wrist and attempt to extend their arm: "Don't let me straighten your arm!"
- *Extension* (C7): Patient holds position above as you resist extension at the elbow by pushing on their distal forearm or wrist: "Push me away!"

Wrist

- *Flexion* (C6, C7): With arms supinated, the patient should flex their wrist and hold as you try to extend it by pulling from your own wrists.
- *Extension* (C6, C7): The opposite of flexion. The patient holds their hand out straight and resists your attempts to bend it.

Fingers

- *Flexion* (C8): Ask the patient to squeeze your fingers or (better) ask the patient to grip your fingers palm to palm (see Fig. 10.13c) and resist your attempts to pull their hand open.
- *Extension* (C7, C8): Ask the patient to hold their fingers out straight. You support their wrist with one hand and try to push their fingers down with the side of your hand over their first interphalangeal joints.
- *Abduction* (T1): Ask the patient to splay their fingers out and resist your attempts to push them together.
- *Adduction* (T1): Holding the patient's middle, ring, and little finger with one hand and their index finger with the other, ask the patient to pull their fingers together or place a piece of paper between their outstretched fingers and ask them to resist your attempts to pull it away.

Pronator drift

This is a useful test of subtle weakness. The patient is asked to hold their arms outstretched in front, palms upward and eyes closed. If one side is weak, the arm will pronate and slowly drift downward.

Box 10.4 Muscle strength testing classifications

- 5 = Normal power
- 4 = Movement against resistance but not normal
- 3 = Movement against gravity, but not against resistance
- 2 = Movement with gravity eliminated (e.g., can move leg from side to side on bed but not lift it)
- 1 = Contractions but no movement seen
- 0 = No movement

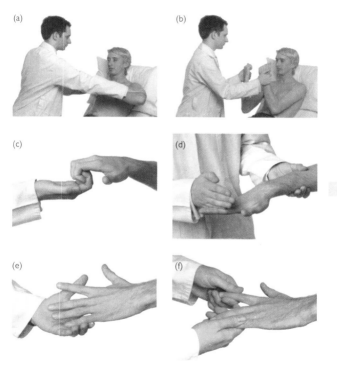

Fig. 10.13 Testing power in the upper limbs. (a) Shoulder movements. (b) Elbow movements. (c) Finger flexion. (d) Finger extension. (e) Finger abduction. (f) Finger adduction.

Motor: lower limb power

The patient should be seated on an exam table or bed with legs out-stretched in front of them. The limbs should be exposed as much as possible so that contractions of the muscles can be *seen*.

Again, power is tested for each muscle group on one side and then the other (Fig. 10.14). Comparing left with right and score results according to the scale in Box 10.4 (📖 p. 299).

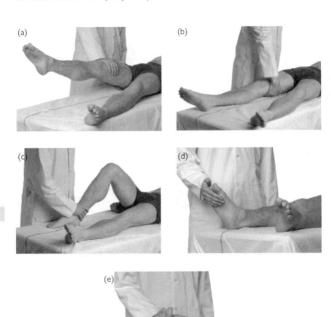

Fig. 10.14 Testing power in the lower limb against resistance. (a) Flexing the hip. (b) Extending the hip. (c) Flexing and extending the knee. (d) Plantar flexion at the ankle. (e) Dorsiflexion at the ankle.

Hip

- *Flexion* (L1, L2, L3): With the lower limbs lying on the bed or couch, the patient raises each leg, keeping the knee straight. Oppose the movement by pushing down on the thigh just above the knee: "Stop me from pushing down!"
- *Extension* (L5, S1): Ask the patient to keep their leg pressed against the bed as you attempt to lift it, either with a hand beneath the calf or the ankle: "Stop me from lifting your leg up!"
- *Abduction* (L4, L5, S1): Ask the patient to move their leg out to the side as you oppose the movement with a hand on the lateral thigh: "Stop me pushing your legs together!"
- *Adduction* (L2, L3, L4): With the legs central, put your hand on the medial thigh and attempt to pull the leg out to the side against resistance: "Don't let me pull your legs apart!"

Knee

- *Flexion* (L5, S1): Take hold of the patient's knee with one hand and their ankle with the other and flex the leg to about 60°. (The patient may think you want them to resist this, so often a quick instruction of "bend at the knee" is required.) Ask the patient to bend their leg further ("stop me straightening your leg out") and oppose the movement at their ankle.
- *Extension* (L3, L4): With the patient's leg in the flexion position, have the patient extend their leg ("push me away," "straighten your leg out") as you oppose it. Alternatively, attempt to bend the patient's leg from a straightened starting position.

Ankle

- *Plantar flexion* (S1, S2): With the patient's leg out straight and ankle relaxed, put your hand on the ball of the foot and ask the patient to push you away: "Push down and stop me pushing back!"
- *Dorsiflexion* (L4, L5): From the starting position for plantar flexion, hold the patient's foot just above the toes and ask them to pull their foot backward. Patients often attempt to move their entire leg here, so tell them, "Pull your foot back and stop me pushing your foot down," along with an accompanying hand gesture.

Tendon reflexes

Theory

The sudden stretch of a muscle is detected by the muscle spindle, which initiates a simple two-neuron reflex arc, causing that muscle to contract. Tendons are struck with a reflex hammer (causing a sudden stretch of the muscle) and the resultant contraction is observed. In LMN lesions or myopathies, the reflex is diminished or absent, but is hyperactive or brisk in UMN lesions.

Technique

The tendons are tapped with a reflex hammer (Fig. 10.15). For each reflex, test the right, then left, and compare. The hammer should be held at the far end of the handle and swung in a loose movement from the wrist. The patient should be relaxed (see 📖 p. 303).

Record deep tendon results according to the scale in Box 10.5.

Examination

Biceps(C5, C6)

With the patient seated, lay their arms across their abdomen. Place your thumb across the biceps tendon and strike it with the reflex hammer as above. Watch the biceps for contraction.

Supinator (C5, C6)

The muscle tested is actually the brachioradialis. With the patient's arms lying loosely across their abdomen, put your fingers on the radial tuberosity and tap with the hammer. The arm will flex at the elbow. If brisk, the fingers may also flex.

Triceps (C7)

Taking hold of the patient's wrist, flex their arm to ~90°. Tap the triceps tendon about 5 cm superior to the olecranon process of the ulna. Watch the triceps.

Fingers (C8)

This is only present if tone is pathologically ↑. With your palm up and the patient's arm pronated, lay their fingers on yours. Strike the back of your fingers. The patient's fingers will flex.

Knee (L3, L4)

With the patient's leg extended, use one hand behind their knee to lift their leg to ~60°. Tap the patella tendon and watch the quadriceps. If brisk, proceed to testing for clonus here.

Knee clonus

With the patient's leg extended, place your thumb and index finger over the superior edge of the patella. Create a sudden downward (toward the feet) movement and *hold*. Watch the quadriceps. *Any* beat of clonus here is abnormal.

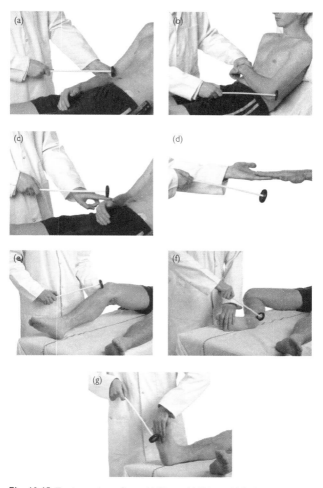

Fig. 10.15 Testing tendon reflexes. (a) Biceps. (b) Triceps. (c) Supinator. (d) Fingers. (e) Knee. (f) Ankle. (g) Alternative method for ankle.

Box 10.5 Recording deep tendon reflexes

These are usually recorded as a list, or often by applying the numbers below to the appropriate area of a stick-man sketch.
- 0 = absent
- ± = present only with reinforcement
- 1+ = less than normal
- 2+ = normal
- 3+ = hyperactive without clonus.
- 4+ = hyperactive with clonus.

Ankle (S1, S2)

With the hip flexed and externally rotated and the knee flexed to ~90°, hold the foot and tap the Achilles tendon. Watch the calf muscles for contraction and ankle flexion.

Alternatively, with the leg extended and relaxed, place your hand on the ball of the foot and strike your hand with the hammer.

Augmentation

If the reflex is absent, it can sometimes be elicited by asking the patient to perform an augmenting action, which acts to increase the activity of neurons in the spinal cord. This effect is short-lived, however, so you should aim to test the reflex in the first 10 seconds of the augmentation.
- For upper limb reflexes, ask the patient to clench their teeth.
- For lower limb reflexes, ask the patient to lock their fingers together, pulling in opposite directions.

Other reflexes

In normal practice, the plantar response is the only one of the following routinely tested.

Abdominal reflex

This test relies on observing the abdominal muscles. It is therefore not easy in those with a covering of fat. It is also less obvious in children, the elderly, multiparous patients, or those who have had abdominal surgery.
- The patient should lie on their back, relaxed, with abdomen exposed.
- Using a tongue depressor or something similar, stroke each of the 4 segments of the abdomen in a brief movement toward the umbilicus.
- As each segment is stroked, the abdominal muscles will reflexively contract.
- Summarize the findings diagrammatically using a simple 2 x 2 grid and indicating the presence or absence of a response by marking "+" and "–", respectively ("9" for an intermediate response).

The upper segments are supplied by T8–T9; the lower, by T10–T11.

Cremasteric reflex (L1, L2)

Given its nature, this reflex is very rarely tested and requires a full expla-nation and consent from the patient first.
- With the male patient standing and naked from the waist down, lightly stroke the upper aspect of their inner thigh.
- The ipsilateral cremaster muscle contracts and the testicle will briefly rise.

Plantar response (L5, S1, S2)

This is sometimes, inappropriately, called the *Babinski reflex*.
- The patient should be lying comfortably, legs outstretched.
- Warn the patient that you are about to touch the sole of their foot (this may prevent a startled withdrawal response).
- Stroke the patient's sole with a tongue depressor or similar disposable item (many people use their fingernail, but this has obvious implications for sterility).
- Stroke from the heel, up the lateral aspect of the sole to the base of the fifth toe (Fig. 10.16). If there is no response, the stroke can be continued along the ball of the foot to the base of the big toe.
- Watch the big toe for its *initial* movement.
  - Normal response is plantar flexion of the big toe.
  - UMN lesions will cause the big toe to dorsiflex. This is the Babinski response.
- Document your findings using arrows:
  - ↓ for plantar flexion
  - ↑ for dorsiflexion
  - – for an absent response
- If the leg is withdrawn and the heel moves in a ticklish reaction, this is called a *withdrawal* response and the test should be repeated.

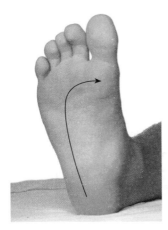

Fig. 10.16 Testing the plantar response. The arrow shows the direction that the stroke should take.

Ankle clonus
A rhythmical contraction of a muscle when suddenly stretched is a sign of hyperreflexia due to a UMN lesion. With the patient lying on the bed, knee straight, and thigh slightly externally rotated, suddenly dorsiflex the foot. More than three beats of clonus—as long as the foot is held dorsiflexed—is abnormal.

Primitive reflexes

These are reflexes seen in the newborn, but they may still be present in a few normal adults. They return somewhat in the elderly but are seen mainly in frontal lobe disease and encephalopathy.

The primitive reflexes are not routinely tested unless the examiner is looking specifically for frontal lobe signs or Parkinson's disease.

Glabellar tap
- Using your index finger, repeatedly tap (gently) the patient's forehead between the eyebrows.
- If normal, the patient will blink only with the first three or four taps.

Palmomental reflex
- Stroke the patient's palm, using sharp, firm pressure from the radial side to the ulnar side.
- Watch the patient's chin.
- If the reflex is present, there will be a contraction of the ipsilateral mentalis seen in the neck and chin.

Grasp reflex
- Gently stroke your fingers over the patient's palm in a radial–ulnar direction, telling the patient *not* to grip your hand.
- If present, the patient will involuntarily grasp your hand and seemingly refuse to let go.

Snout (or pout) reflex
- With the patient's eyes closed, gently tap their lips with your fingers or (very cautiously) with a patellar hammer.
- An involuntary puckering of the lips is a positive reflex.

Suckling reflex
With the patient's eyes closed, gentle stimulation at the corner of their mouth will result in a suckling action at the mouth. The patient's head may also turn toward the stimulus.

Sensory: applied anatomy

The sensory system, like the rest of the nervous system, is vastly complex. The following is a simplified explanation that should provide enough background to make sense of the examination technique and findings.

Spinal roots and dermatomes

At each spinal level, a spinal nerve arises that contains sensory and motor neurons serving a specific segment of the body. The area of skin supplied by the sensory neurons corresponding to each spinal level can be mapped out—each segment is called a *dermatome*. See Figs. 10.18 and 10.19 on 📖 p. 310, 311.

There is considerable overlap such that loss of sensation in just one dermatome is usually not testable (and textbooks show a marked variation in dermatome maps). Health sciences students should become familiar with the dermatomal distribution at an early stage.

Somatic sensory pathways

There are two main spinal pathways for sensory impulses. The clinical importance of these can be seen in spinal cord damage and is summarized on 📖 p. 326.

Posterior columns

These convey light touch, proprioception, and vibration sense, as well as stereognosis (the ability to recognize an object by touch), weight discrimination, and kinesthesia (the perception of movement).

Nerves from receptors extend up the ipsilateral side of the spinal cord to the medulla, their axons forming the posterior columns (fasciculus gracilis and fasciculus cuneatus). The second-order neurons decussate (cross over) at the medulla and travel in the medial lemniscus to the thalamus. From there, the impulse is conveyed to the sensory cortex.

Spinothalamic tract

This carries pain and temperature sensation. From a clinical point of view, the important difference here is that the first-order neurons synapse in the posterior gray horn on joining the spinal cord. The second-order neurons then cross over and ascend the contralateral side of the cord in the spinothalamic tract to the thalamus.

Sensory cortex

This is located at the postcentral gyrus, just posterior to the motor cortex. Much like the motor strip, the areas receiving stimuli from various parts of the body can be mapped out (see Fig. 10.17). A lesion affecting one area will cause sensory loss in the corresponding body area on the contralateral side (see Somatic Sensory Pathways, above).

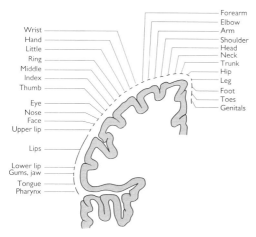

Fig. 10.17 Sensory cortex map showing areas corresponding to the different parts of the body. Note the large areas given over to the fingers and lips.

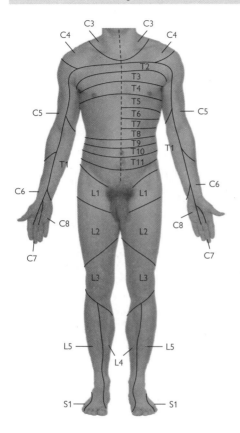

Fig. 10.18 The dermatomes (anterior view). Students should be familiar with these diagrams, particularly the limbs. Note important landmarks to aid recall (C7 covers the middle finger, T4 lies at the level of the nipples, T10 is over the umbilicus).

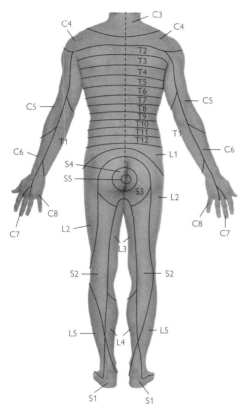

Fig. 10.19 The dermatomes (posterior view).

Sensory examination

This examination can be difficult, as it requires concentration and co-operation on the part of both the patient and the examiner. The results depend on the patient's response and are thus partly subjective. Many patients prove unreliable witnesses from a lack of understanding or attempts to please the examiner. Education, explanation, and reassurance are important at all times.

Often, sensory loss (particularly vibration and temperature) is not noticed by the patient, and revealing them during the course of an examination may be upsetting. Keep this in mind as you proceed.

Technique

The examination should be influenced by the history. In practice, only light touch is tested as a quick screening exam if no deficit is expected.

If you are testing vibration sense and proprioception, it may be best to test these first, as they require the least concentration and can be used to assess the patients' reliability as a witness, before testing the other sensory modalities.

For each modality, begin at any area of supposed deficit and work outward, mapping the affected area, then move to a systematic examination from head to toe. Always test one side, then the other for each limb and body area. Aim to test one spot in each dermatome.

Light touch

With the patient's eyes closed, touch their skin with a wisp of cotton wool and ask them to say "yes" when it is felt. The interval between each touch should be irregular and unpredictable.

- In practice, a gentle touch with a finger is often used. However, this risks testing pressure, not light-touch sensation—it is also harder to ensure that equal force is applied in all areas.
- Do not make tiny stroking movements on the skin—this stimulates hair fibers and is not a test of light touch.
- Be aware of areas where decreased sensation is expected (foot calluses, etc.).
- After testing each limb and body area, double check with the patient: "Did that feel the same all over?" Explore any areas of abnormal sensation more thoroughly before moving on.

Sensory inattention

- This is a subtle but often clinically important sign of parietal lobe dysfunction. The patient feels a stimulus on the affected part, but *not* when there is competition from a stimulus on the opposite side.
- Ask the patient to close their eyes and tell you if they feel a touch on their left or right—use any body part—commonly hands and feet as a quick screen.
- Touch the right hand, then the left hand, then both.
- The touches should be repeated randomly to confirm the result.

- For example, with a right-sided parietal lesion, the patient will feel both left and right stimuli, but when both sides are touched, they will not be able to feel the stimulus on the left.

Vibration sense

A 128 Hz tuning fork (compare with CN VIII) is used.

- Ask the patient to close their eyes, tap the tuning fork, and place the base on a bony prominence. Ask if the patient can feel the *vibration*.
- If yes, then confirm by taking hold of the tuning fork with your other hand to stop the vibration after asking the patient to tell you when the vibration ceases.
- As always, compare left to right and work in a systematic fashion, testing bony prominences:
  - Fingertip, wrist, elbow, shoulder, anterior superior iliac spine, tibial tuberosity, matatarsophalangeal joint, and toes

Proprioception

Testing of proprioception in the manner described below provides a rough gauge, thus results must be interpreted with the rest of the history and examination.

Loss of position sense is usually distal. Start by testing the patient's big toe as follows. This technique can be used at any joint.

- With the patient's eyes closed and leg relaxed, grasp the distal phalanyx of the big toe from the sides.
- While stabilizing the rest of the foot, move toe up and down at joint.
- Ask the patient if they can feel any movement and in which direction.
- Flex and extend the joint, stopping at intervals to ask the patient whether the toe is up or down.
- If proprioception is absent, test other joints, working proximally.
- The toe is gripped from the *sides*—if held incorrectly, pressure on the nail may suggest that the toe is pressed down.
- Normal proprioception should allow the patient to identify very subtle movements that are barely visible.

Box 10.6 Romberg's sign

This is a further test of joint position sense. When proprioception is lost in the limbs, patients can often stand and move normally as long as they can see the limb in question.

🔹Perform with care, only if you are able to safely catch the patient in the event of a fall!

- Ask the patient to stand, and you stand facing them.
- Ask the patient to close their eyes.
- If there is loss of proprioception, the patient will lose their balance and fall. If so, catch them with care, asking them to open their eyes again immediately if they haven't already done so.

Pin-prick

Use a disposable pin or safety pin—not a hypodermic needle, as these break the skin (a line of tiny wounds up a patient's arm or weeping edema up a shin is an infection risk and very embarrassing).

- Test as you would for light touch, gently pressing the pin on the skin.
- Test each dermatome in a systematic way, mapping out abnormalities.
- On each touch, ask the patient to say whether it feels *sharp* or *dull*.
- Occasionally, test the patient's reliability as a witness with a negative control by using the opposite (blunt) end of the pin.

Temperature

- This is not routinely tested outside of specialist clinics. Loss of temperature sensation may be evident from the history (accidental burns?).
- When tested, test tubes or similar vessels containing hot and ice-cold water are used, and each dermatome is tested as with pin-prick.
- Remember to ensure the exterior of the tube is dry.

Coordination

Coordination should be tested in conjunction with gait (📖 p. 321).
Cerebellar lesions cause incoordination on the ipsilateral side (📖 p. 327).
For each of the following, compare performance on the left and right.

Upper limbs

Finger–nose test

- Ask the patient to touch the end of their nose with their index finger.
- Hold your own finger out in front of them—at arm's reach from
  the patient—and ask them to then touch the tip of your finger with
  theirs.
- Ask them to move between their nose and your finger (Fig. 10.20).
- Look for intention tremor (worse as it approaches the target) and
  past-pointing (missing the target entirely).
- The test can be made more difficult by moving the position of your
  finger each time the patient touches their nose.

Rapid alternating movements

- This is hard to describe and should be demonstrated to the patient.
  Ask the patient to repeatedly supinate and pronate their forearm,
  keeping the other arm still such that they clap their hands palm to
  palm, then back to palm, and so on (see Fig. 10.21).
- Alternatively, ask them to mimic screwing in a lightbulb.
  - Slow and clumsy = dysdiadokokinesis
  - ⓘ Dysdiadokokinesis is the *inability* to perform rapidly alternating
    movements (diadoke = Greek for "succession"). It is not, as many
    students think, the actual test.

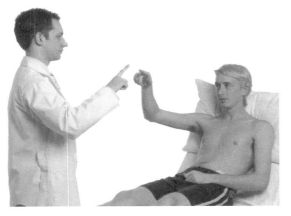

Fig. 10.20 Finger–nose testing.

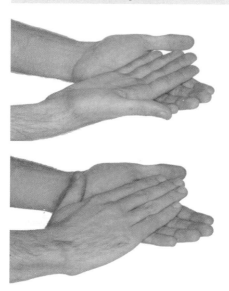

Fig. 10.21 Testing rapidly alternating movements. This can be hard to describe to a patient—a brief demonstration is usually required.

Rebound

- From a resting (arms at their side) position, ask the patient to quickly abduct their arms and stop suddenly at the horizontal level.
  - In cerebellar disease, there will be a delay in stopping and the arm will oscillate about the intended final position.
- Alternatively, pull on the patient's flexed arms (as if testing elbow flexion power) and suddenly let go. If lacking coordination, the patient will hit his- or herself in the face. This test does little for provider–patient trust and is rarely performed for obvious reasons.

Lower limbs

Heel–shin test

- With the patient sitting, legs outstretched, ask them to slide the heel of one foot up and down the shin of the other leg at a moderate pace.
  - A lack of coordination will manifest as the heel moving side to side about the intended path.
  - In sensory, in contrast to cerebellar, ataxia (lack of proprioception), patients will perform worse with their eyes closed.

Foot tapping

- The patient taps your hand with their foot as fast as possible.
  - The nondominant side performs poorly in normal individuals.

Some peripheral nerves

Peripheral nerve lesions may occur in isolation (e.g., trauma, compression, neoplasia) or as part of a wider pathology (e.g., mononeuritis multiplex). The following pages describe the signs associated with lesions of a selection of peripheral nerves.

Upper limb

Median nerve (C6–T1)

- *Motor:* muscles of the anterior forearm, except flexor carpi ulnaris, and LOAF (lateral 2 lumbricals, opponens pollicis, abductor pollicis brevis and flexor pollicis brevis)
- *Sensory:* thumb, anterior index and middle fingers, as well as some of the radial side of the palm (see Fig. 10.22)

Examining a lesion

- Weakness and wasting of the thenar eminence
- With the hand lying flat, palm up, hold your pen above the thumb and ask the patient to move their thumb vertically to touch it (pen-touching test)—they will not be able to.
- Often power is good here despite symptoms and obvious carpel tunnel syndrome.
- For lesions of the nerve at the cubital fossa, perform Ochsner's clasping test for weakness of flexor digitorum superficialis. Ask the patient to clasp their hands together. If a lesion is present, the index finger will fail to flex.

Ulnar nerve (C8–T1)

- *Motor:* all of the small muscles of the hand except LOAF and flexor carpi ulnaris
- *Sensory:* ulnar side of the hand, little finger, and half of ring finger (see Fig. 10.22).

Examining a lesion

- This is hard to test. There may be visible wasting of the small muscles of the hand, with clawing of the fingers (extension at the phalangeometacarpal joints and flexion at the interphalangeal joints).
- Froment's sign: ask the patient to grasp a piece of paper between their thumb and forefinger. Alternatively, ask them to make a fist. The thumb is unable to adduct and so will flex instead (see Fig. 10.23).

Radial nerve (C5–C8)

- *Motor:* triceps, brachioradialis, and extensors of the hand
- *Sensory:* a small area over the anatomical snuffbox—hard to test

Examining a lesion

- Look for wrist drop. If not obvious, ask the patient to flex at the elbow, pronate the forearm, and extend the wrist (you may need to demonstrate). Wrist weakness will become clear. See also Box 10.7 for testing nerve compression.

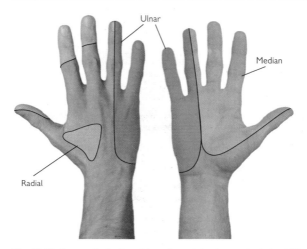

Fig. 10.22 Sensory distribution of the major peripheral nerves in the hand. There is considerable overlap and the small area supplied by the radial nerve may not be detectable clinically.

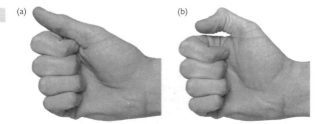

Fig. 10.23 Froment's sign. (a) Normal. (b) Froment's positive.

Box 10.7 Tinel's sign

This is a test for nerve compression. It is commonly used at the wrist to test for median nerve compression in carpal tunnel syndrome.
- Percuss the nerve over the site of possible compression (at the wrist, gently tap centrally near the flexor palmaris tendon).
- If the nerve is compressed, the patient will experience tingling in the distribution of the nerve on each tap.

Lower limb

Lateral cutaneous nerve of the thigh (L2–L3)
- *Motor:* none
- *Sensory:* lateral aspect of the thigh (see Fig. 10.24a)

Examining a lesion
There may be some sensory loss as indicated, but in practice this is very hard to test. Although sensory loss to this nerve is rare, conditions such as meralgia paresthetica can result in a complete or partial loss of sensation in this nerve distribution.

Common peroneal nerve (L4–S2)
- *Motor:* anterior and lateral compartments of the leg
- *Sensory:* dorsum of the foot and anterior aspect of the leg

Examining a lesion
- Foot drop with corresponding gait (📖 p. 321). Weakness of foot dorsiflexion (📖 p. 297) and eversion. Preserved inversion (Fig. 10.24b)
- In an L5 lesion there will be a similar deficit but will also display a weakness of inversion, hip abduction, and knee flexion.

Femoral nerve (L2–L4)
- *Motor:* quadriceps
- *Sensory:* medial aspect of the thigh and leg (see Fig. 10.24d)

Examining a lesion
- Weakness of knee extension is only slightly affected—hip adduction is preserved (📖 p. 356).
- Stretch: With the patient lying prone, abduct the hip, flex the knee and plantar-flex the foot. The stretch test is positive if pain is felt in the thigh/inguinal region.

Sciatic nerve (L4–S3)
- *Motor:* all the muscles below the knee and some hamstrings.
- *Sensory:* posterior thigh, ankle and foot (see Fig. 10.24c).

Examining a lesion
- Foot drop and weak knee flexion (📖 p. 321).
- Knee jerk reflex (📖 p. 302) is preserved but ankle jerk and plantar response (📖 p. 302) are absent.
- Stretch test: with the patient lying supine, hold the ankle and lift the leg, straight, to 90°. Once there, dorsiflex the foot. If positive, pain will be felt at the back of the thigh.

(a)

(b)

(c)

(d)

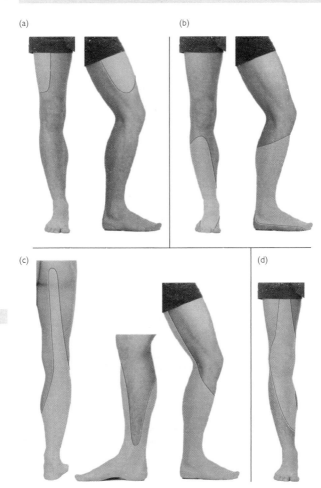

Fig. 10.24 Distribution of the sensory component of some lower limb nerves.
(a) Lateral cutaneous nerve of the thigh. (b) Common peroneal nerve. (c) Sciatic
nerve. (d) Femoral nerve.

Gait

This is easily missed from the neurological examination. Gait is often difficult to test in a crowded ward or cramped exam room. However, you should try to incorporate it into your assessment.

Gait can be observed informally as the patient makes their way to the clinic room or returns to their chair on the ward. Watch the patient stand, and use the same opportunity for Romberg's test (Box 10.6, 📖 p. 313).

The patient may be simply lacking in confidence, and this will be evident later. Do not test if you suspect a severe problem with balance.

Examination

- Ask the patient to walk a few yards, turn, and walk back to you.
- Note especially the following:
  - Use of walking aids
  - Symmetry
  - Length of paces
  - Lateral distance between the feet
  - How high the feet and knees are lifted
  - Bony deformities
  - Disturbance of normal gait by abnormal movements
- You may want to consider asking the patient to
  - Walk on tiptoes (inability = S1 or gastrocnemius lesion)
  - Walk on their heels (inability = L4/L5 lesion—foot drop)

Findings

- **Hemiplegia:** One side will be obviously weaker than the other with the patient tilting the pelvis to lift the weak leg, which may swing out to the side. Gait may be unsafe without the use of walking aid.
- **Scissoring:** If both legs are spastic (cerebral palsy, MS), toes drag on floor, trunk sways from side to side, and legs cross over on each step.
- **Parkinsonism:** flexed posture with small, shuffling steps. No or little arm swing. Difficulty starting, stopping, and turning. Gait seems hurried (festinant) as legs attempt to prevent the body from falling forward.
- **Cerebellar ataxia:** broad-based (legs wide) gait with lumbering body movements and variable distance between steps. The patient has difficulty turning (be there to catch them).
- **Sensory ataxia** (loss of proprioception): The patient requires more sensory input to be sure of leg position so lifts legs high (high-stepping) and stamps the feet down with a wide-based gait. They may also watch their legs as they walk. Romberg's is positive (see Box 10.6, 📖 p. 313).
- **Waddling** (weakness of proximal lower limb muscles): The patient fails to tilt the pelvis as normal and then rotates to compensate, also at the shoulders. You may also see i lumbar lordosis.
- **Foot drop** (L4/L5 lesion, sciatic, or common peroneal nerves): Failure to dorsiflex the foot leads to a high-stepping gait with ↑ flexion at the hip and knee. If bilateral, this may indicate peripheral neuropathy.
- **Apraxic** (usually frontal lobe pathology such as normal pressure hydrocephalus or cerebrovascular disease): Problems with gait occur even if all other movements are normal. The patient may appear

frozen to the spot and be unable to initiate waking. Movements are disjointed once walking.

- *Marche à petits pas* (diffuse cortical dysfunction): There is upright posture and small steps with a normal arm swing.
- *Painful gait:* The cause will normally be obvious from the history. The patient limps with an asymmetrical gait due to painful movement.
- *Functional* (also known as hysterical): Gait problems will be variable and inconsistent, often with bizarre and elaborate consequences. The patient may fall without causing injury. Gait is often worse when watched.

Important presenting patterns

Neck stiffness

This is caused by a number of conditions provoking painful extensor muscle spasm, including bacterial and viral meningitis, subarachnoid hemorrhage, parkinsonism, raised intracranial pressure, cervical spondylosis, cervical lymphadenopathy, and pharyngitis.

   None of the following tests should be conducted if there is suspicion of cervical injury or instability.

Testing stiffness
- Lay the patient flat.
- Taking their head in your hands, gently rotate it to the sides in a "no" movement, feeling for stiffness.
- Lift the head off the bed and watch the hips and knees—the chin should easily touch the chest.

Brudzinski's sign
When the head is flexed by the examiner, the patient briefly flexes at the hips and knees. This is a test for meningeal inflammation.

Kernig's sign
- A further test of meningeal inflammation
- With the patient lying flat, flex their hip and knee, holding the weight of the leg yourself (Fig. 10.25).
- With the hip flexed to 90°, extend the knee joint so as to point the leg at the ceiling.
- If positive, there will be resistance to leg-straightening (caused by hamstring spasm as a result of inflammation around the lumbar spinal roots) and pain felt at the back of the neck.

Lhermitte's phenomenon
- A test for intrinsic lesion in the cervical cord (not meningeal irritation)
- When the neck is flexed as for testing stiffness, the patient feels an electric shock–like sensation down the center of their back.

Upper motor and lower motor nerve lesions

Upper motor neuron (UMN) lesions
These are defined as damage above the level of the anterior horn cell—anywhere from the spinal cord to the primary motor cortex.
- No muscle wasting (although patients will have disuse atrophy in long-term weakness)
- ↑Tone. Spasticity (clasp-knife) due to stretch reflex hypersensitivity
- The typical pattern of weakness (Box 10.8) is termed *pyramidal:*
  - Upper limbs: weak abductors and extensors
  - Lower limbs: weak adductors and flexors
- ↑Tendon reflexes and clonus. Up-going plantar response

(a)

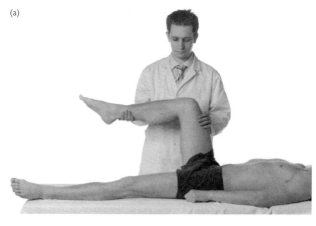

(b)

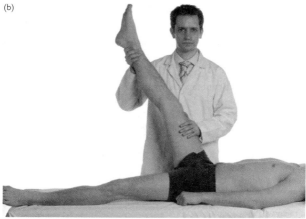

Fig. 10.25 Testing for Kernig's sign. The patient's leg is flexed at the hip and knee, then extended at the knee as above. If positive, there is resistance to knee extension in this position and pain is felt at the back of the neck.

Box 10.8 Some definitions of weakness

- *Monoplegia:* one limb affected
- *Hemiplegia:* one side of the body (left or right).
- *Paraplegia:* both lower limbs affected.
- *Quadriplegia:* all 4 limbs

Lower motor neuron (LMN) lesions

- Muscle wasting. Fasciculation
- Diminished tone
- Flaccid weakness
- Diminished deep tendon reflexes. Plantar response may be down-going or absent.

Motor neuron disease (MND)

There is damage to anterior horn cells, medulla, and spinal tracts.

- UMN and LMN pattern of weakness
- Fasciculations almost always present
- Reflexes normal or i until later in the disease
- Plantar response is up-going
- External ocular muscles almost never involved
- No sensory disturbance (distinguishing presentation from a polyneuropathy)

Parkinsonism

This is a pattern of symptoms comprising an akinetic-rigid syndrome. Parkinsonism has a number of causes, including drug-induced and other intracranial pathologies. Diagnosis of Parkinson's disease (loss of dopaminergic neurons in the subtantia nigra) is often inaccurate; there is no single test.

- Triad of resting tremor, bradykinesia, and rigidity
- *Face:* mask-like and expressionless facies, little blinking, positive glabellar tap reflex (📖 p. 307)
- *Gait:* flexed posture with ↓ arm swing. Gait is *festinant*, meaning hurried, often in small, shuffling steps, with feet barely lifted off the ground. The patient is slow to start and has difficulty stopping.
- *Tone:* ↑ tone with cogwheel or lead-pipe rigidity (📖 p. 297).
- *Tremor:* pill-rolling flexion at the thumb and forefinger at 4–8 Hz
- *Speech:* extrapyramidal dysarthria; soft, quiet, and hesitant speech. You may have to wait some time for the answer to a question.
- *Writing:* writing is small and neat—micrographia.

Abnormal movements defined

- *Akathisia:* motor restlessness with a feeling of muscle quivering and an inability to remain in a sitting position
- *Athetosis:* slow, writhing involuntary movements, often with flexion, extension, pronation, and supination of the fingers and wrists
- *Blepharospasm:* intermittent spasm of muscles around the eyes
- *Chorea:* nonrhythmical, dance-like, spasmodic movements of the limbs or face. Movements appear pseudopurposeful (the patient often hides

the condition by turning a spasm into a voluntary movement—e.g., the arm suddenly lifts up and the patient pretends they were adjusting their hair).

- *Dyskinesia:* repetitive, automatic movements that stop only during sleep
- *Tardive dyskinesia:* dyskinetic movements, often of the face (lip-smacking, twisting of the mouth). This is often a permanent side effect of neuroleptic therapy.
- *Dystonia:* markedly ↑ tone, often with spasms causing uncomfortable-looking postures
- *Hemiballismus:* violent involuntary flinging movements of the limbs on one side, like severe chorea
- *Myoclonus:* brief, shock-like movement of a muscle or muscle group
- *Pseudoathetosis:* writhing limb movements (often finger or arm) much like athetosis but caused by a loss of proprioception. The arm returns to the normal position when the patient notices it straying.
- *Myokymia:* continuous quivering and rippling movements of muscles at rest, like a bag of worms. Facial myokymia occurs especially near the eyes.
- *Tic:* repetitive, active, habitual, purposeful contractions causing stereotyped actions. It can be suppressed for brief periods, with effort.
- *Titubation:* rhythmical contraction of the head. There may be either yes–yes or no–no movements.
- *Tremor:* repetitive, alternating movements, usually involuntary

Spinal cord lesions

As neurons in some spinal cord tracts relate to the contralateral side of the body, others the ipsilateral side, certain types of spinal cord damage will give predictable patterns of motor and sensory loss.

Complete section of the cord

There is loss of all modalities below the level of the lesion.

Hemisection of the cord

This is also known as Brown-Sequard syndrome.*

- *Motor:* below the level of the lesion, UMN pattern of weakness on ipsilateral side
- *Sensory:* below the level of the lesion:
  - Contralateral loss of pain and temperature sensation
  - Ipsilateral loss of light touch, vibration sense, and proprioception
  - Light touch may remain intact, as some fibers travel in the spinothalamic tract.

Posterior column loss

There is loss of vibration sense and proprioception on both sides below the level of the lesion.

---

* Charles Edward Brown-Sequard discovered this while studying victims of failed murder attempts among traditional cane cutters in Mauritius.

Subacute combined degeneration of the cord
Posterolateral column syndrome is often due to vitamin B$_{12}$ deficiency.
- Loss of vibration sense and proprioception on both sides below the level of the lesion
- UMN weakness in lower limbs, *absent* ankle reflexes
- Also peripheral sensory neuropathy, optic atrophy, and dementia

Anterior spinal artery occlusion
- Loss of pin-prick and temperature sensation below the lesion
- Intact light-touch, vibration sense, and proprioception

Central lesions
These include syringomyelia—longitudinal cavities in the central part of the spinal cord and brainstem.
- Loss of pain and temperature sensation over the neck, shoulders, and arms in a 'cape' distribution.
- Intact vibration sense, proprioception, and light touch.
- Atrophy and areflexia in the arms.
- UMN weakness in the lower limbs.
- Look also for scoliosis due to weakness of paravertebral muscles.

Cerebellar lesions
Signs are *ipsilateral* to the lesion and may include the following:
- Nystagmus (p. 276)
- Speech is staccato, scanning (p. 260).
- Diminished tone, drift and tremor in limbs (upper especially, p. 256)
- Finger–nose testing (p. 315) may reveal intention tremor and past-pointing.
- Dysdiadokokinesis (p. 315)
- Rebound (p. 316)
- Pendular jerks—best seen in knee. Test tendon reflex at knee as normal. If pendular, the extensor response will continue to several beats.
- Poor sitting balance
- Ataxic gait

Disturbance of higher functions
This includes a selection of testable consequences of cortical lesions.

Parietal lobe
- Sensory and visual inattention (p. 312 and p. 265).
- Visual field defects (p. 264).
- *Gerstmann's syndrome:* right–left dissociation, finger agnosia, dysgraphia (writing defect), dyscalculia (test with serial 7s; instruct the patient to count backwards from 100 in increments of seven. For instance 100, 93, 86 ect.).

Agnosias (lack of sensory perceptual abilities)
- *Hemi-neglect*—patient ignores one side of their body
- *Asomatagnosia*—patient fails to recognize own body part
- *Anosagnosia*—patient is unaware of neurological deficits
- *Finger agnosia*—patient is unable to show you different fingers when requested (e.g., "show me your index finger")

- *Astereognosis*—inability to recognize an object by touch alone
- *Agraphaesthesia*—inability to recognize letters or numbers when traced on the back of the hand
- *Prosopagnosia*—inability to recognize faces (test with faces of family members or famous faces from a nearby magazine)

Apraxias (inability to perform movements or use objects correctly)
- *Ideational apraxia*—unable to perform task but understands what is required
- *Ideomotor apraxia*—performs task but makes mistakes (e.g., puts tea into kettle and pours milk into cup)
- *Dressing apraxia*—inability to dress correctly (test with a dressing gown). This is one of a number of apraxias named after the action tested.

Temporal lobe
- Memory loss—confabulation (invented stories and details)

Frontal lobe
- Primitive reflexes
- Concrete thinking (unable to explain proverbs—e.g., ask to explain what "a bird in the hand is worth two in the bush" means)
- Loss of smell sensation
- Gait apraxia (□ p. 321)

Myopathies

Muscle disease causes a weakness similar to that of LMN lesions with no sensory loss. Tendon reflexes are reduced or absent. The causes and types are numerous.

Myotonias

These are characterized by continued, involuntary muscle contraction after voluntary effort has ceased.

Myotonic dystrophy

This is a defect of skeletal muscle Cl⁻ channels caused by a trinucleotide repeat, usually. It becomes evident at age 20–50.
- Distal limb weakness
- Weak sternomastoids (evident by weakness of neck flexion with normal power on neck extension)
- Weak facial muscles (expressionless face)
- Test by shaking the patient's hand—they may be unable to let go.
- It is also associated with frontal baldness, cataracts (look for thick glasses), mild intellectual impairment, cardiomyopathy, hypogonadism, and glucose intolerance.

Percussion myotonia
- Tap the patient's thenar eminence. This will cause contraction and very slow relaxation of abductor pollicis brevis.

Myasthenia gravis

This is an autoimmune disease with antibodies against acetylcholine receptors.

- Complex palsies, including extraocular muscles. Weakness is proximal and often includes the eyelids (ptosis) and muscles of mastication.
- Weakness increases with use. Patients report ↑ severity of symptoms at the end of the day.
- In the early stages, patients will feel tired as they expend extra energy in performing routine tasks. Friends may notice ptosis (see Fig. 10.25).

Test for fatiguability:

- Ask the patient to look to the ceiling and hold the position. Watch for ptosis.
- Ask the patient to hold their arms above their head, or out to the sides—watch for ↑ weakness.

Some characteristic headaches summarized

Tension headache

- Bilateral—frontal, temporal
- Sensation of tightness radiating to neck and shoulders
- Can last for days
- No associated symptoms

Subarachnoid hemorrhage

- Sudden, dramatic onset like being hit with a brick
- Occipital initially—may become generalized
- Associated with neck stiffness and sometimes photophobia

Sinusitis

- Frontal, felt behind the eyes or over the cheeks
- Ethmoid sinusitis is felt deep behind the nose.
- Overlying skin may be tender.
- Worse on bending forward
- Lasts 1–2 weeks. Associated with coryza

Temporal (giant cell) arteritis

- Diffuse, spreading from the temple—unilateral
- Tender overlying temporal artery (painful brushing hair)
- Jaw claudication while eating
- Blurred vision—can lead to loss of vision if severe and untreated

Meningitis

- Generalized
- Associated with neck stiffness and signs of meningism (p. 323)
- Nausea, vomiting, photophobia
- Purpuric rash is caused by septicemia, not meningitis per se.

Cluster headache

- Rapid onset, usually felt over one eye
- Associated with a bloodshot, watering eye and facial flushing
- May also have rhinorrhea (runny nose)
- Last for a few weeks at a time

Raised intracranial pressure

- Generalized headache, worse when lying down, straining, coughing, on exertion or in the morning

- Headache may wake the patient in the early hours.
- It may be associated with drowsiness, vomiting, and focal neurology.

Migraine
- Unilateral—rarely crosses the midline*
- Throbbing and pounding headache
- Associated with photophobia, nausea, vomiting, and neck stiffness
- May have preceding aura

* Hence the name. *Migraine* is a shortened version of *hemicranium* (say the second and third syllables out loud), meaning "half the head."

The unconscious patient

History
- Is there an eyewitness account? State of clothing—loss of continence?
- Look for alert necklace or bracelet. Look in patient's wallet or purse.

Examination

ABC (Airway, Breathing, Circulation)
- Is the airway patent? Should the patient be in the recovery position?
- Measure the respiratory rate, note pattern of breathing. Is O_2 needed?
- Is there cyanosis? Feel the pulse. Listen to the chest. Measure heart rate and blood pressure (BP).

Skin
- Look for injury, petechial hemorrhage, and evidence of intravenous (IV) drug use.

Movements and posture
- Watch! Is the patient still or moving? Are all four limbs moving equally?
- Are there any abnormal movements—fitting, myoclonic jerks?
- Test tone and compare both sides.
- Squeeze the nail bed to test the response to pain (all four limbs).
- Test tendon reflexes and plantar response.
- *Decorticate posture* (lesion above the brainstem): flexion and internal rotation of the arms, extension of the lower limbs
- *Decerebrate posture* (lesion in the midbrain): extension at the elbow, pronation of the forearm, and extension at the wrist. Lower limbs are extended.

Consciousness
- Attempt to wake the patient by sound. Ask them their name. If responsive, are they able to articulate appropriately? Note the best response. Be aware of possible dysphasia or aphasia that may cause an inappropriate response in an otherwise alert individual.
  - Score level of consciousness according to GCS (Box 10.9).

Neck
- Do not examine the neck if there may have been trauma. Test for meningeal irritation (📖 p. 323)—these signs ↓ as coma deepens.

Head
- Inspect for signs of trauma and facial weakness. Test pain sense.
  - Battle's sign: bruising behind the ear = a base of skull fracture.

Ears and nose
- Look for CSF leakage or bleeding. Test any clear fluid for glucose (positive result = CSF). Inspect eardrums.

Tongue and mouth
- Look for cuts on the tongue (seizures) and corrosive material around the mouth. Smell breath for alcohol or ketosis. Test the gag reflex; it is absent in brainstem disease or deep coma.

Eyes
- Pupils: measure size in mm. Are they equal (📖 p. 273)? Test direct and consensual light responses. Pupils ↑ with atropine, tricyclic antidepressants, and amphetamine; ↓ with morphine and metabolic coma.
- Test corneal reflex.
- Fundi: look especially for papilledema and retinopathy.
- Doll's head maneuver: take the patient's head in your hands and turn it from side to side. The eyes should move to stay fixed on an object; this indicates an intact brainstem.

Box 10.9 Glasgow Coma Scale (GCS)

This is an objective score of consciousness. Repeated testing is useful for judging whether coma is deepening or lifting. There are three categories. Note that the lowest score in each category is 1, meaning that the lowest possible GCS = 3 (even if the patient is dead).

Eye opening (max 4 points)

Spontaneously open	4
Open to (any) verbal stimulus	3
Open in response to painful stimulus	2
No eye opening at all	1

Best verbal response (max 5 points)

Conversing and orientated (normal)	5
Conversing but disorientated and confused	4
Inappropriate words (random words, no conversation)	3
Incomprehensible sounds (moaning, etc.)	2
No speech at all	1

Best motor response (max 6 points)

Obeying commands (e.g., "raise your hand")	6
Localizing to pain (moves hand toward site of stimulus)	5
Withdraws to pain (pulls hand away from stimulus)	4
Abnormal flexion to pain (decorticate posturing)	3
Abnormal extension to pain (decerebrate posturing)	2
No response at all	1

Box 10.10 AVPU

This is a more simplified score used in rapid assessment of consciousness and by nonspecialist nurses in monitoring consciousness level.

A = Alert
V = responds to **V**oice
P = responds to **P**ain
U = Unresponsive

Rest of the body

- Brief but thorough exam. Look especially for trauma, fractures, signs of liver disease (📖 p. 246), and added heart sounds.

Other bedside tests

- Test urine, capillary glucose, and temperature.

The elderly patient

Diagnosing and managing neurological illness can be complex; the combination of cognitive failure and the effects of an aging neurological system can present additional significant challenges for clinicians.

Presentations of neurological disease are varied, and the range of diagnoses diverse. Epilepsy, Parkinsonism, and dementia are all common problems in older age, so resist the temptation to restrict your diagnoses to stroke or TIA.

History

Witness histories

These are vital. Many patients may attend with vague symptoms that may be underplayed. Partial complex seizures may be very difficult to diagnose, so pursue witness histories from families, neighbors, and home care staff, etc. Inquire not just about the present incident but also prior function and any decline.

Drug history

Falls are a common presentation and often multifactorial. Always remember to ask about any drugs that may lower blood pressure, even if the primary cause of the fall is due to neurological disease.

Intercurrent illness

This may precipitate further seizures or make pre-existing neurological signs seem worse. Don't rush to diagnose a worsening of the original problem—careful assessment pays dividends.

Cognition and mood disorders

These often complicate presentations. Look for clues in the history, and ask witnesses.

Functional history

This is a key part of the neurological history. The disease itself may be incurable—functional problems often are not.

Examination

Observe

Nonverbal clues may point to mood or cognitive disorders. Handshakes and facial expressions are an important part of the examination

Think

Think about patterns of illness and attempt to identify if there are single or multiple lesions. There may often be more than one diagnosis—e.g., cerebrovascular disease and peripheral neuropathy due to diabetes.

Assess cognition

Use a scale that you are comfortable with, such as the Abbreviated Mental Test Score (AMTS, p. 262; Mini-Mental State Examination [MMSE]), but remember, no half marks!

Gait

Even simple observation of a patient's walking can reap rewards. Always include it in your examination where practicable and note why, if unable.

Therapy colleagues

Sharing observations is a useful practice. Therapists are a huge source of knowledge and experience, so seek them out to learn from them.

Additional points

Communicating diagnoses

Many diagnoses—e.g., dementia and motor neuron disease—can be devastating, so be thoughtful in your approach. Clarify what the patient knows and what has already been said. Learn first from your senior colleagues how to explain the diagnosis and, more importantly, talk about its impact. It is also vital to reassure patients—many with benign essential tremors are terrified that they may have Parkinson's disease

Managing uncertainty

Many diagnoses are not clear, especially in the early stages of diseases. Try to resist labeling your patients when a diagnosis is unclear; be open about uncertainty—patients often cope with it better than their doctors.

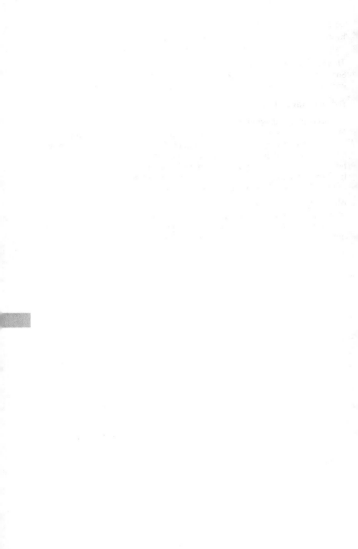

Musculoskeletal system

The hand examination is described in Chapter 3, 🕮 p. 62

Applied anatomy and physiology

The joint

A *joint* (articulation) is a connection or point of contact between bones or between bone and cartilage.

Joints are classified according to the type of material uniting the articulating bones as well as the degree of movement they allow. There are three types:

- **Fibrous joints:** held together by fibrous (collagenous) connective tissue and are fixed or immoveable. They do not have a joint cavity. Examples include the connections of the skull bones.
- **Cartilagenous joints:** held together by cartilage, are slightly moveable and have no cavity. An example is the vertebral joints.
- **Synovial joints:** covered by cartilage with a synovial membrane enclosing a joint cavity. These joints are freely moveable and the most common type of joint functionally, being typical of nearly all joints of the limbs.

Synovial joints

Articular cartilage covers the surface of the bones and ↓ friction at the joint and facilitates shock absorption. A sleeve-like bag (fibrous capsule lined with a synovial membrane) surrounds the synovial joint (Fig. 11.1).

The inner synovial membrane secretes synovial fluid, which has a number of functions, including lubrication and supply of nutrients to the cartilage. The fluid contains phagocytic cells that remove microbes and debris within the joint cavity.

Synovial joints are usually supported by accessory ligaments and muscle. There are different types of synovial joints. Some of the more important types are as follows:

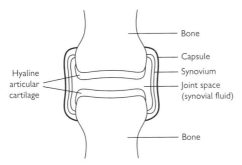

Fig. 11.1 Diagram of cross-section through a typical synovial joint.

- *Hinge:* movement occurs primarily in a single plane (e.g., elbow, knee, and interphalangeal joints) (see Box 11.1).
- *Ball and socket:* allows movement around three axes (flexion/extension, abduction/adduction, and rotation). Examples are the shoulder and hip.
- *Pivot:* a ring of bone and ligament surrounds the surface of the other bone, allowing rotation only (e.g., atlantoaxial joint at C1 and C2 vertebrae and the connection between the radius and ulna).
- *Gliding:* flat bone surfaces allow side-to-side and backward and forward movements (e.g., between carpals, tarsals, sternum and clavicle and the scapula and clavicle).
- *Saddle:* similar to a hinge joint but with a degree of movement in a second plane (e.g., base of thumb).

Box 11.1 Some movements at synovial joints

Angular movements
- *Flexion:* a decrease in angle between the articulating bones (e.g., bending the elbow = elbow flexion)
- *Extension:* an increase in angle between the articulating bones (e.g., straightening the elbow = elbow extension)
- *Abduction:* movement of a bone away from the midline (e.g., moving the arm out to the side = shoulder abduction)
- *Adduction:* movement of a bone toward the midline (e.g., bringing the arm in to the side of the body = shoulder adduction)

Rotation
This involves movement of a bone about its longitudinal axis.
- *Internal or medial rotation:* rotating a bone toward the midline (e.g., turning the lower limb such that the toes point inward = internal rotation at the hip)
- *External or lateral rotation:* rotating a bone away from the midline (e.g., turning the lower limb such that the toes point outward = external rotation at the hip)

Special movements
These occur at specific joints only.
- *Pronation:* moving the forearm as if turning a doorknob counterclockwise (internal rotation of the forearm in anatomical position)
- *Supination:* moving the forearm as if turning a doorknob clockwise (external rotation of the forearm in anatomical position)
- *Dorsiflexion:* moving the ankle to bring the dorsum of the foot toward the tibia
- *Plantar flexion:* moving the ankle to bring the plantar surface in line with the tibia (e.g., pointing toes or depressing a pedal)
- *Inversion:* tilting soles of the feet inward to face each other
- *Eversion:* tilting soles of the feet outward away from each other
- *Protraction:* moving the mandible forward
- *Retraction:* moving the mandible backward.

Important locomotor musculoskeletal symptoms

As with any system, but especially the musculoskeletal system, a carefully and accurately compiled history can be very informative and may point to a diagnosis even before examination or laboratory tests.

Pain

Pain is the most common symptom with problems of the musculoskeletal system and should be approached in the same way as any other type of pain (☐ p. 33). Determine its character, nature of onset, site, radiation, severity, periodicity, exacerbating and relieving factors (particularly how it is influenced by rest and activity), and diurnal variation.

- Pain in a joint is called *arthralgia*.
- Pain in a muscle is called *myalgia*.

Character

- Bone pain is typically experienced as boring and penetrating and is often worse at night. Causes include tumor, chronic infection, avascular necrosis, and osteoid osteoma.
- Pain associated with a fracture is usually sharp and stabbing and is often exacerbated by movement.
- Shooting pain is suggestive of nerve entrapment (e.g., disc protrusion).

Onset

- Acute onset of pain is often a manifestation of infection, such as septic arthritis or crystal arthropathies (e.g., gout).
- Osteoarthritis and rheumatoid arthritis (RA) can cause chronic pain.

Site

Determine the exact site of maximal pain, if possible, and any associated lesser pains. Remember that the site of pain is not necessarily the site of pathology; often pain is referred. Referred pain is due to the inability of the cerebral cortex to distinguish between sensory messages from embryologically related sites. See Boxes 11.2 and 11.3.

Box 11.2 Some causes of knee arthralgia

Chondromalacia patellae
This is from softening of the patellar articular cartilage and is felt as a patellar ache after prolonged sitting. It is usually seen in young people.

Osteochondritis dissecans
This is usually associated with trauma resulting in osteochondral fracture that forms a loose body in the joint, with underlying necrosis.

Osgood–Schlatter's disease
This arises as a result of a traction injury of the tibial epiphysis, which is classically associated with a lump over the tibia.

Box 11.3 Some causes of arthralgia in adults

Knee
- Osteoarthritis
- Referred from the hip
- Chondromalacia patellae
- Trauma
- Osteochondritis dissecans
- Bursitis
- Tendonitis
- Osgood–Schlatter's disease
- Rheumatoid arthritis
- Infection
- Malignancy

Hip
- Osteoarthritis
- Referred pain—e.g., from a lumber spine abnormality
- Trauma
- Rheumatoid arthritis
- Infection
- Hernia
- Tendonitis
- Bursitis

Shoulder
- Rotator cuff disorders (e.g., tendonitis, rupture, adhesivecapsulitis or frozen shoulder)
- Referred pain—e.g., cervical, mediastinal, cardiac
- Arthritis—glenohumeral, acromioclavicular

Elbow
- Lateral epicondylitis (tennis elbow)
- Medial epicondylitis (golfer's elbow)
- Olecranon bursitis
- Referred pain from neck or shoulder (e.g., cervical spondylosis)
- Osteoarthritis
- Rheumatoid arthritis

Mechanical or degenerative back pain
- Arthritis
- Trauma
- Disc prolapse
- Osteoporosis
- Infection
- Ankylosing spondylitis
- Spondylolisthesis
- Lumbar spinal or lateral recess stenosis
- Spinal tumors—especially metastases from the lung, breast, prostate, thyroid, and kidney
- Metabolic bone disease

Stiffness

This is a subjective symptom that must be explored in detail to establish exactly what the patient means.

Stiffness is the inability to move the joints after a period of rest. It may be due to mechanical dysfunction, local inflammation of a joint, or a combination of both.

▶ If stiffness predominates over pain, consider spasticity or tetany. Look for hypertonia and other upper motor neuron signs (📖 p. 297).

Ask the patient the following:
- When is the stiffness worst?
  - Early-morning stiffness is seen in inflammatory conditions (e.g., rheumatoid arthritis), whereas mechanical joint disease will become worse as the day progresses.
- Which joints are involved? Or is the stiffness generalized?
  - A generalized stiffness may be seen in rheumatoid arthritis and ankylosing spondylitis.
- How long does it take the patient to get going in the morning?
- How is the stiffness related to rest and activity?
  - Mechanical joint diseases will be exacerbated by prolonged activity.

Locking

This is the sudden inability to complete a certain movement and suggests a mechanical block or obstruction, usually caused by a loose body or torn cartilage within the joint (often secondary to trauma).

Swelling

Joint swelling can be due to a variety of factors, including inflammation of the synovial lining, an increase in volume of synovial fluid, hypertrophy of bone, or swelling of structures surrounding the joint.

This symptom is particularly significant in the presence of joint pain and stiffness. Establish the following:
- Which joints are affected (small or large)?
- Is the distribution symmetrical or not?
- What was the nature of onset of the swelling?
  - Rapid onset: hematoma or hemarthrosis (exacerbated by anticoagulants or any underlying bleeding disorder)
  - Slow onset is suggestive of a joint effusion.
- Are the joints always swollen or does it come and go (and when)?
- Is there any associated pain?
- Do the joints feel hot to touch?
- Is there erythema? (This is common in infective, traumatic, and crystal arthropathies.)
- Have the joints in question sustained any injuries?

Deformity

Establish the following:
- Time frame over which the deformity has developed
- Any associated symptoms, such as pain and swelling
- Any resultant loss of function? (What is the patient now unable to do with the joint in question?)

Acute deformity may arise with a fracture or dislocation. Chronic deformity is more typical of bone malalignment and may be partial/subluxed or complete/dislocated. Some common deformities are discussed later in this chapter (see also Box 11.4).

Weakness

Always inquire about the presence of localized or generalized weakness, which suggests a peripheral nerve lesion or systemic cause, respectively.

Consider that the weakness may be neurogenic or myopathic in origin.

Sensory disturbance

Ask about the exact distribution of any numbness or paraesthesia and document any exacerbating and relieving factors.

Loss of function

Loss of function is the inability to perform an action (disability) and is distinguished from the term *handicap*, which is the social and functional result or impact that disability has on the individual's life.

Loss of function can be caused by a combination of muscle weakness, pain, mechanical factors, and damage to the nerve supply.

The questions you ask will depend partly on the patient's occupation. It is also essential to gain some insight into the patient's mobility: Can they use stairs? How do they cope with personal care such as feeding, washing and dressing? Can they manage shopping and cooking?

Extra-articular features

Several musculoskeletal disorders (e.g., rheumatoid arthritis) cause extra-articular or multisystem features, some of which are outlined below:

- Systemic symptoms: fever, weight loss, fatigue, lethargy
- Skin rash
- Raynaud's phenomenon
- Gastrointestinal (e.g., diarrhea and resultant reactive arthritis or enteropathic arthritis secondary to inflammatory bowel disease)
- Urethritis (Reiter's syndrome)
- Eye symptoms
- Cardiorespiratory: breathlessness (pulmonary fibrosis?), pericardial and pleuritic chest pain, aortic regurgitation, and spondyloarthropathies.
- Neurological: nerve entrapment, migraine, depression, stroke

Box 11.4 Some terminology of joint deformity

Valgus

The bone or part of limb distal to the joint is deviated laterally. For example, a valgus deformity at the knees would give "knock knees" that tend to meet in the middle, despite the feet being apart.

Varus

Here, the bone or part of limb distal to the joint is deviated medially. For example, a varus deformity at the knees would give "bow legs" with a gap between the knees, even if the feet are together.

The rest of the history

Past medical history
Ask about all previous medical and surgical disorders and inquire specifically about any previous history of trauma or musculoskeletal disease.

Family history
It is important to note any FH of illness, especially those musculoskeletal conditions with a heritable element:
• Osteoarthritis
• Rheumatoid arthritis
• Osteoporosis
Note that the seronegative spondyloarthropathies (e.g., ankylosing spondylosis) are more prevalent in patients with the HLA B27 haplotype.

Drug history
Take a full drug history, including all prescribed and over-the-counter medications. Assess the efficacy of each treatment, past and present.
Ask about side effects of any drugs taken for musculoskeletal disease:
• Gastric upset associated with nonsteroidal anti-inflammatory drugs (NSAIDs)
• Long-term side effects of steroid therapy, such as osteoporosis, myopathy, infections, and avascular necrosis
Ask also about medication with known adverse musculoskeletal effects:
• Statins: myalgia, myosistis, and myopathy
• ACE inhibitors: myalgia
• Anticonvulsants: osteomalacia
• Quinolone: tendinopathy
• Diuretics, aspirin, alcohol: gout
• Procainamide, hydralazine, isoniazid: systemic lupus erythematosus (SLE)
▶ Bear in mind that illicit drugs may increase the risk of developing infectious diseases, such as TB, HIV, and hepatitis, all of which can cause musculoskeletal complaints.

Smoking and alcohol
As always, full smoking and alcohol histories should be taken (📖 p. 37 and 38).

Social history
This should form a natural extension of the functional inquiry and include a record of the patient's occupation if not already noted and ethnicity.
• *Certain occupations* predispose to specific musculoskeletal problems—e.g., repetitive strain injury, hand-vibration syndrome, and fatigue fractures seen sometimes in dancers and athletes.
• *Ethnicity* is relevant, as there is an overrepresentation of lupus and TB in Asian populations. Both of these disorders are linked to a variety of musculoskeletal complaints.

- If the patient is an older person, make a note about the activities of daily living (ADL), how mobile the patient is, and if there are any home adaptations, such as a chair lift or railings.
- Remember to ask about home care or other supports.
- Where appropriate, take a sexual history. This is important because reactive arthritis or Reiter's syndrome may be caused by sexually transmitted diseases, such as chlamydia and gonorrhea.

The outline examination

A full examination of the entire musculoskeletal system can be long and complicated (but see Box 11.5 for framework). In this chapter, we have broken down the examination into the following joints and regions: elbow, shoulder, spine, hip, knee, ankle, and foot.

> **Box 11.5 Examination framework**
>
> Examination of each joint should follow the standard format:
> - Look
> - Feel
> - Move*
>   - Passive
>   - Active
> - Measure
> - Special tests
> - Function
>
> ▶ In a thorough locomotor examination, examine the joints above and below the symptomatic one. For example, for an elbow complaint, also examine the shoulder and wrist.
>
> * Limitation of active movement reflects underlying pathology of the tendons and muscle surrounding the joint, but limitation of both active and passive movement suggests an intrinsic joint problem.

▶ The hand examination is discussed in Chapter 3, 📖 p. 62.

GALS screen

The overall integrity of the musculoskeletal system can be screened very quickly by using the GALS method of assessment.

You may use this method to make a quick, screening examination of the whole musculoskeletal system in order to identify the joints or regions that need to be examined in more detail (see also Box 11.6).

The GALS screen consists of four components:

- **G** = gait
- **A** = arms
- **L** = legs
- **S** = spine

Box 11.6 Modified GALS screen

The GALS screen was originally devised as a quick screen for abnormality without symptoms. Our slightly modified version follows:

Gait

- Watch the patient walk.
  - There should be symmetry and smoothness of movement and arm swing with no pelvic tilt and with normal stride length. The patient should be able to start, stop, and turn quickly.

Arms (sitting on couch)

- *Inspection:* Look for muscle wasting and joint deformity at the shoulders, elbows, wrists, and fingers. Squeeze across the second to fifth metacarpals—there should be no tenderness.
- *Shoulder abduction:* Ask the patient to raise their arms out sideways, above their head. Normal range is 170–180°.
- *Shoulder external rotation:* Ask the patient to touch their back between their shoulder blades.
- *Shoulder internal rotation:* Ask the patient to touch the small of their back. They should touch above T10.
- *Elbow extension:* Ask patient to straighten out arms. Normal is 0°.
- *Wrist and finger extension:* the prayer sign (📖 p. 65).
- *Wrist flexion and finger extension:* reverse prayer sign (📖 p. 65).
- *Power grip:* Ask patient to make a tight fist, hiding fingernails.
- *Precision grip:* Ask patient to put their fingertips on their thumb.

Legs (lying on couch)

- *Inspection:* Look for swelling or deformity at the knee, ankle, and foot, as well as quadriceps muscle wasting. Squeeze across the metatarsals—there should be no tenderness.
- *Hip and knee flexion:* Test passively and actively. Normal hipflexion is 120°, normal knee flexion is 135°.
- *Hip internal rotation:* Normal is 90° at 45° flexion. See 📖 p. 356.
- *Knee:* bulge test (📖 p. 358) and patellar tap (📖 p. 358)
- *Ankle:* Test dorsiflexion (normal 15°) and planarflexion (normal 55°).

Box 11.6 (Cont'd.)

Spine (standing)
- *Inspection from behind:* Look for scoliosis, muscle bulk at the paraspinals, shoulders, and gluteals, and level iliac crests.
- *Inspection from the side:* Look for normal thoracic kyphosis and lumbar and cervical lordosis.
- *Tenderness:* Feel over the mid-supraspinatus—there should be no tenderness.
- *Lumbar flexion:* Ask patient to touch their toes. Normal is finger-floor distance <15 cm. Lumbar expansion (Schober's test 📖 p. 355)
- *Cervical lateral flexion:* Ask the patient to put their ear on their shoulder.

Republished with permission from Doherty et al. (1992). Ann Rheum Dis 51:1165–1169.

Elbow

Look

Look around the bed for any mobility aids or other clues. Ask the patient to stand. Make sure both upper limbs are exposed and look at the patient from top to toe.

Inspect the elbow joint from the front, side, and behind, noting:
- Malalignment of the bones
- Scars
- Skin change (e.g., psoriatic plaques)
- Skin or subcutaneous nodules
- Deformities
  - Varus (cubitus varus) can be caused by a supracondylar fracture.
  - Valgus (cubitus valgus) can be caused by nonunion of a lateral condylar fracture.
- Muscle wasting
- Swelling

Feel

▶ Always ask about pain before getting started.

Palpate the joint posteriorly and feel for the following:
- Temperature
- Subcutaneous nodules
- Swelling
  - Soft swelling may be due to olecranon bursitis.
  - Hard swelling suggests a bony deformity.
  - Boggy swelling suggests synovial thickening (e.g., secondary to RA).
- If fluid is present, attempt to displace it on either side of the olecranon.
- Carefully palpate the joint margin for tenderness and note if it is localized to the medial epicondyle (golfer's elbow) or the lateral epicondyle (tennis elbow).

Move

◑ Check that there is good shoulder function before attempting to assess elbow movements.

▶ Remember to test passive movements (you do the moving) and active movements (the patient does the moving) at each stage.
- Ask the patient to place their arms on the back of their head.
- Next assess elbow flexion and extension with the upper arm fixed.
  - Remember to compare with the opposite side.
- With the elbows tucked into the sides and flexed to a right angle, test the radioulnar joints for pronation (palms toward floor) and supination (palms toward the sky) (Fig. 11.2).

Measure

Measure elbow flexion and extension in degrees from the neutral position (i.e., consider a straight elbow joint to be 0°).

Function

Observe the patient pouring a glass of water and then putting on a jacket.

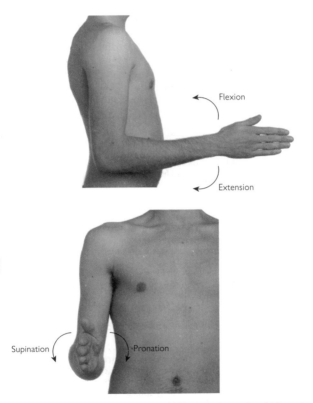

Fig. 11.2 Movements at the elbow joint. (a) Flexion and extension. (b) Pronation and supination (remember that pronation and supination require movement at the elbow as well as at the wrist).

Shoulder

Look

Look for any aids or adaptations. Ask the patient to remove any covering clothing and have them expose the upper limbs, neck, and chest. Scan the patient from top to toe. Inspect from the front, side, and behind.

Look especially for the following:

- Contours
  - Make note of any obvious asymmetry or deformity, such as winging of the scapula, prominence of the acromioclavicular joint, and wasting of the deltoid or short rotators that overlie the upper and lower segments of the scapula.
- Joint swelling
  - This is more obvious from the front and may be a clue to acute bleeds, rheumatoid effusions, pseudogout, or sepsis.
- Scars
- Bruising or other skin or subcutaneous tissue changes
- Position of both shoulders, looking for evidence of dislocation
  - Posterior dislocation can be seen when the arm is held in an internally rotated position.
  - Anterior dislocation can be seen easily when the arm is displaced in a forward and downward position.
- ▶ Remember to inspect the axillary regions.

Feel

▶ Always ask about pain before getting started.

Make note of any temperature changes, tenderness, or crepitus. Standing in front of the patient:

- Palpate the soft tissues and bony points in the following order: sternoclavicular joint, clavicle, acromioclavicular joint, acromial process, head of humerus, coracoid process, spine of scapula, greater tuberosity of humerus.
- Check the interscapular area for pain.
- Palpate the supraclavicular area for lymphadenopathy.

Move

▶ Remember to test *passive* movements (you do the moving) and *active* movements (the patient does the moving) at each stage. Quantify any movement in degrees *(measure)*.

ⓘ To test true glenohumeral movement, anchor the scapula by pressing firmly down on the top of the shoulder. After about 70° of abduction, the scapula rotates on the thorax—movement is scapulothoracic.

- *Flexion:* Ask the patient to raise their arms forward above their head.
- *Extension:* Straighten the arms backward as far as possible.
- *Abduction:* Move the arm away from the side of the body until the fingertips are pointing to the ceiling.
- *Adduction:* Ask the patient to move the arm inward toward the opposite side, across the trunk.

- *External rotation:* With the elbows held close to the body and flexed to 90°, ask the patient to move the forearms apart in an arc-like motion, to separate the hands as widely as possible.
- *Internal rotation:* Ask the patient to bring the hands together again across the body. (Loss of rotation suggests a capsulitis.)
- *Compound movements:* These types of movements may be employed as screening tests to assess shoulder dysfunction, taking the place of a fuller examination if no abnormalities are detected. See Fig. 11.3.
  - Ask the patient to put both hands behind their head (external rotation in abduction).
  - Ask the patient to reach up their back with the fingers to touch a spot between their shoulder blades (internal rotation in adduction).

Special tests

Testing for a rotator cuff lesion or tendonitis: the painful arc
Ask the patient to abduct the shoulder against light resistance.

Pain in early abduction suggests a rotator cuff lesion and usually occurs between 40° and 120°. This is due to a damaged and inflamed supraspinatus tendon being compressed against the acromial arch.

Testing for acromioclavicular arthritis
If there is pain during a high arc of movement (starting around 90°) and the patient is unable to raise their arm straight up above their head to 180°, even passively, this suggests acromioclavicular arthritis.

Function
Ask the patient to scratch the center of their back or to put on a jacket.

(a)   (b)

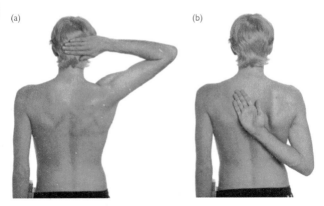

Fig. 11.3 Compound movements. (a) External rotation and abduction.
(b) Internal rotation and adduction

Box 11.7 A word about winging of the scapula

This is due to weakness of the serratus anterior, from damage to the long thoracic nerve, injury to the brachial plexus, injury or viral infections of C5–7 nerve roots, and muscular dystrophy.

Winging only becomes obvious when the serratus anterior contracts against resistance, such as pushing outstretched hands against a wall.

Spine

Look

Scan around the room for any clues, such as a wheelchair or walking aids. Watch how the patient walks into the room or moves around the bed area. Study their posture, paying particular attention to the neck.

Ask the patient to strip down to their underwear. Inspect from in front, the side, and behind, in both the standing and sitting positions.

Look especially for the following:
- Scars
- Pigmentation
- Abnormal hair growth
- Unusual skin creases
- Asymmetry, including abnormal spinal curvature
  - *Kyphosis:* convex curvature—normal in the thoracic (T) spine
  - *Lordosis:* concave curvature—normal in the lumbar (L) and cervical (C) spines
  - *Scoliosis:* side-to-side curvature away from the midline

▶ A question-mark spine with exaggerated thoracic kyphosis and a loss of lumbar lordosis is a classic sign of ankylosing spondylitis.

Feel

Palpate each spinous process, noting any prominence or step, and feel the paraspinal muscles for tenderness.

You should also make a point of palpating the sacroiliac joints.

Move

C-spine

Assess active movements of the C-spine first. These include flexion, extension, lateral flexion, and rotation. It is often helpful to demonstrate these movements yourself.
- *Flexion:* Ask the patient to put their chin on their chest.
- *Extension:* Ask the patient to look up to the ceiling.
- *Lateral flexion:* Ask the patient to lean their head sideways, placing an ear on their shoulder.
- *Rotation:* Ask the patient to look over each shoulder.

T- and L-spine

Movements at the thoracic and lumbar spine include flexion, extension, lateral flexion, and rotation.
- *Flexion:* Ask the patient to touch their toes.
- *Extension:* Ask the patient to lean backward.
- *Lateral flexion:* Ask the patient to bend sideways, sliding each hand down their leg as far as possible.
- *Rotation:* Anchor the pelvis (put a hand on either side) and ask the patient to twist at the waist to each side in turn.

Measure

Schober's test

This is a useful measurement of lumbar flexion.

- Ask the patient to stand erect with normal posture. Identify the level of the posterior superior iliac spines on the vertebral column.
- These are located at ~ L5.
- Make a small pen mark at the midline 5 cm below and 10 cm above this point.
- Now instruct the patient to bend at the waist to full forward flexion.
- Measure the distance between the two marks, using a tape measure.
- The distance should have increased to >20 cm (an increase of >5 cm). If not, there is a limitation in lumbar flexion (e.g., found in ankylosing spondylitis).

Special tests

Sciatic nerve stretch test

- This test is used to look for evidence of nerve root irritation (see also Box 11.8).
- With the patient lying supine, hold the ankle and lift the leg, straight, to 90°. Once there, dorsiflex the foot (Bragard test). If positive, pain is felt at the back of the thigh. The pain may be relieved by knee flexion.
- A positive stretch test suggests tension of the nerve roots supplying the sciatic nerve (L5–S2), commonly over a prolapsed disc (L4/5 or L5/S1).
- This test is partially age dependent. Most elderly people will struggle to flex their hip beyond 70°.

Femoral nerve stretch test

With the patient lying prone, abduct and extend the hip, flex the knee, and plantarflex the foot. The stretch test is positive if pain is felt in the thigh or inguinal region. See p. 319.

Box 11.8 Neurological examination

Don't forget the neurological aspects of the examination. The femoral and sciatic stretch tests may uncover root irritation, but you should also examine for the neurological and functional consequences as in Chapter 10.

Hip

Look

Expose the whole lower limb. Look around the room for any aids or devices such as orthopedic shoes or walking aids. If they have not done so already, ask the patient to walk, and note the gait. Note if there is evidence of a limp or obvious pain.

With the patient in standing position, inspect from the front, side, and behind. Look for the following:

- Scars
- Sinuses
- Asymmetry of skin creases
- Swelling
- Muscle wasting
- Deformities

Pay attention to the position of limbs (e.g., external rotation, pelvic tilting, standing with one knee bent or foot held plantarflexed or in equinus).

Feel

Feel for bony prominences, such as the anterior superior iliac spines and greater trochanters. Check that they are in the expected position.

Palpate the soft tissue contours and feel for any tenderness in and around the joint.

Move

Ask the patient if they have any pain before you examine them.

▶ Fix the pelvis by using your left hand to stabilize the contralateral anterior superior iliac spine, since any limitation of hip movement can easily be hidden by movement of the pelvis. With the patient *supine:*

- **Flexion:** Ask the patient to flex the hip until the knee meets the abdomen. Normal is around ~120°.
- **Abduction:** With the patient's leg held straight, ask them to move it away from the midline. Normal is 30–40°.
- **Adduction:** With the patient's leg held straight, ask them to move it across the midline. Normal is ~30°.

With the patient *prone:*

- **Extension:** Ask the patient to raise each leg off the bed. Normal is only a few degrees.
- **Internal rotation:** Ask the patient to keep the knees tight together and spread the ankles as far as possible.
- **External rotation:** Ask the patient to cross the legs over.

Passive movements

Most of these movements should be assessed by the examiner as for active movements while the patient is in a relaxed state.

- *Passive external and internal rotation:* With the patient supine, flex the knee, stabilizing it with one hand while the other hand moves the heel laterally or medially so that the heel either moves away or toward the midline (internal and external rotation respectively).

Measure (limb length)

True shortening, in which there is loss of bone length, must not be confused with apparent shortening due to a deformity at the hip, in which there is no loss of bone length.

Technique

- With the patient supine, place the pelvis square and the lower limbs in comparable positions in relation to the pelvis.
- Measure the distance from the anterior superior iliac spine to the medial malleolus on each side *(true length)*.
  - *Apparent length* is measured from a midline structure, such as the xiphisternum or umbilicus, to the medial malleolus.

Special tests

Trendelenberg test

This is useful as an overall assessment of the function of the hip and will expose dislocations or subluxations, weakness of the abductors, shortening of the femoral neck, or any painful disorder of the hip.

- Ask the patient to stand up straight without any support.
- Ask them to raise their left leg by bending the knee.
- Watch the pelvis (normally it should rise on the side of the lifted leg).
- Repeat the test with the patient standing on the left leg.
- A *positive test* is when the pelvis falls on the side of the lifted leg, indicating hip instability on the supporting side (i.e., the pelvis falls to the left = right hip weakness).

Thomas test

A fixed flexion deformity of the hip (often seen in osteoarthritis) can be hidden when the patient lies supine by tilting the pelvis and arching the back. The Thomas test will expose any flexion deformity.

- With the patient lying supine, feel for lumbar lordosis (palm upward).
- With the other hand, flex the opposite hip and knee fully to ensure that the lumbar spine becomes flattened.
- If a fixed-flexion deformity is present, the opposite leg flexes too (measure the angle relative to the bed).
- Remember to repeat the test on the other hip.

Function

Assess gait. See Chapter 10, p. 321.

Knee

Look

Scan the room for any walking aids or other clues and inspect the patient standing. The lower limbs should be completely exposed except for underwear so that comparisons can be made.

Compare one side to the other and look for the following:
- Deformity (valgus, varus, or flexion)
- Scars or wounds to suggest infection past or present
- Muscle wasting (quadriceps)
- Swelling (including posteriorly)
- Erythema
- Look for loss of the medial and lateral dimples around the knees, which suggests the presence of an effusion.

Feel

▶ Always ask about pain before getting started. Always compare sides. With the patient lying supine:
- Palpate for temperature using the back of the hand.
- Ask if the knee is tender on palpation.
- Feel around the joint line while asking the patient to bend the knee slightly.
- Palpate the collateral ligaments (either side of the joint).
- Feel the patellofemoral joint (by tilting the patella).

Examining for a small effusion—the bulge sign
- Holding the patella still, empty the medial joint recess using a wiping motion of your index finger (Fig. 11.4a).
  - This will milk any fluid into the lateral joint recess.
- Now apply a similar wiping motion to the lateral recess and
- Watch the medial recess (Fig. 11.4b).
  - If there is fluid present, a distinct bulge should appear on the flattened, medial surface and it is milked out of the lateral side.

Examining for a large effusion—the patellar tap
If the effusion is large, the bulge sign is absent, as you will be unable to empty either recess of fluid—use the patellar tap instead.
- Move any fluid from the medial and lateral compartments into the retropatellar space.
  - Apply firm pressure over the suprapatellar pouch with the flat of the hand and use your thumb and index finger placed on either side of the patella to push any fluid centrally (see Fig. 11.5a).
- With the first one or two fingers of the other hand, push the patella down firmly (see Fig. 11.5b).
- If fluid is present, the patella will bounce off the lateral femoral condyle behind. You will feel it being pushed down and then "tap" against the femur.

Move

▶ Remember to test *passive* movements (you do the moving) and *active* movements (the patient does the moving) at each stage. Quantify any movement in degrees *(measure)*.

- Begin by moving the joint passively and feel over the knee with one hand for any crepitus.
- *Flexion:* Ask the patient to maximally flex the knee. Normal ≈135°.
- *Extension:* Ask the patient to straighten the leg at the knee.
- *Hyperextension:* Assess by watching the patient lift the leg off the bed and then holding the feet stable in both hands above the bed or couch, and ask the patient to relax. Ensure that you are not causing the patient any discomfort.

Measure

The visual impression of wasting of the quadriceps can be confirmed by measuring the circumference of the thighs at the same level using a fixed bony point of reference e.g., 2.5 cm above the tibial tubercle.

(a)   (b)

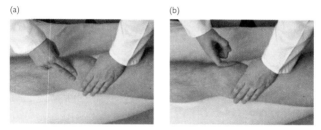

Fig. 11.4 Examining for the bulge sign. (a) Wipe any fluid from the medial joint recess. (b) Wipe the fluid back out of the lateral joint recess and watch the medial side.

(a)   (b)

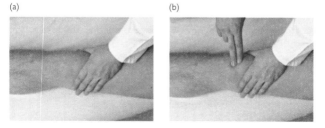

Fig. 11.5 Testing for patellar tap. (a) Use the palmar surface, thumb, and index finger of one hand to move any fluid into the retropatellar space. (b) Attempt to tap the patella on the femur using the other hand.

Special tests

Testing for medial and lateral collateral ligament instability

- Take the patient's foot with your right hand.
- Hold the patient's extended knee firmly with your left hand (Fig. 11.6).
- Attempt to bend the distal leg medially (varus)
  • This tests the lateral collateral ligament.
- Attempt to bend the distal leg laterally (valgus).
  • This tests the medial collateral ligament.
- Repeat the above with the knee at 30° of flexion.
  • Normally, the joint should move no more than a few degrees. Excessive movement suggests torn or stretched collateral ligament.

Anterior and posterior drawer tests

These test the anterior and posterior cruciate ligaments, which prevent the distal part of the knee from moving anteriorly and posteriorly.

- Ensure that the patient is lying in a relaxed supine position.
- Ask the patient to flex the knee to 90°.
- You may wish to position yourself perched on the patient's foot to stabilize the leg. Warn the patient about this first!
- Wrap your fingers around the back of the knee, using both hands, positioning the thumbs over the patella pointing toward the ceiling (Fig. 11.7).
- Push up with your index fingers to ensure the hamstrings are relaxed.
- The upper end of the tibia is then pulled forward and pushed backward in a rocking motion.
  • Normally, there should be very little or no movement seen.
  • Excessive anterior movement reflects anterior cruciate laxity.
  • Excessive posterior movement denotes posterior cruciate laxity.

McMurray test

This is a test for detecting meniscal tears (Fig. 11.8a).

- With the patient lying supine, bend the hip and knee to 90°.
- Grip the heel with your right hand and press on the medial and lateral cartilage with your left hand.
- Internally rotate the tibia on the femur and slowly extend the knee.
- Repeat, but externally rotate the distal leg while extending the knee.
- Repeat with varying degrees of knee flexion.
  • If there is a torn meniscus, a tag of cartilage may become trapped between the articular surfaces, causing pain and an audible click. You may also be able to feel the click with your left hand.

Apley test

This is another test for meniscal tears (Fig. 11.8b).

- Position the patient *prone* with the knee flexed to 90°.
- Stabilize the thigh with your left hand.
- With your right hand, grip the patient's foot.
- Rotate or twist the foot and press downward in a grinding motion.
  • This test should produce symptoms if a meniscus is torn.

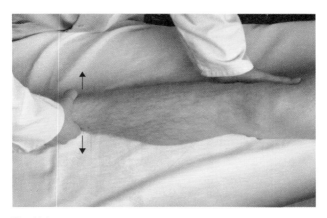

Fig. 11.6 Testing collateral ligament stability.

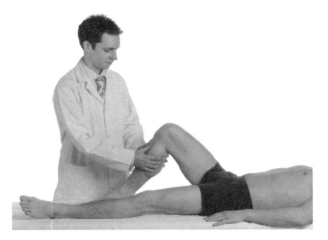

Fig. 11.7 Performing the anterior drawer test.

(a)

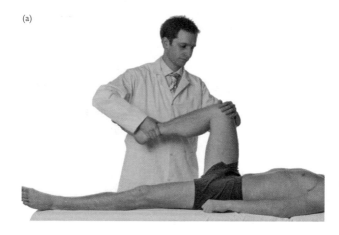

(b)

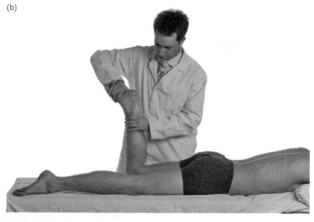

Fig. 11.8 Testing for meniscal tears. (a) McMurray test. (b) Apley grinding test.

Ankle and foot

Look

Expose the lower limbs and make note of any walking or other aids present. Take a moment to also examine the shoes carefully for any abnormal wear or stretching.

Examine feet and ankles when the patient is standing and, more carefully, with the patient lying on a couch or bed. Look for the following:

- Skin or soft tissue lesions, including calluses, swellings, ulcers, and scars
- Muscle wasting at the calf and lower leg
- Deformities, especially those involving the arch
  - Pes planus (flat foot)
  - Pes cavus (high-arched foot)
- Look for a bunion (bony deformity) at the first metatarsophalangeal (MTP) joint.
- Look for a bunionette at the fifth MTP joint.
- Examine nails carefully for any abnormalities, such as fungal infections or in-growing toenails.

▶ Don't forget to look between the toes. You may also wish to inspect for evidence of other abnormalities, such as hammertoes, claw toes, or clubbing of the feet (talipes equinovarus).

Feel

▶ Always ask about pain before getting started.
- Assess the skin temperature and compare over both the feet.
- Look for areas of tenderness, particularly over bony prominences (lateral and medial malleoli, MTP joints, interphalangeal joints, and heel) as well as the metatarsal heads.
- Squeeze across the MTP joints and assess pain and movement.
- Remember to palpate any swelling, edema, or lumps.

Move

The ankle and foot constitute a series of joints that function as a unit.

▶ Remember to test *passive* movements (you do the moving) and *active* movements (the patient does the moving) at each stage.

Active movements should be performed with the patient's legs hanging over the edge of the bed.
- *Ankle dorsiflexion:* Ask the patient to point their toes at their head.
- *Ankle plantarflexion:* Ask the patient to push their toes down toward the floor, like pushing on a pedal.
- *Inversion:* (subtalar joint between the talus and calcaneus): Grasp the ankle with one hand and, with the other, grasp the heel, thereby fixing the calcaneus, and turn the sole inward toward the midline (Box 11.9).
- *Eversion:* as inversion but turn sole outward, away from the midline.
- *Midtarsal joints:* Grasp the heel with one hand and attempt to move the tarsus up and down and from side to side with the other.
- *Toe flexion:* Ask the patient to curl their toes.
- *Toe extension:* Ask the patient to straighten their toes.
- *Toe abduction:* Ask the patient to fan out their toes as far as possible.
- *Toe adduction:* Ask patient to hold a piece of paper between the toes.

Measure

Calf circumference can be measured bilaterally to check for any discrepancies that may highlight muscle wasting or hypertrophy (e.g., 10 cm below the tibial tuberosities).

Special tests

Thompson or Simmond test

This test is used to assess for a ruptured Achilles tendon.

- Ask the patient to kneel on a chair with their feet hanging over the edge. Squeezes both calves
- Normally the feet should plantarflex. If the Achilles tendon is ruptured, there will be no movement on the affected side.

Function

It is also helpful to observe the patient's gait with and without shoes. Be sure to ask the patient if they are able to do this.

Box 11.9 A word on inversion and eversion

Orthopedic purists will say that the ankle cannot invert or evert as it is mainly a simple hinge—the eversion and inversion tests are, therefore, "failure only" tests. You should note that some eversion and inversion is possible in the normal state at the tarsal joints, as tested by neurologists.

Orthopedic practitioners test pathological inversion and eversion by watching the heels from behind as the patient stands on tiptoes.

Important presenting patterns

Rheumatoid arthritis (RA)

RA is a chronic inflammatory, multisystem, autoimmune disease mediated by proinflammatory cytokines, such as tumor necrosis factor alpha (TNF-α), and in some cases is characterized by the presence of rheumatoid factor (RF).

There is a strong association with HLA-DR4, and patients with DR4 tend to have more severe disease. It affects around 1–3% of the population in all racial groups, with peak age of onset in the fourth and fifth decades and a female–male ratio of 3:1.

The usual pattern of disease is insidious but can also be episodic with complete resolution between attacks (palindromic) or acute. The clinical features of RA can be divided into articular and extra-articular features and are summarized below.

Articular features

RA usually presents as a symmetrical polyarthritis affecting the wrists and small joints of the hands and feet. Occasionally, a patient presents with a monoarthritis of a larger joint, such as the knee or shoulder. Common presenting symptoms are joint pain, stiffness, and swelling that are typically worse in the mornings and improve as the day progresses. The disease eventually leads to varying degrees of functional loss.

Signs of RA in the hands and wrist

There is synovitis involving the wrists and metacarpophalangeal (MCP) and proximal interphalangeal (PIP) joints, with sparing of the distal interphalangeal (DIP) joints.

- Ulnar deviation of fingers (subluxation or dislocation at MCP joints)
- Swan neck deformity: hyperextension of PIP joints with flexion of MCP and DIP joints.
- Boutonniere's deformity: flexion deformity of PIP joints with extension of DIP and MCP joints
- Z-deformity of thumb: flexed MCP joint with extended interphalangeal joint of thumb
- Triggering of finger
- Generalized wasting of small muscles of hand
- Cutaneous vasculitis

Signs of RA in the feet

- Forefoot synovitis with proximal phalangeal subluxation dorsally
- Metatarsal head erosion and displacement toward the floor. The patient experiences this as like walking on marbles.
- Valgus deformities
- Collapse of longitudinal arch

Signs of RA in the spine

- Atlantoaxial subluxation ± spinal cord compression

Extra-articular features of RA
- Rheumatoid nodules: common at sites of pressure (elbows and wrists). They are associated with more severe disease and always RF positive.
- Tenosynovitis and bursitis
- Carpal tunnel syndrome
- Amyloidosis (proteinuria, hepatosplenomegaly)
- Systemic features (fever, malaise, weight loss, and lymphadenopathy)

Anemia

Causes include the following:
- Anemia of chronic disease
- GI bleeding associated with NSAID use
- Bone marrow suppression secondary to disease-modifying antirheumatic drugs, such as gold and penicillamine
- Megaloblastic anemia from folic acid deficiency (also secondary to methotrexate) or pernicious anemia
- Felty's syndrome (RA, splenomegaly, and leucopenia)

Lung features
- Pleuritic pain
- Pleural effusions
- Pulmonary fibrosis
- Pulmonary nodules
- Obliterative bronchiolitis
- Caplan syndrome (massive lung fibrosis in patients with pneumoniosis)

Neurological features
- Peripheral nerve entrapment
- Mononeuritis multiplex
- Peripheral neuropathy
- Cervical myelopathy due to atlantoaxial subluxation

Cardiac features
- Pericarditis
- Pericardial effusions

Eye features
- Painless episcleritis
- Painful scleritis
- Scleromalacia perforans
- Keratoconjunctivitis sicca
- Sjögren's syndrome
- Cataracts (chloroquine, steroids)

Vasculitis
- Nail fold infarcts
- Cutaneous ulceration
- Digital gangrene
- Cerebral and mesenteric infarction
- Coronary and renal vasculitis (rare)

Skin lesions
- Palmar erythema
- Pyoderma gangrenosum

Osteoarthritis

Osteoarthritis is a chronic disorder of synovial joints that is characterized by focal cartilage loss and an accompanying reparative bone response.

It represents the single-most important cause of musculoskeletal disability with a prevalence that increases with age and has a female preponderance.

The joints commonly affected include the hips, knees, spine, and first carpometacarpal, first metatarsal, and DIP joints.

Secondary causes include trauma, RA, infection, neuropathic (Charcot's) joints, and metabolic disorders (e.g., Paget's disease, acromegaly, hemachromatosis, avascular necrosis, and hypoparathyroidism).

Clinical features

Common symptoms include swelling, deformity, stiffness, weakness, and pain that is normally worse after activity and relieved by rest.

Common signs include the following:

- Hard, bony swellings of the DIP joints (Heberden's nodes)
- Bony nodules at the PIP joints (Bouchard's nodes)
  - These are bony outgrowths at the joint margins (osteophytes).
- "Square hand" deformity due to subluxation of the base of the thumb
- Valgus and varus deformities
- Crepitus
- Wasting and weakness (especially of the quadriceps and glutei)
- Tilting of the pelvis

Crystal arthropathies

Gout

Gout is a disorder of purine metabolism. It is characterized by hyper-uricemia due to either overproduction or underexcretion of uric acid (Box 11.10). Prolonged hyperuricemia leads to the formation of urate crystals in the synovium, other connective tissues, and the kidney.

Clinical features of acute gout

- Severe pain and swelling classically in the great toe MTP joint, worse at night and associated with redness (Box 11.11)
- Occasionally multiple joints are involved.
- ± Systemic symptoms

Clinical features of chronic (tophaceous) gout

- Tophus formation (soft tissue deposits of urate found especially in digits, helix of the ear, bursae, and tendon sheaths)
  - ± Overlying necrotic skin with chalky exudate of urate crystals

Pseudogout

This is caused by deposition of calcium pyrophosphate crystals in the synovium, joint capsule, and tendons. It is the most common cause of an acute monoarthritis in older adults and may present as either an acute synovitis or a chronic arthritis.

It is linked to chondrocalcinosis (calcification of articular cartilage). On examination, you may find a swollen, erythematous, and tender joint (often knees, wrist, elbow, ankle, or shoulder, and MCP joints, especially the index and middle) associated with systemic upset.

Box 11.10 Causes of hyperuricemia

- Drugs: diuretics, ethanol, low-dose salicylates, pyrazinamide, ethambutol, nicotinic acid, and cyclosporine
- Chronic renal failure
- Myeloproliferative and lymphoproliferative disorders (↑ purine metabolism)
- Obesity
- Hypertension
- Hypothyroidism
- Hyperthyroidism
- Familial
- Excessive dietary purines
  ▶ It is more common in the summer months because of reduced fluid intake and increased fluid loss.

Box 11.11 Conditions associated with gout

- Obesity
- Type IV hyperlipidemia
- Hypertension
- Impaired glucose tolerance or diabetes
- Ischemic heart disease

Spondyloarthropathies

These include ankylosing spondylitis, psoriatic arthritis, reactive arthritis, and enteropathic arthritis. This is a group of related and overlapping forms of inflammatory arthritis that characteristically lack rheumatoid factor and are associated with HLA-B27. They present at any age, though young males are primarily affected.

They also share a number of key features:
- Enthesitis (An *enthesis* is the insertion of a tendon, ligament, or capsule into a bone.)
- Synovitis
- Sacroiliitis
- Dactylitis
- Peripheral arthritis affecting predominantly the large joints

Ankylosing spondylitis

Ankylosing spondylitis usually develops in early adulthood with a peak age of onset in the mid-20s and is three times more common in males.

Common symptoms
- Lower back pain and stiffness that is typically worse in the morning and after long periods of rest
- Chest pain as a result of T-spine involvement as well as enthesitis at the costochondral joints
- Tender sacroiliac joints

- Pain in peripheral joints, such as the shoulders and knees

Musculoskeletal features and signs
- Question-mark posture (loss of lumbar lordosis, fixed kyphoscoliosis of the T-spine, compensatory extension of the C-spine)
- Protuberant abdomen
- Schober's test is positive (see 📖 p. 354)
- Achilles tendonitis
- Plantar fasciitis

Some extraskeletal features
- Anterior uveitis
- Aortic regurgitation
- Apical lung fibrosis
- AV block
- Amyloidosis (secondary)
- Atlantoaxial dislocation
- Traumatic fracture of a rigid spine
- Hypoxia
- Fever
- Weight loss

Psoriatic arthritis

Psoriatic arthropathy affects up to 10% of patients with psoriasis and may precede or follow the skin disease.

▶ The arthropathy does not correlate with the severity of skin lesions. There are five main subtypes of psoriatic arthropathy:
- Asymmetrical distal interphalangeal joint arthropathy
- Asymmetrical large joint mono- or oligoarthropathy
- Spondyloarthropathy and sacroiliitis
- Rheumatoid-like hands (clinically identical to RA but seronegative)
- Arthritis mutilans (a severely destructive form with telescoping of the fingers)

Associated clinical features
- Psoriatic plaques (classically found on the extensor surfaces and scalp, behind the ears, and in the navel and natal cleft)
- Nail involvement (pitting, onycholysis, discoloration, and thickening)
- Dactylitis (sausage-shaped swelling of the digits due to tenosynovitis)

Reactive arthritis
- An aseptic arthritis, strongly linked to a recognized episode of infection. Common causes are gut and genitourinary pathogens.
- It mainly affects young adults and usually presents with asymmetric and oligoarticular arthritis with symptoms starting a few days to a few weeks after the infection.
- Enthesitis and dactylitis are other common features. Patients may experience pain in the articular joints.

Associated extraskeletal features
- Urethritis
- Conjunctivitis
- Skin and mucosal lesions

Reiter's syndrome
This is a form of reactive arthritis associated with the classic triad of
- Arthritis
- Urethritis
- Conjunctivitis

It often follows dysenteric infections such as *Shigella*, *Salmonella*, *Campylobacteria*, and *Yersinia* or infections of the genital tract. Other findings that may be encountered are mouth ulceration, circinate balanitis, keratoderma blennorrhagica (pustular-like lesions found on the palms or soles), and persistent plantar fasciitis.

Enteropathic arthritis
Enteropathic arthritis is a peripheral or axial arthritis occurring in association with inflammatory bowel disease (IBD) and does not typically correlate with the severity of bowel disease. However, the peripheral arthritis has been shown to improve if the affected bowel is resected.

Osteoporosis

Osteoporosis is a systemic skeletal disorder involving ↓ bone mass (osteopenia) and microarchitectural deterioration, resulting in an ↑ risk of fracture. Classification (and treatment) is based on measurement of bone mineral density (BMD), with comparison to that of a young healthy adult.

The underlying pathology is related to an imbalance between osteoblast cells producing bone and osteoclast cells removing bone, which ultimately produces a net loss of bone. See Box 11.12 for risk factors.
- *Type I:* accelerated (mainly trabecular) bone loss secondary to estrogen deficiency and leads to fracture of vertebral bodies as well as the distal forearm in women in their late 60s and 70s
- *Type II:* age-related cortical and trabecular bone loss occurring in both sexes and leads to fractures of the proximal femur in the elderly

Clinical features
The process leading to established osteoporosis is asymptomatic and the condition usually presents only after bone fractures.

Features differ according to the fracture site. The most common clinical features include the following:
- Marked kyphosis
- Loss of height
- Protuberant abdomen
- Spinal tenderness

Paget's disease

This disorder of bone remodeling is characterized by ↑ osteoclastic and osteoblastic cell activity, leading to accelerated but disorganized bone resorption and formation.

Paget's disease is the second most common disease of bone after osteoporosis, is more common in males, and affects around 3% of the population >40 years of age. It occurs more commonly in Britain than anywhere else in the world; there are thought to be up to one million sufferers in the UK.

While the exact etiology remains unknown, a number of factors have been implicated, including a slow viral infection. Some 30% of Paget's patients have an affected first-degree relative.

Important clinical features and complications

- Enlargement of the skull
- Hearing loss (ossicles are involved and VIII nerve compression)
- Optic atrophy and angioid streaks
- Cardiac failure
- Kyphosis, anterior bowing of the tibia, lateral bowing of the femur
- ↑ Bone warmth
- ↓ Mobility
- Fractures
- Sarcomatous change (rare)
- Cord compression
- Cerebellar signs
- Hypercalcemia

Box 11.12 Risk factors for osteoporosis

- Smoking
- High alcohol consumption
- BMI <19
- Family history
- Premature menopause
- Prolonged immobilization
- Prolonged secondary amenorrhea
- Primary hypogonadism
- Low dietary calcium and vitamins
- Older age
- Female gender
- Sedentary lifestyle
- Caucasian or Asian origin

Chronic disorders, such as the following:

- Anorexia nervosa
- Malabsorption syndromes
- Primary hyperthyroidism
- Post-transplantation
- Cushing's syndrome
- Chronic renal failure

Box 11.13 Some important causes of a swollen knee

- RA
- Ruptured Baker's cyst
- Pseudogout
- Gout
- Edematous states (e.g., CHF, nephrotic syndrome)

- Trauma
- Charcot's knee
- Septic arthritis
- Hemarthrosis

The elderly patient

Rheumatological diseases represent a huge spectrum of illness in older people, often complicating and concurrent with other diseases—e.g., the impact of severe arthritis on COPD or heart failure or the effect of hip or knee arthritis on recovery after acute stroke.

Arthritis and osteoporosis are two major factors in the geriatric giants of immobility and instability—pertinent reminders of the widespread effect of musculoskeletal illness with advancing age.

History

Method of presentation

This can vary, ranging from the fall that leads to a femoral neck fracture or a referral "off legs" or with declining mobility. Older people will often have an existing diagnosis of some form of arthritis—the difficulty is not in the diagnosis but in understanding the impact on everyday life.

Musculoskeletal illnesses are a key part of such presentations, and attention to these illnesses is vital. However, it is important to remember that presentations such as falls are multifactorial—try to work out how musculoskeletal illness contributes to mobility or risk of falls.

Intercurrent illness

This may often precipitate gout or particularly pseudogout. Equally important are those illnesses that disturb carefully balanced homeostasis, leading to a fall and fracture. Your task is to not just treat the consequence of the fall but look at why it happened in the first place

Septic joints

They can be notoriously difficult to diagnose at times. Unilateral large joint swelling and acute arthritis should ring alarm bells, especially if the patient is unwell. A myriad of causes contribute to back pain, but never forget deep-seated infection, such as discitis or osteomyelitis, which may be a consequence of something as innocuous as a urinary infection.

Drug history

This is a keystone of any assessment. Consider the side-effect profile of NSAIDs or whether gout has been precipitated by the effects of diuretics or low-dose aspirin. If the patient has sustained a fragility fracture due to osteoporosis, are they on appropriate treatment?

Never forget the ↑ number of older people whose arthritis is successfully treated with disease-modifying drugs, and understand the effects of such drugs (and the need to prescribe concurrent folic acid with methotrexate).

Activities, occupation, and interests

These overlap with the functional history. Multidisciplinary assessment is vital for tailoring rehabilitation, physical aids, and future care, where appropriate. Ask about hobbies and interests—improving balance, minimizing pain, and maximizing function may allow patients to carry on with activities that are a key part of their lives (and might represent an opportunity for continued exercise or rehabilitation).

Examination

General

The signs are often very clear but despite this, easily overlooked. The need here is for a careful and thoughtful assessment of function as well as disease activity. Always ask about your patient's comfort, and examine carefully, explaining what you wish to do, to avoid misunderstanding and pain.

Pattern of disease

Look for typical patterns of disease and single-joint pathology. Look at the ankles, feet, and back. It takes only a little more time to undertake a good examination, but is depressingly common to see patients with poor balance and a history of falls whose files detail no musculoskeletal assessment.

Disease activity

Be careful when palpating, but look to see if an acute exacerbation of joint disease may well have contributed to the current presentation.

Gait and balance

These are often overlooked but are a vital part of the examination. Learn (e.g., from the ward physiotherapist) how to undertake the get up and go test, a well-validated test of gait and balance (see Box 11.14). This assessment should overlap with neurological assessment when appropriate.

Box 11.14 Get up and go

This is an easy test to do and one that gives a wealth of information. In essence, ask the patient to rise to standing from a chair, walk 10 feet, then turn and return to the chair. The clinician's role is not that of a pure observer—you must make an assessment of safety and be on hand to support the patient, if needed.

Male reproductive system

Applied anatomy and physiology

Anatomy

The male reproductive system consists of a pair of testes, a network of excretory ducts (epididymis, ductus deferens, and ejaculatory tracts), seminal vesicles, prostate, bulbourethral glands, and the penis.

Penis

The penis consists of erectile tissue contained within two dorsally placed corpora cavernosa and the corpus spongiosum, which lies on their ventral surface. The corpora are attached proximally to the inferior pubic rami. The corpus spongiosum expands distally to form the glans penis and surrounds the urethra.

The three corpora are contained within a fibrous tubular sheath of fascia and covered by freely mobile (and elastic) skin. A loose fold of skin, the prepuce or foreskin, extends distally to cover the glans penis.

Scrotum

This is a muscular out-pouching of the lower part of the anterior abdominal wall. It contains the testes, epididymis, and lower ends of the spermatic cords. The scrotum acts as a climate-control system for the testes. Muscles in the wall of the scrotum, in conjunction with muscle fibers in the spermatic cord, allow it to contract and relax, moving the testicles closer or further away from the body.

Testes

These are paired, ovoid organs measuring ~4 x 3 x 2 cm, found within the scrotal sac. The testes are made up of masses of seminiferous tubules that are responsible for producing spermatozoa. Interstitial or Leydig cells lying between these tubules produce the male sex hormones.

In the fetus, the testes develop close to the kidneys in the abdomen, then descend caudally through the inguinal canal to reach the scrotum at ~38 weeks gestation.

Each testis is covered by an outer fibrous capsule (tunica albuginea). Laterally and medially lies the visceral layer of the tunica vaginalis (a closed serous sac—an embryonic derivative of the processus vaginalis, which normally closes before birth). The posterior surface of the testis is devoid of tunica vaginalis and is pierced by numerous small veins that form the pampiniform plexus. The seminiferous tubules converge here to form the efferent tubules, which eventually give rise to the epididymis.

Spermatic cord

This suspends the testis in the scrotum and contains structures running between the testis and the deep inguinal ring (the ductus deferens, arteries, veins, testicular nerves, and epididymis).

The cord is surrounded by the layers of the spermatic fascia (internal spermatic fascia) formed from the transversalis fascia, the cremasteric fascia formed from fascia covering the internal oblique, and the external spermatic fascia formed from the external oblique aponeurosis.

The cremasteric fascia is partly muscular. Contraction of the cremaster muscle draws the testis superiorly. The raising and lowering of the testis acts to keep it at a near-constant temperature.

Epididymis
This is a convoluted duct ~6 cm in length lying on the posterior surface of the testis. It is a specialized part of the collecting apparatus where spermatozoa are matured before traveling up the vas deferens to join the ducts draining the seminal vesicles, known as the ejaculatory ducts.

The seminal vesicles are paired organs that lie on the posterior surface of the bladder and contribute most of the fluid that makes up semen, along with fructose, ascorbic acid, amino acids, and prostaglandins.

Prostate gland
This is a firm, walnut-sized structure that lies inferior to the bladder, encircling the urethra. Many short ducts produce fluid that is emptied into the urethra and makes up a proportion of semen.

Bulbourethral glands
These are small, pea-sized glands located near the base of the penis.

In response to sexual stimulation, the bulbourethral glands secrete an alkaline mucus-like fluid that neutralizes the acidity of the urine in the urethra and provides a small amount of lubrication for the tip of the penis during intercourse.

Sex hormones
Three hormones are the regulators of the male reproductive system:
- Follicle-stimulating hormone (FSH) is produced in the anterior pituitary gland and stimulates spermatogenesis by its action on Sertoli cells.
- Luteinizing hormone (LH) is produced in the anterior pituitary gland and stimulates the production of testosterone from Leydig cells.
- Testosterone is produced in the testis and adrenal gland and aids in development of male secondary sexual characteristics and spermatogenesis.

Male sexual response
There are four stages of the sexual response:
- *Excitement or arousal* is under control of the parasympathetic nervous system. During this stage, the penis becomes engorged with blood and stands out from the body. Other changes include an i in heart rate, blood pressure, respiratory rate, and skeletal muscle tone.
- *Plateau:* Continued sexual stimulation maintains the changes made in the arousal phase. This can last from a few seconds to many minutes.
- *Orgasm:* In males, this is the briefest stage and mediated by the sympathetic nervous system. Rhythmic contractions of the perineal muscles and accessory glands and peristaltic contraction of the seminal ducts result in ejaculation. This is usually followed by a refractory period during which another erection cannot be achieved. This varies between individuals, from minutes to hours, and lengthens with advancing age.
- *Resolution:* Blood pressure, heart rate, respiratory rate, and muscle tone return to the unaroused state. This is accompanied by a sense of relaxation.

Sexual history

This can be awkward for both the patient and the history-taker. It should be undertaken in a sensitive, confident, and confidential manner. Before the discussion takes place, the patient should be reassured about the levels of privacy and confidentiality and that they are free to openly discuss their sexual life and habits.

Make no assumptions, remain professional, and try to use the patient's own words and language. Be aware of cultural and religious differences surrounding sex and talking about it. See 📖 p. 48 for further guidance.

You should approach a sexual history in a structured way, as below.

Sexual activity

This should include an assessment of the risk of acquiring a sexually transmitted infection (STI).

Determine the number and gender of the patient's sexual partners, their risk of having an STI, and the precautions (if any) that were taken. Try asking the following questions:

- Do you have sex with men, women, or both?
- In the past 2 months, how many people have you had sex with?
- When did you last have sexual intercourse?
- Was it with a man or a woman?
- Were they a casual or regular partner?
- Where were they from?
- Do they use injected drugs?
- Do they have any history of sexually transmitted infections?
- How many other partners do you think they've had recently?
- In what country did you have sex?
- What kind of sex did you take part in? (e.g., vaginal, anal, oral)
- For each type of sex, did you use a condom?
- Does your partner have any symptoms?
- Have you had any other partners in the last 6 weeks?
  - If so, repeat the questions above for each partner.

Previous history

You also need to establish the history of STIs for the patient:
- Have you had any other STIs?
- Have you ever had a sexual check-up?
- Have you ever been tested for HIV, hepatitis, or syphilis?
- Have you ever been vaccinated against hepatitis A or B?

Psychological factors

Concerns over loss of libido and sexual function may point to a complex psychological cause for symptoms. Explore this delicately and ask about
- History of sexual abuse
- Problems with the relationship
- Sexual partners outside the relationship
- Any other cause for anxiety
- History of depression or anxiety

Symptoms

Urethral discharge

If the patient complains of discharge or "mucus" from the end of their penis, establish the following:

* Amount
* Color
* Presence of blood?
* Relation between the discharge and urination or ejaculation
* Is there any pain?
* Are there any other symptoms, such as conjunctivitis or arthralgia?
* Has the patient recently had symptoms of gastroenteritis?

You should also determine when this symptom was first noticed and how that relates to any sexual contacts that the patient has had and the possibility of exposure to STIs (see previous pages).

Rashes, warts, ulcers

Treat a genital skin lesion as you would any other rash (📖 p. 80). Also ask about the following:

* Similar lesions elsewhere (mouth, anus)
* Foreign travel

Determine the risk of recent exposure to STIs as previously.

Testicular pain

This is often felt as deep, burning pain and accompanied by nausea. Treat as pain in any other location, as on 📖 p. 33. Also ask about associated genital symptoms, such as testicular swelling, dysuria, or hematuria (see Box 12.1).

Common causes include testicular torsion, mumps, orchitis, andepididymitis. Remember the possibility of cancer.

Erectile dysfunction

The term *impotence* should be avoided by health-care providers because of its negative social implications. Patients may use the term *impotence*

Box 12.1 The rest of the history

A full history needs to be taken in all cases, as described in Chapter 2. The following may have particular relevance here.

PMH

Ask especially about the following:

* Sexually transmitted infections (as previously)
* Orchitis or a history of mumps
* Inguinal, scrotal, and testicular injury or surgery
* Urethral injury

Smoking and alcohol

Detailed histories should be taken as described in 📖 Chapter 2 (p. 41).

for a number of different sexual problems. Ask specifically if the patient means the following:
- Difficulty in achieving or maintaining an erection (erectile dysfunction)
- Difficulty with premature ejaculation (ejaculatory dysfunction)
- Difficulty in reaching orgasm (orgasmic dysfunction)

Remember that an erection is not necessary for men to reach orgasm or to ejaculate. *Erectile dysfunction* is the inability to gain and maintain an erection for satisfactory completion of sexual activities.

If a patient complains of impotence, this needs to be explored in more detail. Establish particularly if the lack of function is related to a particular partner or situation or is constant. Ask the following questions:
- Are you able to get an erection at all?
- Do you wake with an erection in the morning?
- Are you able to get an erection to masturbate?

If the cause is psychological, the patient will often still wake with an erection (the so-called morning glory) but not be able to perform in a sexual situation. This can be tested with a sleep study, if necessary. Psychological factors should be explored with sensitivity.

Organic causes for erectile dysfunction include atherosclerosis, diabetes mellitus, multiple sclerosis, pelvic fractures, urethral injury, or other endocrine dysfunction.

Drug history is important. Drugs associated with erectile dysfunction include barbiturates, benzodiazepines, phenothiazines, lithium, antihypertensives (e.g., B-blockers), alcohol, estrogens, methadone, and heroin.

Loss of sexual desire (libido)

This can be an early sign of a pituitary tumor, but the cause is more often deeply rooted in the patient's psychology. Ask the following questions:
- How often do you shave your face?
- Has this changed recently?
- Do you have any muscle wasting or pain?
- Explore any issues about the sexual partner and the patient's relationship with them.

Infertility

Around 10% of couples have difficulty with conception. Male infertility accounts for 1/3 of childless relationships. This is a complex topic and not within the scope of this book.

Relevant information to ascertain includes the following:
- Age of both partners
- Length of time they have been trying to conceive
- Presence of existing children belonging to both partners, and children of each partner from prior relationships
- Frequency and timing of intercourse
- Any erectile, ejaculatory, or orgasmic dysfunction
- Drug history of both partners
- Factors suggestive of endocrine malfunction, as under Loss of Sexual Desire
- Smoking and alcohol consumption
- Menstrual history from partner

Examining male genitalia

Explain to the patient that you would like to examine the penis and testes and reassure them that the procedure will be quick and gentle.

You should have a chaperone present, particularly if you are female. A chaperone, however, is often desirable even in circumstances where the examiner is male.

Ensure that the examination room is warm and that you are unlikely to be disturbed. With the patient on a bed or couch, raised to a comfortable height, ask them to pull their clothing down. You should be able to see the genitalia and lower part of the patient's abdomen at the very least.

Penis

Inspection

Make a careful inspection of the organ, noting the following:

- Size
- Shape
- Presence or absence of a foreskin
- Color of the skin
- The position and caliber of the urethral meatus (see Box 12.2)
- Any discharge
- Any abnormal curvature
- Any lesion, scaling, scabbing or other superficial abnormality such as erythema or ulceration, particularly at the distal end (glans)

Palpation

Palpate the whole length of the penis to the perineum and note the state of the dorsal vein, which is usually easily seen stretching the length of the penis at the dorsal midline. Note also any abnormalities of the underlying tissues (e.g., firm areas) that may not be visible—this may represent the plaques of Peyrone's disease.

Retract the foreskin to expose the glans penis and urethral meatus. The foreskin should be supple, allowing smooth and painless retraction. Look especially for any secretion or discharge and collect a specimen, if possible. The patient may be able to milk the shaft of the penis to express the secretion.

Box 12.2 Hypospadias

Hypospadias is the abnormal, ventral, positioning of the urethralmeatus. It is seen in 1 in 250 males. In the vast majority, the hypospadias is slight.

Patients may have a hooded foreskin with the meatus at the very edge of the glans or a very slightly ventral meatus that iscompletely covered by a normal foreskin.

Slight hypospadias has no effect on sexual function but may be a cause of anxiety and embarrassment resulting in psychosexual problems once the patient is aware that his penis is "different."

There is often a trace of smegma underlying the foreskin. This is a normal finding.

ⓘ Remember to replace the foreskin at the end of the examination.

Note that in the presence of phimosis, the foreskin will be nonretractile and attempts may cause considerable pain.

Scrotum and contents

Reminder
Before touching the genitalia, consider assessing the patient for the presence of the cremasteric reflex when evaluating complaints of testicular pain. Please note, however, that the assessment of the cremasteric reflex can be unreliable in a patient who is tense or anxious.

Examining the scrotum and scrotal contents is best done with the patient standing up.

Inspection
Make a careful examination of the scrotal skin. It is usually wrinkled and slightly more pigmented than the rest of the patient's body and should be freely mobile of the testis. One testis usually hangs lower than the other. Remember to lift the scrotum, inspecting the inferior and posterior aspects.

Look especially for the following:
• Edema
• Sebaceous cysts
• Ulcers
• Scabies
• Scars

Palpation
The scrotal contents should be *gently* supported with your left hand and palpated with the fingers and thumb of your right hand. It may help to ask the patient to hold their penis to one side (see Fig. 12.1).
• Check that the scrotum contains two testes.
  • Absence of one or both testes may be due to previous excision, failure of the testis to descend, or a retractile testis.
  • If there appears to be a single testis, carefully examine the inguinal canal for evidence of a discrete swelling that could be an undescended testis.
• Make careful note of any discrete lumps or swellings in the body of the testis.
  • Any swelling in the body of the testis must be considered to be suggestive of a malignancy.
• Compare the left and right testes, noting the size and consistency.
  • The testes are normally equal in size, and smooth, with a firm, rubbery consistency. If there is a significant discrepancy, ask the patient if he has ever noticed this.
• Feel for the epididymis, which lies at the posterolateral aspect of each testis.
• The vas can be distinguished from the rest of the cord structures, lying along the posterior aspect of the bundle, and feels firm and wire-like. It runs from the epididymis to the external inguinal ring.

(a)

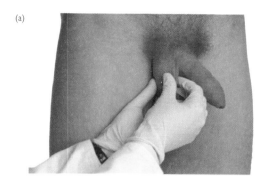

(b)

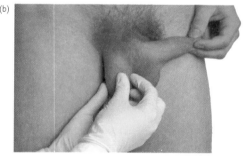

Fig. 12.1 (a) Examine the scrotum with the patient standing and use both hands. It is sometimes preferable to ask the patient to hold their penis aside (b).

Scrotal swellings

If a lump is palpated:

- Decide if the lump is confined to the scrotum. Are you able to feel above it? Does it have a cough impulse? Is it fluctuant? (You will be unable to get above swellings that descend from the inguinal canal.)
- Define the lump as any other mass, as described on 📖 p. 88.
- Transillumination is often important here. Darken the room and shine a small torch through the posterior part of the swelling (see Fig. 12.2).
  - A solid mass remains dark, whereas a cystic mass or fluid will transilluminate.

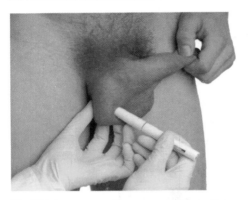

Fig. 12.2 Attempt to transilluminate any swelling by shining a small penlight through it. Unlike the figure above, the room should be darkened.

Perineum and rectum
Don't overlook the perineum, anal canal, and rectum. In particular, a digital rectal examination should be performed as described on 📖 p. 241, with particular attention to feeling the prostate and seminal vesicles.

Local lymphatics
- Lymph from the skin of the penis and scrotum drains to the inguinal lymph nodes.
- Lymph from the covering of the testes and spermatic cord drains initially to the internal, then common, iliac nodes.
- Lymph from the body of the testes drains to the para-aortic lymph nodes—these are impalpable.
- Your examination is not complete without a careful palpation of the inguinal lymph nodes (Fig. 12.3). This is best done with the patient lying comfortably on a bed or couch.
- If any swelling is found, it should be described in the same way as any lump (📖 p. 88).

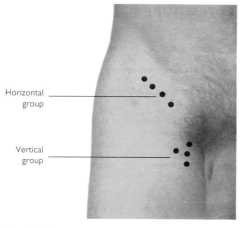

Horizontal group

Vertical group

Fig. 12.3 Diagrammatic representation of the inguinal lymph nodes.

Important presenting patterns

Phimosis

This is a narrowing of the end of the foreskin that prevents its retraction over the glans penis. It can cause difficulty with micturition and lead to recurrent balanitis. It may cause interference with erections and sexual intercourse.

• *Causes*: congenital, infection, trauma, inflammation (balanitis)

Paraphimosis

In this case, the foreskin can be retracted but then cannot be replaced over the glans. This results in edema, which limits its movement still further. If left in this condition, it can become necrotic or gangrenous.

This condition commonly occurs in men 15–30 years old. It is a frequent complication of urinary catheterization if the practitioner fails to replace the foreskin after the procedure is performed.

Hypospadias

See also Box 12.2, 🕮 p. 384. *Hypospadias* is a congenital abnormality in which the urethra opens on the ventral surface of the penis. Minor degrees result in a hooded or dorsal foreskin and spraying of the urine during micturition.

Openings on the ventral surface of the shaft of the penis (secondary hypospadias) or openings at the scrotum or perineum (tertiary hypospadias) may cause serious difficulties with micturition and sexual function.

Balanitis and balanoposthitis

Balanitis is inflammation of the glans penis. *Balanoposthitis* is inflammation of the glans and the foreskin. Such inflammation presents as redness, swelling, and pain of the affected parts, often with difficulty retracting the foreskin.

• *Causes:* Candida albicans (especially in patients with diabetes), herpes infection, carcinoma, drug eruptions, poor hygiene

Priapism

This is a painful, persistent erection and a serious feature of sickle crisis.

Other causes include leukemia, drugs (e.g., erectile dysfunction treatments or psychotropics), and neurogenic (e.g., diseases of spinal cord).

Penile ulcers

Conditions causing ulceration of genitalia include herpes simplex (vesicles followed by ulceration), syphilis (nontender ulceration), malignancy (e.g., squamous cell carcinoma—nontender), and Behçet's syndrome.

Hydrocele

This is fluid entrapment in the tunica vaginalis, causing usually painless swelling of the scrotum, the size of which can be considerable. Hydroceles will surround the testis, making it impalpable. It will transilluminate.

As well as congenital abnormalities in the inguinal canal, hydrocele can be caused by trauma, infection, and neoplastic disease.

Epididymal cysts

These are harmless, painless swellings arising behind and separate from the testis itself. The examiner may be unable to feel the rest of the epididymis. The testicle (anteriorly) should be normal. Epididymal cysts will transilluminate.

Varicocele

This involves abnormal dilatation of the veins in the spermatic cord caused by incompetent valves in the testicular vein. They only become apparent when the patient is standing and almost disappear when the patient is supine. These are much more common on the left.

Varicoceles are usually painless (although they can cause a deep ache in some men) and, in themselves, harmless. Varicocele is, however, associated with a reduction in fertility (it makes the testis abnormally warm). They are classically described as feeling like a bag of worms on palpation.

Orchitis

This is inflammation of the testis. The affected organ will hang higher in the scrotum and may be swollen and warm with redness of the overlying skin. It will be very tender to palpation. The patient may be systemically unwell with fever.

Testicular torsion

This presents in a very similar way to orchitis and is often difficult to distinguish, although the onset is much more sudden in torsion. Twisting of the testis on the spermatic cord (torsion) will cause ischemia and severe pain. Frequently, this pain is referred to the abdomen, often mimicking acute abdominal conditions such as appendicitis.

It usually occurs in young adults and teenagers, with a peak age of 14. Torsion is usually inward, toward the midline.

This is a urological emergency, and its presence must initially be confirmed through vascular ultrasonography to confirm the presence of diminished blood flow. If the testicle is left in this condition without being untwisted (with appropriate analgesia), surgical removal of the testis may be necessary. Immediate surgical referral is advised if this is suspected.

Testicular carcinoma

This should be at the top of your list of differential diagnoses in the case of an intrascrotal mass. Teratomas commonly occur between the ages of 20 and 30 years, whereas seminomas are more common at age 30–40 years.

There may be associated pain and tenderness or a dull aching, dragging sensation in the scrotum and groin. Look for constitutional symptoms suggestive of neoplastic disease, such as malaise, wasting, and anorexia, as well as leg swelling (venous or lymphatic obstruction), lymphadenopathy, or an associated abdominal mass.

The elderly patient

Much of the information on this page overlaps with that on the female reproductive system in Chapter 14. We would encourage the reader to regard both sections as a whole.

It is important to recognize that bladder carcinoma and diseases of the prostate are some of the most common urogenital problems faced by older men; remember to screen for such problems in any assessment. For prostate diseases, it is also important to know that patient awareness is high, so you should expect questions and a wish to be involved in treatment decisions. Equally so, many of these problems are faced by patients with cognitive impairment, in whom history may be limited and thorough assessment is vital.

Retain a holistic outlook on male urogenital problems, and you will be less likely to miss delirium because of acute epididymo-orchitis—a not uncommon presentation!

Studies report that half of U.S. adults ages 65–74 and more than 25% of those age 75 or older maintain active sexual lives. Avoiding sexual issues in this population can cause major problems to be overlooked. Many men over the age of 70 experience erectile dysfunction, so try not to make assumptions when seeing older people with sexual health problems.

History

Explore

Explore the history. Even for patients with prostate disease, how will the effects of treatment (e.g., TURP or conventional surgical prostate resection) affect relationships or sexual activity? Keep your thought processes open when assessing continence problems—there may symptoms of both obstruction and incontinence in many men. See also Box 12.3.

Box 12.3 A note on (recurrent) urinary tract infections

Most readers will have already seen many older patients with this common (and often over diagnosed) problem.

While many diagnoses are made on clinical suspicion, it is vital to undertake urinalysis and obtain urine for microscopy and culture to confirm the presence of urinary tract infections (UTIs). The reasoning is twofold: avoiding rushing to a label of UTI as the cause of delirium or mobility decline will reduce the chance of missing the correct diagnosis. Similarly, a proven culture diagnosis of UTI aids in prescribing and helps identify recurrent infections. Recognizing the latter may reveal underlying diagnoses and reduce discomfort or even hospitalization for some patients.

So, when faced with recurrent infections, be assiduous and request urine cytology (to look for bladder cancers) and ultrasound (for structural abnormalities), and discuss the value of cystoscopy and rotating or long-term antibiotics with urology colleagues.

PMH

Vascular diseases, metabolic, and neurological illnesses may all be underpinning diagnoses when faced with impotence. Could the new presentation of balanitis indicate diabetes?

Drug history

Aside from obvious culprits (e.g., diuretics), consider the effects of antidepressants, digoxin, and antihypertensives on both bladder and sexual function.

SH and sexual history

Always take an appropriate functional history, particularly if there are continence problems. Consider alcohol and tobacco in relation to impotence, and undertake a detailed occupational history if the patient presents with hematuria (bladder cancer?).

   Have the confidence to take a sexual history if there are problems with erectile or ejaculatory dysfunction. As indicated earlier, many older people have active sex lives and you're more likely to be embarrassed about taking the history than they are recounting it.

Examination

General

In addition to the detailed examination considered earlier in this chapter, keep in mind the need for a general examination, focusing on mood and neurological assessment in particular.

Cognition

This is a key part of this assessment, particularly for continence and erectile dysfunction problems.

Urogenital

Think subtly: in older men, orchitis may present with declining mobility, delirium, or falls, so don't forget to undertake a thorough examination in older adults, even when there is apparently little to indicate a urogenital problem. For patients with urinary catheters, whether short or long term, examination is a mandatory part of assessment.

Female breast

Applied anatomy and physiology

Anatomy of the breast

The two mammary glands are highly developed apocrine sweat glands. They develop embryologically along two lines extending from the axillae to the groin—the milk lines (see Fig. 13.1). In humans, only one gland develops on each side of the thorax, although extra nipples with breast tissue may sometimes occur.

The breasts extend from the second to the sixth ribs and transversely from the lateral border of the sternum to the mid-axillary line.

For the purposes of examination, each breast may be divided into four quadrants by horizontal and vertical lines intersecting at the nipple. An additional lateral extension of breast tissue (the axillary tail) stretches from the upper outer quadrant toward the axilla (see Fig. 13.2).

Each mammary gland consists of 15–20 lobes separated by loose adipose tissue and subdivided by collagenous septa. Strands of connective tissue called the *suspensory* ligaments of the breast (Cooper's ligaments) run between the skin and deep fascia to support the breast. Each lobe is further divided into a variable number of lobules composed of grape-like clusters of milk-secreting glands termed *alveoli* and is drained by a lactiferous duct that opens onto the nipple. Myoepithelial cells surround the alveoli, which contract and help propel the milk toward the nipples.

The nipple is surrounded by a circular pigmented area called the *areola* and is abundantly supplied with sensory nerve endings. The surface of this area also contains the glands of Montgomery, which act to lubricate the nipple during lactation.

Lymphatic drainage

Lymphatic drainage from the medial portion of the breast is to the internal mammary nodes. The central and lateral portions drain to the axillary lymph nodes, which are arranged into five groups (see Fig. 13.7, p. 403).

Physiology—normal breast changes in women

- *Puberty:* During adolescence, estrogen promotes the development of the mammary ducts and distribution of fatty tissue, while progesterone induces alveolar growth.
- *The menstrual cycle:* Toward the second half of the menstrual cycle, after ovulation, the breasts can become tender and swollen. They return to their resting state after menstruation.
- *Pregnancy:* High levels of placental estrogen, progesterone, and prolactin promote mammary growth in preparation for milk production.
- *Postnatal:* The sharply declining levels of estrogen and progesterone permit prolactin to stimulate the alveoli and produce milk. Suckling stimuli increases the secretion of prolactin as well as releases oxytocin, which stimulates myoepithelial cells to contract.
- *Menopause:* The breasts become softer and more homogenous and undergo involutional changes, including ↓ size, atrophy of the secretory portions, and some atrophy of the ducts.

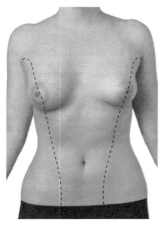

Fig. 13.1 Illustration of the two milk lines along which the nipples form—occasionally extra nipples can be found.

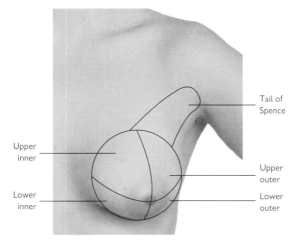

Tail of
Spence

Upper
inner

Upper
outer

Lower
inner

Lower
outer

Fig. 13.2 Illustrations showing the four quadrants of the breast with the axillary tail.

Important symptoms

First steps

Begin by establishing a menstrual history (see Box 13.1 and 📖 Chapter 14). You should also determine the date of the last period of menstruation. Pre-existing disease in the breast is likely to become more noticeable during the second half of the menstrual cycle—lumps often get bigger or become more easily palpable.

▶ Bear in mind that seeking medical attention for a breast lump or tenderness can produce extreme anxiety and embarrassment in patients. Men with gynecomastia are also likely to feel anxious about their breast development (Box 13.2). Be sure that you adopt an appropriately sensitive, sympathetic, and professional approach.

Breast pain (mastalgia)

As for pain at any other site, you should establish the site, radiation, character, duration, severity, exacerbating factors, relieving factors, and associated symptoms. Also ask the following:

• Is the pain unilateral or bilateral?
• Is there any heat or redness at the site?
• Are there any other visible skin changes?
• Is the pain cyclical or constant—and is it related to menstruation?
• Is there a history of any previous similar episodes?
• Is the patient breastfeeding?
• Is the patient on any hormonal therapy (especially perimenopausal)?

The most common cause of mastalgia in premenopausal women is hormone-dependent change. Other benign causes include mastitis and abscesses. One in 100 breast cancers presents with mastalgia as the sole symptom.

Box 13.1 Menstrual history

It is important to take a clear and accurate menstrual history, as outlined in 📖 Chapter 14. Establish the following:

• Age of first menses
• Usual time between menstruation
• Usual duration of menstruation
• Usual quantity of menstruation
• Age of menopause (if applicable)
• Number of pregnancies
• Previous history of breast-feeding
• The date of the beginning of the last menstrual period.

Box 13.2 Male breast

Gynecomastia

This is enlargement of male breast tissue, which should not normally be palpable. There is an ↑ in ductal and connective tissue.

Gynecomastia is a common occurrence in adolescents and the elderly. It is seen in obese men due to increased adipose tissue.

In many patients, gynecomastia is drug related and the full causative list is long. Important drug causes include estrogen receptor binders, such as estrogen, digoxin, and marijuana, as well as anti-androgens, such as spironolactone and cimetidine.

▶ In the history, ask about drug and hormone treatment (e.g., for prostate cancer).

▶ You should also make a full examination of the patient, looking for signs of hypopituitarism, chronic liver disease, and thyrotoxicosis. Remember to carefully examine the genitalia.

Breast cancer in males

The female–male ratio for breast cancer is 100:1.

The appearance and pathology of breast cancer in males is similar to that in females.

The most common presentation in males is a hard, painless lump fixed to the skin or chest wall, followed by nipple discharge.

Nipple discharge

Important causes of nipple discharge include ductal pathology, such as ductal ectasia, papilloma, and carcinoma.

Ask about the following:

• Is the discharge true milk or some other substance?
• What color is the discharge (e.g., clear, white, yellow, blood-stained)?
• Is it spontaneous or nonspontaneous?
• Is the discharge unilateral or bilateral?
• Are there any changes in the appearance of the nipple or areola?
• Mastalgia?
• Are there any breast lumps?
• Periareolar abscesses or fistulae indicating periductal mastitis?
   • This is closely linked to smoking in young women. Periductal mastitis is also associated with hidradenitis suppuritiva. Ask about abscess elsewhere, e.g., axilla and groin. The symptoms are often recurrent.

🌕 Remember that after childbearing, some women continue to discharge a small secretion of milk (galactorrhea). However, in rare instances this can be the first presenting symptom of a prolactin-secreting pituitary adenoma. In the case of true bilateral galactorrhea, you should also ask about

• Headaches
• Visual disturbances, especially visual field deficits

Breast lumps

These are a very important presenting complaint with a number of causes (Box 13.3), the most important one being cancer (see Box 13.4 for risk factors). Establish the following:

• When the lump was first noticed
• Whether the lump has remained the same size or enlarged
• Whether the size of the lump changes according to menstrual cycle
• Is there any pain?
• Are there any local skin changes?
• Is there a history of breast lumps (ask about previous biopsies, diagnoses, and operations)?
• A full systems inquiry should include any other symptoms that might suggest a neoplastic disease (weight loss, loss of appetite, fatigue, etc.) and metastatic spread to other organ systems (shortness of breath, bony pain, etc.).

Age

A good clue as to the likely diagnosis of a lump is the age of the patient:

• Fibroadenomas are common between 20 and 30 years.
• Cysts are common between 30 and 50 years.
• Cancer is very rare <30 years of age but more likely in the >50 age-group.

Box 13.3 Some causes of breast lumps

• Cyst
• Fibroadenoma
• Carcinoma
• Fat necrosis
• Hamartoma
• Lipoma
• Epidermoid cyst
• Cystosarcoma

Box 13.4 Risk factors for breast cancer in females

• Advancing age
• Breast cancer in a first-degree relative
• *BRCA* genes
• Previous cancer in the other breast
• Early menarche (<12 years)
• Late menopause (>55 years)
• Nulliparity (no pregnancies)
• No previous breast-feeding
• Previous radiotherapy—e.g., mantle radiotherapy for Hodgkin's disease
• Oral contraceptive pill or hormone therapy

Inspection of the breast

Before you start
- When examining the female breast, you should have a chaperone present. Ideally, the chaperone should be female.*
- The patient should be fully undressed to the waist and sitting on the edge of the exam table with her arms by her side.
- You should be able to see the neck, breasts, chest wall, and arms.

General inspection
Stand in front of the patient and observe both breasts, noting:
- Size
- Tanner stage
- Symmetry
- Contour
- Color
- Scars
- Venous pattern on the skin
- Any dimpling or tethering of the skin
- Ulceration (describe fully as on 📖 p. 90)
- Skin texture, e.g., any visible nodularity
  - An unusual finding but one that should not be missed is the orange-peel appearance of *peau d'orange* caused by local edema. This is seen in breast carcinoma and following breast radiotherapy.

Nipples
Note whether the nipples are
- Symmetrical
- Everted, flat, or inverted
- Scaling (may indicate eczema or Paget's disease of the breast)
- Associated with any discharge
  - Single-duct discharge can indicate a papilloma or cancer.
  - Multiple-duct discharge at the nipple suggests ductal ectasia.

If abnormalities are present, ask if these are a recent or long-standing appearance. Make note of any additional nipples, which can occur anywhere along the mammary line.

Axillae
Ask the patient to place her hands on her head, and repeat the inspection process. Pay particular attention to any asymmetry or dimpling that is now evident. Examine the axillae for masses or color change.

Maneuvers
Finally, dimpling or fixation can be further accentuated by having the patient perform the following maneuvers (see Fig. 13.3):
- Lean forward while sitting
- Rest her hands on her hips
- Press her hands against her hips (pectoral contraction maneuver)

* Prudent advice is that *all* providers should have a chaperone present when performing an intimate examination and the chaperone should be the same sex as the patient.

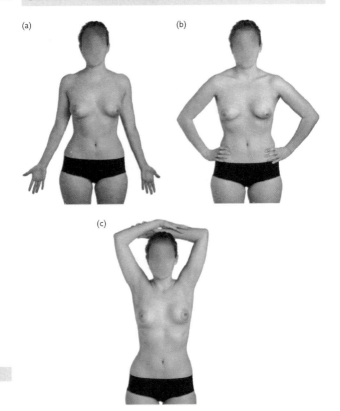

Fig. 13.3 Maneuvers for breast inspection. (a) Anatomical position. (b) Hands on hips. (c) Arms crossed above the head.

Palpation of the breast

Before you start

Palpation of the breast should be performed with the patient lying supine on the exam table. Examination of the breast is best performed with the hand on the side to be examined placed behind her head (Fig. 13.4). A maneuver for flattening a large breast is to have the patient roll onto her contralateral hip, keeping the shoulders flat against the table.[1]

Inform the patient that an adequate breast exam will take approximately 3 minutes per breast; taking this time will help in detecting breast masses.

Palpation

Ask the patient if there is any pain or tenderness, and examine that area last. Also ask her to tell you if you cause any pain during the examination.

Begin the examination on the asymptomatic side; this allows you to determine the texture of the normal breast first.

Ask the patient to point out any areas of tenderness; come to these last.

Breast

Palpation is performed by keeping the hand flat, using the finger pads and applying three levels of pressure as the breast tissue is palpated in a circular pattern against the underlying chest wall.

❶ Most breasts will feel lumpy if pinched.

You should proceed in a systematic way to ensure that the whole breast is examined. There are two regularly used methods (see Fig. 13.5); the authors favor the vertical strip method:

- Start below the areola and work outward in a circumferential pattern, ensuring that all quadrants have been examined.
- Examine breast systematically from the mid-axillary line, palpating up and down between the clavicle and the bra line toward the sternum.

▶ Do not forget to examine the axillary tail of Spence stretching from the upper-outer quadrant to the axilla.

Lumps

- If you feel a lump, describe it according to the method on 📖 p. 88, noting especially the position, color, shape, size, surface, nature of the surrounding skin, tenderness, consistency, temperature, and mobility.
- Next ascertain its relation to the overlying skin and underlying muscle.
- You must decide whether you are feeling a lump or a lumpy area.

Skin tethering

A lump may be described as *tethered* to the skin if it can be moved independently of the skin for a limited distance but pulls on the skin if moved further.

Tethering implies that an underlying lesion has infiltrated Cooper's ligaments, which pass from the skin through the subcutaneous fat.

Tethering may involve the skin itself with cancers or abscesses.

---

[1] Barton MB, Russell H, Fletcher SW (1999). Does this patient have breast cancer? The screening clinical breast examination: should it be done? How?, *JAMA* 282(13):1270–1280.

On inspection at rest, there may be puckering of the skin surface (as if being pulled from within) or there may be no visible abnormality.

To demonstrate tethering:
- Move the lump from side to side and look for skin dimpling at the extremes of movement.
- Ask the patient to lean forward while sitting.
- Ask the patient to raise her arms above her head as in Fig. 13.3.

Skin fixation

This is caused by direct, continuous infiltration of the skin by the underlying disease. The lump and the skin overlying it cannot be moved independently. It is on a continuum with skin tethering. This may be associated with some changes of skin texture.

Relation of a lump to muscle

The lump may be tethered or fixed to the underlying muscle (e.g., pectoralis major).

▶ Lumps attached to the underlying muscle can be moved to some degree if the muscle is relaxed but are less mobile if the muscle is tensed.
- Ask the patient to rest her hand on her hip with the arm relaxed.
- Hold the lump between your thumb and forefingers and estimate its mobility by moving it in two planes at right angles to each other (e.g., up/down and left/right).
- Ask the patient to press her hand against her hip, causing contraction of pectoralis major. Repeat the mobility exercise.

Immobile lumps

If a lump is immobile in all situations, it may have spread to involve the bony chest wall (e.g., in the upper half of the breast or axilla).

Nipple

If the patient complains of nipple discharge, ask her to gently squeeze and express any discharge. Note the color, presence of blood, and odor.

Milky, serous or green-brown discharges are almost always benign. A bloody discharge may indicate neoplasia (e.g., papilloma or cancer).

Although the time typically spent palpating the breast is considered an excellent time to instruct the patient in self-examination, recent recommendations have not supported the usefulness of teaching it. In any case, women should be counseled on breast awareness. Providers should continue to look for further information on this.

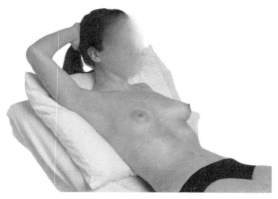

Fig. 13.4 Correct position of the patient for examination of the breast.

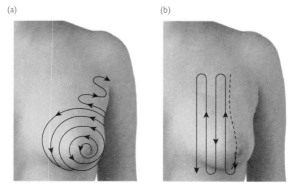

(a)   (b)

Fig. 13.5 Two methods for systematic palpation of the breast. (a) Work circumferentially from the areola. (b) Examine each half at a time, working from bottom to top.

Examining beyond the breast

Lymph nodes

The technique is described in detail on 📖 p. 58.

Support the patient's arm. For example, when examining the right axilla, abduct the patient's right arm gently and support it at the wrist with your right hand while examining the axilla with your left hand.

Examine the main sets of axillary nodes (Fig. 13.6):

- Central
- Lateral
- Medial (pectoral)
- Infraclavicular
- Supraclavicular (Fig. 13.7)
- Apical

If you feel any lymph nodes, consider site, size, number, consistency, tenderness, fixation, and overlying skin changes.

Remember to also palpate for lymph nodes in the lower deep cervical lymph chain at the same time as the supraclavicular nodes.

The rest of the body

If cancer is suspected, perform a full general examination, keeping in mind the common sites of metastasis of breast cancer. Examine especially the lungs, liver, skin, skeleton, and central nervous system.

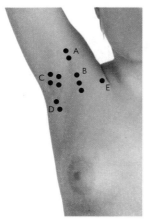

A = Lateral
B = Pectoral
C = Central
D = Subscapular
E = Infraclavicular

Fig. 13.6 Axillary lymph nodes.

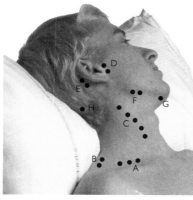

A = Supraclavicular
B = Posterior triangle
C = Jugular chain
D = Preauricular
E = Postauricular
F = Submandibular
G = Submental
H = Occipital

Fig. 13.7 Cervical and supraclavicular lymph nodes.

Important presentations

Fibroadenoma

This is a benign neoplasm of the breast that is composed of both fibrous and glandular tissue. It is usually found in young women <30 years old.

It presents as a painless, solid, mobile, well-circumscribed, rounded breast mass with a smooth surface and rubbery consistency.

They may be multiple and bilateral with no axillary lymphadenopathy. Large fibroadenomas may be found in teenagers.

Fibrocystic disease

This is another common benign breast condition consisting of fibrous (rubbery) and cystic changes in the breast.

It usually presents with pain or tenderness that varies with the menstrual cycle. Cysts and fibrous nodular fullness can be found on examination. A solitary cyst is usually smooth, spherical, and tense. It is rarely possible to elicit fluctuation or to transilluminate. The axillary lymph nodes should not be palpable.

Fat necrosis

This can occur after trauma. The physical signs can mimic cancer (e.g., a firm, hard lump with skin tethering).

Abscesses

These occur mainly during childbearing years and are often associated with trauma to the nipple during breast-feeding.

They present with a painful, spherical lump with surrounding edema. Breast often shows additional signs of inflammation (hot, red). The patient may have constitutional symptoms, including malaise, night sweats, hot flushes, and rigors.

Most recurrent or chronic breast abscesses occur in association with duct ectasia or periductal mastitis. The associated periductal fibrosis can often lead to nipple retraction.

Abnormal nipple and areola

Diseases of the nipple are important because they must be differentiated from malignancy and they cause concern to patients.

Unilateral retraction or distortion of a nipple is a common sign of breast carcinoma, as is blood-stained nipple discharge. The latter suggests an intraductal carcinoma or benign papilloma.

A unilateral red, crusted, and scaling areola suggests an underlying carcinoma (Paget's disease of the breast) or, more commonly, eczema. Ask the patient if she has eczema at other sites and examine appropriately.

Breast cancer

After non-melanoma skin cancers, breast cancer is the most common form of cancer affecting women in the United States. It is second to lung cancer as a cause of cancer mortality.* It is rare under the age of 35, with the incidence steadily increasing per decade.

There are a number of risk factors (see 📖 Box 13.4, p. 396). Several on-line risk calculators are available for use by patients and clinicians to estimate breast cancer risk (www.nci.nih.gov; Gail model).

There are two main types, which may be invasive or in situ:
• Ductal
• Lobular

In situ cancer is usually not palpable and diagnosed on mammography or biopsy. Clinicians should remember that mammography does not detect all breast cancers. It is estimated that 4–10% of cancers will be detected on clinician exam alone.

There are a number of prognostic factors in breast cancer, mostly related to the histological presentation of the tumor.

Presenting symptoms

The presenting symptoms may be related to the primary lesion. For example:
• Palpable mass
• Pain (1/100 cancers present with mastalgia only)
• Nipple discharge, retraction, or rash
• Dimpling of the breast tissue
• Local edema

The presenting symptom may be related to the effects of secondary spread. For example:
• Arm swelling (lymphatic or venous obstruction)
• Backache (skeletal infiltration)
• Malaise
• Loss of weight
• Dyspnea
• Cough
• Nodules in skin
• Jaundice
• Mental changes
• Seizures
• Symptoms of hypercalcemia (e.g., thirst)

---

* http://www.cdc.gov/cancer/breast/statistics/

Female reproductive system

Applied anatomy

Pelvis

The bony pelvis is composed of the two pelvic bones with the sacrum and coccyx posteriorly. The pelvic brim divides the "false pelvis" above (part of the abdominal cavity) and the "true pelvis" below.

- *Pelvic inlet:* also known as the pelvic brim. It is formed by the sacral promontory posteriorly, the iliopectineal lines laterally, and the symphysis pubis anteriorly.
- *Pelvic outlet:* formed by the coccyx posteriorly, ischial tuberosities laterally, and pubic arch anteriorly. The pelvic outlet has three wide notches. The sciatic notches are divided into the greater and lesser sciatic foramina by the sacrotuberous and sacrospinous ligaments, which can be considered part of the perimeter of the outlet clinically.
- *The pelvic cavity:* lies between the inlet and the outlet. It has a deep posterior wall and a shallow anterior wall giving a curved shape.

The contents of the pelvic cavity

The pelvic cavity contains the rectum, sigmoid colon, coils of the ileum, ureters, bladder, female reproductive organs, fascia, and peritoneum.

Female internal genital organs

Vagina

The vagina is a thin-walled distensible, fibromuscular tube that extends up and backward from the vestibule of the vulva to the cervix. It is ~8 cm long and lies posterior to the bladder and anterior to the rectum.

The vagina serves as an eliminatory passage for menstrual flow, forms part of the birth canal, and receives the penis during sexual intercourse.

Fornix

This is the vaginal recess around the cervix and is divided into anterior, posterior, and lateral regions, which, clinically, provide access points for examining the pelvic organs.

Uterus

The uterus is a thick-walled, hollow, pear-shaped muscular organ consisting of the cervix, body, and fundus. In the nulliparous female, it is 7–8 cm long, ~5 cm wide, and ~2.5 cm deep. The uterus is covered with peritoneum that forms an anterior uterovesical fold, a fold between the uterus and rectum termed the *pouch of Douglas*, and broad ligaments laterally.

The uterus receives, retains, and nourishes the fertilized ovum.

Uterine orientation

In most females, the uterus lies in an anteverted and anteflexed position.
- *Anteversion:* the long axis of the uterus is angled forward.
- *Retroversion:* The fundus and body are angled backward and therefore lie in the pouch of Douglas. This occurs in about 15% of the female population. A full bladder may result in retroversion clinically.

- *Anteflexion:* The long axis of the body of the uterus is angled forward on the long axis of the cervix.
- *Retroflexion:* The body of the uterus is angled backward on the cervix.

Fallopian tubes

The fallopian, or uterine, tubes are paired tubular structures ~10 cm long. The fallopian tubes extend laterally from the cornua of the uterine body, in the upper border of the broad ligament, and open into the peritoneal cavity near the ovaries. The fallopian tube is divided into four parts:

- *Infundibulum:* distal, funnel-shaped portion with finger-like fimbriae
- *Ampulla:* widest and longest part of tube outside the uterus
- *Isthmus:* thick-walled with a narrow lumen and, therefore, least distensible part. The isthmus enters the horns of the uterine body.
- *Intramural:* that part which pierces the uterine wall

The main functions of the uterine tube are to receive the ovum from the ovary, provide a site where fertilization can take place (usually in the ampulla), and transport the ovum from the ampulla to the uterus. The tube also provides nourishment for the fertilized ovum.

Ovaries

The ovaries are whitish-gray, almond-shaped organs measuring ~4 cm x 2 cm that are responsible for production of the female germ cells, ova, and female sex hormones, estrogen and progesterone.

They are suspended on the posterior layer of the broad ligament by a peritoneal extension (mesovarium) and supported by the suspensory ligament of the ovary (a lateral extension of the broad ligament and meso-varium) and the round ligament, which stretches from the lateral wall of the uterus to the medial aspect of the ovary.

Perineum

The perineum lies inferior to the pelvic inlet and is separated from the pelvic cavity by the pelvic diaphragm.

Seen from below with the thighs abducted, it is a diamond-shaped area bounded anteriorly by the pubic symphysis, posteriorly by the tip of the coccyx, and laterally by the ischial tuberosities.

The perineum is artificially divided into the anterior urogenital triangle, containing the external genitalia in females, and an anal triangle, containing the anus and ischiorectal fossae.

Female external genital organs

These are collectively known as the *vulva.* It consists of the following:

- *Labia majora:* a pair of fat-filled folds of skin extending on either side of the vaginal vestibule from the mons towards the anus.
- *Labia minora:* a pair of flat folds containing a core of spongy connective tissue with a rich vascular supply. Lie medial to the labia majora.
- *Vestibule of the vagina:* between the labia minora, contains the urethral meatus and vaginal orifice. Outlet for mucous secretions from the greater and lesser vestibular glands.

- ***Clitoris:*** short, erectile organ; the female homologue of the male penis. Like the penis, a crus arises from each ischiopubic ramus and join in the midline forming the 'body' capped by the sensitive 'glans'.
- ***Bulbs of vestibule:*** 2 masses of elongated erectile tissue, ~3 cm long, lying along the sides of the vaginal orifice.
- ***Bulbs of vestibule:*** Greater and lesser vestibular glands.

Applied physiology

Menstrual cycle

Menstruation is the shedding of the functional superficial 2/3 of the endometrium after sex hormone withdrawal. This process, consisting of three phases, is typically repeated ~300–400 times during a woman's life. Coordination of the menstrual cycle depends on a complex inter-play between the hypothalamus, pituitary gland, ovaries, and uterine endometrium.

Cyclical changes in the endometrium prepare it for implantation in the event of fertilization and menstruation in the absence of fertilization. It should be noted that several other tissues are sensitive to these hormones and undergo cyclical change (e.g., the breasts and the lower part of the urinary tract).

The endometrial cycle can de divided into three phases.

Phases of the menstrual cycle

The first day of the menses is considered day 1 of the menstrual cycle.

Proliferative or follicular phase

This begins at the end of the menstrual phase (usually day 4) and ends at ovulation (days 13–14). During this phase, the endometrium thickens and ovarian follicles mature.

The hypothalamus is the initiator of the follicular phase. Gonadotrophin-releasing hormone (GnRH) is released from the hypothalamus in a pulsa-tile fashion to the pituitary portal system surrounding the anterior pituitary gland. GnRH causes release of follicle-stimulating hormone (FSH). FSH is secreted into the general circulation and interacts with the granulosa cells surrounding the dividing oocytes.

FSH enhances the development of 15–20 follicles each month and interacts with granulosa cells to enhance aromatization of androgens into estrogen and estradiol.

Only one follicle with the largest reservoir of estrogen can withstand the declining FSH environment, while the remaining follicles undergo atresia at the end of this phase.

Follicular estrogen synthesis is essential for uterine priming but is also part of the positive feedback that induces a dramatic preovulatory lutein-izing hormone (LH) surge and subsequent ovulation.

Luteal or secretory phase

The luteal phase starts at ovulation and lasts through day 28 of the men-strual cycle.

The major effects of the LH surge are the conversion of granulosa cells from predominantly androgen-converting cells to predominantly progesterone-synthesizing cells. High progesterone levels exert negative feedback on GnRH, which in turn ↓ FSH/LH secretion.

At the beginning of the luteal phase, progesterone induces the endome-trial glands to secrete glycogens, mucus, and other substances. These glands become tortuous and have large lumina due to ↑ secretory activity. Spiral arterioles extend into the superficial layer of the endometrium.

In the absence of fertilization by day 23 of the menstrual cycle, the superficial endometrium begins to degenerate, and consequently ovarian hormone levels ↓. As estrogen and progesterone levels fall, the endometrium undergoes involution.

If the corpus luteum is not sustained by human chorionic gonadotrophin (hCG) hormone from the developing placenta, menstruation occurs 14 days after ovulation. If conception occurs, placental hCG maintains luteal function until placental production of progesterone is well established.

Menstrual phase
In this phase, there is a gradual withdrawal of ovarian sex steroids, which causes slight shrinking of the endometrium, thus the blood flow of spiral vessels is reduced. This, together with spiral arteriolar spasms, leads to distal endometrial ischemia and stasis. Extravasation of blood and endometrial tissue breakdown lead to the onset of menstruation.

The menstrual phase begins as the spiral arteries rupture, releasing blood into the uterus and the apoptosing endometrium is sloughed off.

During this period, the functionalis layer of the endometrium is completely shed. Arteriolar and venous blood, remnants of endometrial stroma and glands, leukocytes, and red blood cells are all present in the menstrual flow. Shedding usually lasts ~4–7 days.

History-taking in gynecology

It is important to remember that many females can be embarrassed by having to discuss their gynecological problems, so it is vital to appear confident, remaining open to questions or concerns, and be nonjudgmental.

Although there are parts particular to this history, most of it is the same as the basic outline described in 📖 Chapter 2. We suggest that readers review that chapter before going on.

Patient profile
This includes the patient's name, age, date of birth, and occupation.

Chief complaint
Ask the patient to tell you in her own words what she perceives as being the main symptoms. Document each in order of severity.

History of presenting illness
More detailed questioning will depend on the presenting complaint (see following pages). As described on 📖 p. 33, ascertain the following:
- Exact nature of the symptom
- Onset
  - When and how it began (e.g., suddenly, gradually—over how long?)
  - If long-standing, why is the patient seeking help now?
- Periodicity and frequency
  - Is the symptom constant or intermittent?
  - If intermittent, how long does it last each time?
  - What is the exact manner in which it comes and goes?
  - ► How does it relate to the menstrual cycle?
- Change over time
- Exacerbating and relieving factors
- Associated symptoms
- Degree of functional disability caused

Menstrual history
- Age of menarche (first menstrual period)
  - Normally at about 12 years, but can be as early as 9 or as late as 16
- Date of last menstrual period (LMP)
- Duration and regularity of periods (cycle)
  - Normal menstruation lasts 4–7 days.
  - The average length of the menstrual cycle is 28 days (i.e., the time between first day of one period and the first day of the following period), but it can vary between 21 and 42 days in normal women.
- Menstrual flow: whether light, normal, or heavy (see 📖 p. 415)
- Menstrual pain: whether it occurs prior to or at the start of bleeding
- Irregular bleeding
  - E.g., intermenstrual blood loss, postcoital bleeding
- Associated symptoms
  - Bowel or bladder dysfunction, pain
- Hormonal contraception or hormone therapy (HT)
- Age at menopause (if this has occurred)

Past gynecological history

Record all details of the following:
- Previous cervical smears, including date of last Pap smear, any abnormal smear results, and treatments received
- Previous history and results of human papillomavirus (HPV) testing
- Previous history of HPV vaccination
- Previous gynecological problems and treatments, including surgery and pelvic inflammatory disease (PID)

Contraception

It is essential to ask women of reproductive age who are sexually active with men about contraception, including the methods used, duration of use and acceptance, current method, and future plans.

Past obstetric history

- Gravidity and parity: see ▢ p. 434 for a full explanation.

Document the specifics of each pregnancy:
- Current age of the child and age of the mother when pregnant
- Birth weight
- Complications of pregnancy, labor, and puerperium
- Miscarriages and terminations. Note gestation time and complications. Ask if Rhogam was given if Rh negative.

Past medical history

This is as described in ▢ Chapter 2. Pay particular attention to any history of chronic lung or heart disease, and note all previous surgical procedures.

Drug history

This is as described in ▢ Chapter 2. Ask about all medication and drugs taken (prescribed, over the counter, herbs, vitamins, and illicit drugs). Record dosage and frequency, as well as any known drug allergies.
▶ Make particular note to ask about use of the oral contraceptive pill (OCP), patch, implant, vaginal ring, or hormone-releasing intrauterine device (IUD) and of HT if not done so already.

Family history

Note especially any history of genital tract cancer, breast cancer, or diabetes.

Smoking and alcohol

As always, document this fully, as described on ▢ p. 37.

Social history

Take a standard SH, including living conditions and marital status.

This is also an extra chance to explore the impact of the presenting problem on the patient's life, in terms of her social life, employment, home life, and sexual activity (see Sexual History, ▢ p. 378). This discussion may lead to issues far beyond the presenting complaint.

It is important to obtain a history regarding sexual abuse (rape, incest, childhood molestation). Women who have a history of sexual abuse may have flashbacks during an exam or may be unable to tolerate a full exam.

Abnormal bleeding in gynecology

Menorrhagia

This is defined as >80 mL of menstrual blood loss per period (normal = 20–60 mL) and may be caused by a variety of local, systemic, or iatrogenic factors. Menorrhagia is hard to measure, but periods are considered heavy if they lead to frequent changes (every 1–2 hours) of sanitary products and there are clots >1 inch in diameter. Causes are listed in Box 14.1

In the absence of structural uterine disease or other pathology, menorrhagia can also be described as *dysfunctional uterine bleeding* (DUB). This is often found in adolescence or in the perimenopausal period.

In addition to the standard questions for any symptom, ask about the following:

- Number of sanitary pads or tampons used per day and the strength (absorbency) of those products
- Bleeding through to clothes or onto the bedding at night (flooding)
- The need to use two pads at once
- The need to wear double protection (i.e., pad and tampon together)
- Any clots in the menstrual flow (compare to the size of coins)
- Interference with normal activities

▶ Remember to ask about symptoms of iron-deficiency anemia, such as lethargy, breathlessness, and dizziness.

Dysmenorrhea

This is pain associated with menstruation and is thought to be caused by ↑ levels of endometrial prostaglandins during the luteal and menstrual phases of the cycle, resulting in uterine contractions (Box 14.2). The pain is typically cramping, localized to the lower abdomen and pelvic regions and radiating to the thighs and back.

Dysmenorrhea may be primary or secondary:

- *Primary:* occurring from menarche

Box 14.1 Some causes of menorrhagia

- Hypothyroidism
- IUD
- Fibroids
- Endometriosis
- Polyps—cervix, uterus
- Uterine cancer
- Infection (STIs)
- Previous sterilization
- Warfarin therapy
- Aspirin
- NSAIDs
- Clotting disorders (e.g., von-Willebrand's disease)

Box 14.2 Some causes of secondary dysmenorrhea

- Pelvic inflammatory disease
- Endometriosis
- Uterine adenomyosis
- Fibroids
- Endometrial polyps
- Premenstrual syndrome
- Cessation of OCP

Box 14.3 Some causes of intermenstrual bleeding

- **Obstetric:** pregnancy, ectopic pregnancy, gestational trophoblastic disease
- **Gynecological:** vaginal malignancy, vaginitis, cervical cancer, adenomyosis, fibroids, ovarian cancer
- **Iatrogenic:** anticoagulants, corticosteroids, antipsychotics, tamoxifen, selective serotinin reuptake inhibitors (SSRIs), rifampicin, antiepileptic drugs (AEDs)

- **Secondary:** occurring in females who previously had normal periods (often caused by pelvic pathology)

When taking a history of dysmenorrhea, take a full pain history as on p. 33 and detailed menstrual history (p. 413), and ask about the relationship of the pain to the menstrual cycle. Remember to ask about the functional consequences of the pain—how does it interfere with normal activities?

Intermenstrual bleeding (IMB)

Intermenstrual bleeding is uterine bleeding that occurs between the menstrual periods. Causes are listed in Box 14.3

As for all of these symptoms, a full standard battery of questions should be asked (p. 413), as full menstrual history (p. 413), past medical and gynecological histories (p. 414), and sexual history (p. 414).

Ask also about association of the bleeding with hormonal therapy, contraceptive use, and previous cervical smears.

Postcoital bleeding

This is vaginal bleeding precipitated by sexual intercourse. It can be caused by similar conditions to those for intermenstrual bleeding (Box 14.4). Take a full and detailed history, as for IMB.

Amenorrhea

This is the absence of periods and may be primary or secondary.

- **Primary:** failure to menstruate by 16 years of age in the presence of normal secondary sexual development or failure to menstruate by 14 years in the absence of secondary sexual characteristics.

Box 14.4 Some causes of postcoital bleeding

These are similar to those for intermenstrual bleeding, as well as vaginal infection with *Chlamydia*, gonorrhea, trichomoniasis, or yeast. Cervicitis can also result in bleeding.

Box 14.5 Some causes of amenorrhea

- *Hypothalamic:* idiopathic, weight loss, intense exercise
- *Hypogonadism from hypothalamic or pituitary damage:* tumors, craniopharyngiomas, cranial irradiation, head injuries
- *Pituitary:* hyperprolactinemia, hypopituitarism
- *Delayed puberty:* constitutional delay
- *Systemic:* chronic illness, weight loss, endocrine disorders (e.g., Cushing's syndrome, thyroid disorders)
- *Uterine:* mullerian agenesis
- *Ovarian:* PCOS, premature ovarian failure (e.g., Turner's syndrome, autoimmune disease, surgery, chemotherapy, pelvic irradiation, infection)
- *Psychological:* emotional stress at school, home, or work

- *Secondary:* normal menarche, then cessation of menstruation with no periods for at least 6 months.
▶ Amenorrhea is a normal feature in prepubertal girls, pregnancy, during lactation, postmenopausal females, and in some women using hormonal contraception (see Box 14.5).

History-taking

A full and detailed history should be taken as described on 📖 p. 33 and in 📖 Chapter 2. Ask especially about the following:
- Childhood growth and development
- If secondary amenorrhea:
  - Age of menarche
  - Cycle days
  - Day and date of LMP
  - Presence or absence of breast soreness
  - Mood change immediately before menses
- Chronic illnesses
- Previous surgery (including cervical surgery, which can cause stenosis, and, more obviously, oophorectomy and hysterectomy)
- Prescribed medications known to cause amenorrhea, such as phenothiazines and metoclopramide (they produce either hyperprolactinemia or ovarian failure)
- Illicit or recreational drugs
- Sexual history
- Social history, including any emotional stress at school, work, or home, and exercise and diet—include here any weight gain or weight loss.

- Systems review: include vasomotor symptoms, hot flashes, virilizing changes (e.g., ↑ body hair, greasy skin), galactorrhea, headaches, visual field disturbance, palpitations, nervousness, hearing loss

Postmenopausal bleeding

This is vaginal bleeding occurring >6 months after menopause. It requires reassurance and prompt investigation, as it could indicate the presence of malignancy (see Box 14.6). In addition to the points outlined for amenorrhea, ask about the following:

- Local symptoms of estrogen deficiency, such as vaginal dryness, soreness, and superficial dyspareunia (📖 p. 419)
- Itching (pruritus vulvae—more likely in non-neoplastic disorders)
- Presence of lumps or swellings at the vulva

Cervical or endometrial malignancy

This is often present with profuse or continuous vaginal bleeding or with a bloodstained, malodorous discharge.

Box 14.6 Some causes of postmenopausal bleeding

- Cervical carcinoma
- Uterine sarcoma
- Vaginal carcinoma
- Endometrial hyperplasia, carcinoma, or polyps
- Cervical polyps
- Trauma
- Hormone therapy (HT)
- Bleeding disorder
- Vaginal atrophy
- Sexually transmitted infections

Other symptoms in gynecology

Pelvic pain and dyspareunia

As with any type of pain, pelvic pain may be acute or chronic (see also Box 14.7). Chronic pelvic pain is often associated with dyspareunia.

Dyspareunia

This is painful sexual intercourse and may be experienced superficially at the area of the vulva and introitus on penetration or deep within the pelvis (see Box 14.8 for causes). Dyspareunia can lead to failure to reach orgasm, avoidance of sexual activity, and relationship problems.

When taking a history of pelvic pain or dyspareunia, you should obtain a detailed history as for any type of pain (📖 p. 34) including site, radiation, character, severity, mode and rate of onset, duration, frequency, exacerbating factors, relieving factors, and associated symptoms.

You also need to establish the relationship of the pain to the menstrual cycle. Ask about the following:
- Date of LMP
- Cervical (Pap) smears
- Intermenstrual or postcoital bleeding
- Previous gynecological procedures (e.g., IUD, hysteroscopy)
- Previous PID or genitourinary infections
- Previous gynecological surgery (adhesion formation?)
- Vulvovaginal discharge

Box 14.7 Gynecological vs. gastrointestinal pain

Distinguishing between pain of gynecological and gastrointestinal origin is often difficult. This is because the uterus, cervix, and adnexae share the same visceral innervation as the lower ileum, sigmoid colon, and rectum. Be careful in your history to rule out a gastrointestinal problem, and keep an open mind.

Box 14.8 Some causes of dyspareunia

- Scars from episiotomy
- Vaginal atrophy
- Vulvitis
- Vulvar vestibulitis
- PID
- Ovarian cysts
- Endometriosis
- Varicose veins in pelvis
- Ectopic pregnancy
- Infections (STIs)
- Bladder or urinary tract disorder
- Cancer in the reproductive organs or pelvic region

- Bowel habit, nausea, and vomiting (📖 p. 208)
- A detailed sexual history (📖 p. 378) should include contraceptive use and the degree of impact the symptoms have on the patient's normal life and psychological health.

Vaginal discharge

Vaginal discharge is a common complaint during the childbearing years. In addition to the standard questions (📖 p. 413), ask about the following:
- Color, volume, odor, and presence of blood
- Irritation
- Hygiene habits including douching
- Which OTC remedies have been tried

▶ Don't forget to ask about diabetes and obtain a full drug history, including recent antibiotic use; both may precipitate candidal infection.
- Obtain a full sexual history (📖 p. 378). A full gynecological history should include history of cervical (Pap) smear testing, use of ring pessaries, and recent history of surgery (↑ risk of vesicovaginal fistulae).

▶ Lower abdominal pain, backache, and dyspareunia suggest PID.
▶ Weight loss and anorexia may indicate underlying malignancy.

Physiological vaginal discharge

Physiological discharge is usually scanty, mucoid, and odorless. It occurs with the changing estrogen and progesterone levels during the menstrual cycle (clear discharge ↑ in quantity mid-cycle, with subsequent thickening as a physiological sign of ovulation) and pregnancy.

It may arise from vestibular gland secretions, vaginal transudate, cervical mucus, and residual menstrual fluid.

Pathological vaginal discharge

This usually represents infection (trichomonal or candidal vaginitis) and may be associated with pruritus or burning of the vulval area.
- *Candida albicans:* discharge is typically thick and causes itching
- *Bacterial vaginitis:* discharge is gray and watery with a fishy smell. It is seen especially after intercourse.
- *Trichomonas vaginalis:* discharge is typically profuse, opaque, cream-colored, and frothy. It also has a characteristic fishy smell. This may also be accompanied by urinary symptoms, such as dysuria and frequency.

Vulval symptoms

The main symptom to be aware of is itching or irritation of the vulva (pruritis vulvae). It can be debilitating and socially embarrassing. Embarrassment often delays the seeking of advice.

Causes include infection, vulval dystrophy, neoplasia, and other dermatological conditions. Ask especially about the following:
- Nature of onset, exacerbating and relieving factors
- Abnormal vaginal discharge
- History of cervical intraepithelial neoplasia ([CIN] thought to share a common etiology with vulval intraepithelial neoplasia [VIN])
- Sexual history

- Dermatological conditions such as psoriasis and eczema
- Symptoms suggestive of renal or liver problems (📖 p. 210)
- Diabetes
- Use of douching and feminine hygiene products

Urinary incontinence

This is an objectively demonstrable involuntary loss of urine that can be both a social and hygienic problem.

The two most common causes of urinary incontinence in females are *stress incontinence (SI)* and *detrusor overactivity (DO)*. Other less commonly encountered causes include mixed SI and DO, sensory urgency, chronic voiding problems, and fistulae.

When taking a history of urinary incontinence, ascertain under what circumstances the patient experiences symptom. See also 📖 p. 218. Remember to ask about the functional consequences on the patient's daily life.

Stress incontinence

Patients notice small amounts of urinary leakage with a cough, sneeze, or exercise. One-third may also admit to symptoms of DO.

Ask about the following:
- Number of children (↑ risk with ↑ parity)
- Genital prolapse
- Previous pelvic floor surgery

Detruser overactivity

With DO there is urge incontinence, urgency, frequency, and nocturia (see 📖 p. 447). Ask about the following:
- History of nocturnal enuresis
- Previous neurological problems
- Previous incontinence surgery
- Incontinence during sexual intercourse
- Drug history (see note under The Elderly Patient, 📖 p. 447)

Overflow incontinence

Voiding disorders can result in chronic retention, leading to overflow incontinence and ↑ predisposition to infection. The patient may complain of hesitancy, straining, poor flow, and incomplete emptying in addition to urgency and frequency.

Fistulae

Suspect these if incontinence is continuous during the day and night.

Genital prolapse

Genital prolapse is descent of the pelvic organs through the pelvic floor into the vaginal canal (possible causes are listed in Box 14.9). In the female genital tract, the type of prolapse is named according to the pelvic organ involved. Some examples include the following:
- Uterine: uterus
- Cystocele: bladder
- Vaginal vault prolapse: apex of vagina after hysterectomy
- Enterocele: small bowel
- Rectocele: rectum

Mild degrees of genital prolapse are often asymptomatic. More extensive prolapse may cause vaginal pressure or pain, introital bulging, a feeling of something coming down, and impaired sexual function.

Uterine descent often gives symptoms of backache, especially in older patients.

There might be associated symptoms of incomplete bowel emptying (rectocele) or urinary symptoms such as frequency or incomplete emptying (cystocele or cystourethrocele).

Box 14.9 Some causes of genital prolapse

- *Estrogen-deficiency states:* advancing age and menopause (atrophy and weakness of the pelvic support structures)
- *Childbirth:* prolonged labor, instrumental delivery, fetal macrosomia, ↑ parity
- *Genetic or congenital factors:* e.g., spina bifida
- *Chronic raised intra-abdominal pressure:* e.g., chronic cough, constipation

---

Box 14.10 Some other common vulval conditions

- *Dermatitis:* atopic, seborrheic, irritant, allergic, steroid induced (itch, burning, erythema, scale, fissures, lichenification)
- *Vulvovaginal candidiasis:* itch, burning, erythema, vaginal discharge
- *Lichen sclerosus:* itch, burning, dyspareunia, white plaques, atrophic wrinkled surface
- *Psoriasis:* remember to look for other areas of psoriasis; scalp, natal cleft, nails
- *Vulval intraepithelial neoplasia:* itch, burning, multifocal plaques
- *Erosive vulvovaginitis:* erosive lichen planus, pemphigoid, pemphigus vulgaris, fixed drug eruption (chronic painful erosion and ulcers with superficial bleeding)
- *Atrophic vaginitis:* secondary to estrogen deficiency (thin, pale, dry vaginal epithelium; superficial dyspareunia, minor vaginal bleeding, pain)

Outline gynecological examination

The gynecological examination should include a full abdominal examination before proceeding to pelvic, speculum, and bimanual examinations.

Explain to the patient that you would like to examine their genitalia and reproductive organs, and reassure them that the procedure will be quick and gentle. You should have a chaperone present, particularly if you are male.*

As always, ensure that the room is warm and well lit, preferably with a moveable light source, and that you will not be disturbed.

The examination should follow an orderly routine. The authors' suggestion is shown in Box 14.11. It is standard practice to start with the cardiovascular and respiratory systems—this not only gives a measure of the general health of the patient but also establishes a physical rapport before you examine more sensitive areas.

General inspection and other systems

Always begin with a general examination of the patient (as described in 📖 Chapter 3), including temperature, hydration, coloration, nutritional status, lymph nodes, and blood pressure. Note especially the following:

- Distribution of facial and body hair, as hirsutism may be a presenting symptom of various endocrine disorders
- Height and weight
- Examine the cardiovascular and respiratory systems in turn(see 📖 Chapters 7 and 8).
- Examine the breast in a systematic approach. Although the value of teaching and performing breast self-exam is debated, patient education on breast awareness during the exam is a good use of time and should be done (see 📖 Chapter 13).

Abdominal examination

A full abdominal examination should be performed (see 📖 Chapter 9). Look especially in the periumbilical region for scars from previous laparoscopies and in the suprapubic region, where transverse incisions from caesarean sections and most gynecological operations are found.

Box 14.11 Framework for gynecological examination

- General inspection
- Cardiorespiratory examination
- Breast examination
- Abdominal examination
- Pelvic examination
  - External genitalia—inspection
  - External genitalia—palpation
  - Speculum examination
  - Bimanual examination

---

* Attitudes regarding chaperones vary. Official advice is that *all* providers should have a chaperone when performing an intimate examination and the chaperone should be the same sex as the patient. In practice, male providers performing an examination on a female and females performing an examination on a male should always have a chaperone present; the need for a chaperone in other situations is judged at the time.

Pelvic examination

The patient should be allowed to undress in privacy and, if necessary, to empty her bladder first.

Setup and positioning

Before starting the examination, explain to the patient what will be involved. Keep the abdomen covered. Ensure good lighting, and always wear disposable, latex-free gloves.

Ask the patient to lie on her back on an examination table with both knees bent up; the head of the table can be raised for comfort. The buttocks should be at the edge of the main table surface, with the heels placed in stirrups or the feet on the table extension. Her knees should fall to the side when the exam starts. In many clinical settings, it is standard to use stirrups to support the heels; however, keeping the feet on the table extension during the exam has been found to increase comfort and decrease the patient's sense of vulnerability during the exam.[1]

Examination of the external genitalia

- Uncover the mons to expose the external genitalia, making note of the pattern of hair distribution.
- Separate the labia from above with the forefinger and thumb of your gloved left hand.
- Inspect the clitoris, urethral meatus, and vaginal opening.
- Look especially for any of the following:
  - Discharge
  - Redness
  - Ulceration
  - Atrophy
  - Old scars
- Ask the patient to cough or strain down and look at the vaginal walls for any prolapse.

Palpation

- Palpate length of the labia majora between the index finger and thumb.
  - The tissue should feel pliant and fleshy.
- Palpate for Bartholin's gland with the index finger of the right hand just inside the introitus and thumb on the outer aspect of labium majora.
  - Bartholin's glands are only palpable if the duct becomes obstructed, resulting in a painless cystic mass or an acute Bartholin's abscess. The latter is seen as a hot, red, tender swelling in the posterolateral labia majora.

Speculum examination

Speculum examination is carried out to see further inside the vagina and to visualize the cervix. It also allows the examiner to take a cervical smear or swabs.

---

[1] Seehusen DA, Johnson DR, Earwood JS, et al. (2006). Improving women's experience during speculum examinations at routine gynaecological visits: randomized clinical trial. *BMJ* 333:171.

(a)   (b)

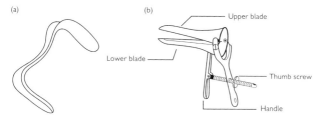

Fig. 14.1 (a) Sim's speculum—used mainly in examination of women with vaginal prolapse. (b) Cusco's speculum.

Box 14.12 A word about specula

Many departments and clinical areas now used plastic or disposable specula. These do not have a thumb-screw but have a ratchet to open and close the blades.

Take care to familiarize yourself with the operation of the speculum-*before* starting the examination. The clicking noise can startle a patient, so it is best to comment on this prior to insertion.

Plastic specula with a light source are very convenient and much easier to use than struggling to properly position a large lamp.

There are different types of vaginal specula (see Fig. 14.1), but the most common is the bivalve speculum (Peders on or Graves). Plastic, disposable speculum are in use in many clinics. It is important that you familiarize yourself with the operation of the speculum before examining a patient so that you can concentrate on the findings (see Box 14.12).

Inserting the speculum
- Explain to the patient that you are about to insert the speculum into the vagina, and provide reassurance that this should not be painful.
- Warm the speculum under running water.
- Test the temperature of the speculum on the inner thigh (warning the patient before this is done).
- Using the left hand, open the lips of the labia minora to obtain a good view of the introitus.
- Hold the speculum in the right hand with the main body of the speculum in the palm (see Fig.14.2) and the closed blades projecting between index and middle fingers.
- Gently insert the speculum into the vagina, held with your wrist turned such that the blades are in line with the opening between the labia.
- The speculum should be angled down and backward due to the angle of the vagina.
- Maintain a posterior angulation and rotate the speculum through 90° to position handles downward.

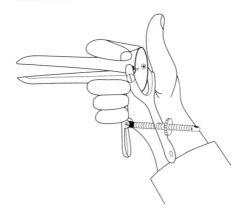

Fig. 14.2 Hold speculum in the right hand such that the handles lie in the palm and the blades project between the index and middle fingers.

- When it cannot be advanced further, maintain a downward pressure and press on the thumb piece to hinge the blades open, exposing the cervix and vaginal walls.
- Once the optimum position is achieved, tighten the thumbscrew or engage the locking mechanism (plastic speculum).

Findings
Inspect the cervix, which is usually pink, smooth, and regular.
- Look for the external os (central opening), which is round in nulliparous women and slit-shaped after childbirth.
- Look for cervical ectopy (eversions), which appear as strawberry-red areas spreading circumferentially around the os and represent extension of the endocervical epithelium onto the surface of the cervix.
- Note the presence of an IUD string if you obtained that history.
- Identify any ulceration or growths that may suggest cancer.
- Cervicitis may give a mucopurulent discharge associated with a red, inflamed cervix that bleeds on contact. Take swabs for culture.

Removing the speculum
▶ This should be conducted with as much care as insertion. You should still be examining the vaginal walls as the speculum is withdrawn.
- Undo the thumbscrew or lock and withdraw the speculum.
- ❶ The blades should be held open until their ends are visible distal to the cervix to avoid causing pain.
- Rotate the open blades in a counterclockwise direction to ensure that the anterior and posterior walls of the vagina can be inspected.

- Near the introitus, allow the blades to close, taking care not to pinch the labia or pubic hairs.

Bimanual examination

Digital examination helps identify the pelvic organs. Ideally, the bladder should be emptied, if not already done so by this stage. In some cases, and with patients over age 50, a rectal exam is done as the last step of the bimanual exam.

Getting started

- Explain to the patient that you are about to perform an internal examination of the vagina, uterus, tubes, and ovaries, and obtain verbal consent.
- The patient should be positioned as described on p. 424.
- Expose the introitus by separating the labia with the thumb and forefinger of the gloved left hand.
- Gently introduce the lubricated index and middle fingers of the gloved right hand into the vagina.
  - Insert your fingers with the palm facing laterally and then rotate 90° so that the palm faces up.
  - The thumb should be abducted and the ring and little finger flexed into the palm (see Fig. 14.3).

Vagina, cervix, and fornices

- Feel walls of the vagina, which are slightly rugated, supple, and moist.
- Locate the cervix—usually pointing down in the upper vagina.
  - The normal cervix has a similar consistency to that of cartilage in the tip of the nose.
- Assess the mobility of the cervix by moving it from side to side and note any tenderness suggesting infection.
- Gently palpate the fornices on either side of the cervix.

Uterus

- Place your left hand on the lower anterior abdominal wall about 4 cm above the symphysis pubis.

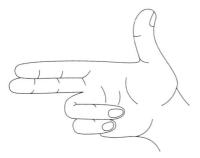

Fig. 14.3 Correct position of fingers of the right hand for *vaginal* examination.

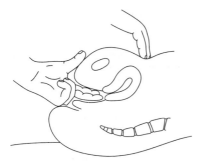

Fig. 14.4 Bimanual examination of the uterus.

- Move the fingers of your right internal hand to push the cervix upward and simultaneously press the fingertips of your left external hand toward the internal fingers (Fig. 14.4).
  - You should be able to capture the uterus between your two hands. Note the following features of the uterine body:
- Size: A uniformly enlarged uterus may represent a pregnancy, fibroid, or endometrial tumor.
- Shape: Multiple fibroids tend to give the uterus a lobulated feel.
- Position
- Surface characteristics
- Any tenderness
- ▶ Remember that an anteverted uterus is easily palpable bimanually, but a retroverted uterus may not be.
- Assess a retroverted uterus with the internal fingers positioned in the posterior fornix or during the rectovaginal exam.

Ovaries and fallopian tubes
- Position the internal fingers in each lateral fornix (finger pulps facing the anterior abdominal wall) and place your external fingers over each iliac fossa in turn.
- Press the external hand inward and down, and the internal fingers upward and laterally.
- Feel the adnexal structures (ovaries and fallopian tubes), assessing size, shape, mobility, and tenderness.
  - Ovaries are firm, ovoid and often palpable. If there is unilateral or bilateral ovarian enlargement, consider benign cysts (smooth and compressible) and malignant ovarian tumors.
  - Normal fallopian tubes are not palpable.
  - There may be marked tenderness of the lateral fornices and cervix in acute infection of the fallopian tubes (salpingitis).

Rectal
- If a rectal exam is done and you want to test any fecal material for blood, change gloves prior to the exam.

- The third finger of the examining hand is inserted into the rectum, with the second finger in the vagina (rectovaginal).
- Palpate the uterus and adnexal structures as described under Uterus, and Ovaries and Fallopian Tubes. Palpate the rectal wall for any masses or abnormalities.

Masses

It is often not possible to differentiate between adnexal and uterine masses. However, there are some general rules:

- Uterine masses may be felt to move with the cervix when the uterus is shifted upward, whereas adnexal masses will not.
- If you suspect an adnexal mass, there should be a line of separation between the uterus and the mass, and the mass should be felt distinctly from the uterus.
- While the consistency of the mass may help distinguish its origin in certain cases, an ultrasound is necessary to further evaluate the mass.

Finishing the examination

- Withdraw your fingers from the vagina.
  - Inspect the glove for blood or discharge.
- Redrape the genital area and allow the patient to get dressed in privacy—offer them tissues to wipe and assistance, if needed.

Taking a cervical smear

Theory

The purpose of the cervical smear is to detect premalignant conditions of the cervix. The U.S. Preventive Services Task Force recommends screening sexually active women with a cervix starting 3 years after initial sexual activity or at age 21. Cervical samples should be taken regularly (at least every 3 years). See Box 14.13 for taking samples during pregnancy.

Routine sampling after age 65 is not recommended for women with adequate, recent negative screening and who are not at high risk for cervical cancer. There is no indication for routine screening in women who have had a hysterectomy for benign disease. Current recommendations indicate that there is insufficient evidence to recommend routine screening for *human papillomavirus* (HPV) as a primary cancer screen. (http://www.ahrq.gov/clinic/USpstf/uspscerv.htm).

A sample of cells from the squamocolumnar junction are obtained and a cytological examination performed to look for evidence of cervical intraepithelial neoplasia (CIN). Early stages of cervical cellular abnormality are easily and successfully treated.

Most clinical settings now use liquid-based cytology (LBC), to minimize the number of inadequate samples.

Box 14.13 Cervical smears in pregnancy

Cervical smears may be performed during pregnancy. However, the broom or brush type sampling devices may cause excessive (and concerning) bleeding, so the more traditional wooden or plastic spatula is often used instead.

Equipment

- Specula of different sizes
- Disposable latex-free gloves
- Request form
- Sampling device—plastic broom, spatula or cytobrush (Fig. 14.5)
- LBC vial—preservative for sample

Before you start

- Ensure that the woman understands the purpose of the examination.
- Discuss how and when she will receive the results.
- Document the date of the last menstrual period.
- Document the use of hormonal treatment (e.g., contraception, HT).
- Record the details of the last smear and previous abnormal results.
- Ask about irregular bleeding (e.g., postcoital or postmenopausal).
- Ask about unusual discharge.
- Where appropriate, offer screening for *Chlamydia* infection (under age 25 years, symptomatic).

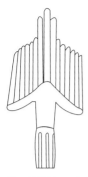

Fig. 14.5 The end of a typical Cervex-Brush®.

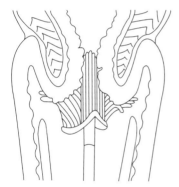

Fig. 14.6 Representation of how to use a Cervex-Brush®. Note that the longer, central bristles are within the cervical canal, while the outer bristles are in contact with the ectocervix.

Procedure

- Prepare the woman as for a vaginal examination, remembering to make her comfortable and allow privacy—see 📖 p. 424.
- Write the patient's identification details on the LBC vial.
- Insert the speculum to identify and visualize cervix as on 📖 p. 425. Record any abnormal features of the cervix.
- Insert the plastic broom so that the central bristles of the brush are in the endocervical canal and the outer bristles in contact with the ectocervix (see Fig. 14.6).
- Using pencil pressure, rotate the brush 5 times in a clockwise direction.
  - The bristles are beveled to scrape cells only on clockwise rotation.

- Rinse the brush thoroughly in the preservative (ThinPrep®) or break off brush into the preservative (SurePath®).
- If using a cytobrush, spatula, and slide, obtain adequate endocervical (cytobrush) and ectocervical (spatula) samples and apply the specimen to the slide (roll the brush across the slide; apply a thin smear of material from the spatula to the slide) and apply fixative.
- Place the slide in transport packaging with a completed request form.
- Remove the speculum as on 📖 p. 426.
- Perform the bimanual exam.
- Allow the patient to get dressed in privacy.

Current practice recommendations and consensus guidelines are available from the American Society of Colposcopy and Cervical Pathology Web site at: http://www.asccp.org/

History-taking in obstetrics

Although some parts are particular to this history, most of this process is the same as the basic outline described in 📖 Chapter 2. We suggest that readers review that chapter before going on.

The parts of the history detailed below are only those that differ from those described in 📖 Chapter 2 and earlier in this chapter (📖 p. 413).

Demographic details
- Name, age, and date of birth
- Gravidity and parity—see Box 14.15

Estimated date of delivery (EDD)
The EDD can be calculated from the last menstrual period (LMP) by Naegele's rule,* which assumes a 28-day menstrual cycle (Box 14.4).

Box 14.14 Calculating the EDD
- Subtract 3 months from the first day of the LMP.
- Add on 7 days and 1 year.

If the normal menstrual cycle is <28 days or >28 days, then an appropriate number of days should be subtracted from or added to the EDD, respectively. For example, if the normal cycle is 35 days, 7 days should be added to the EDD.

It is important to consider at this point any details that may influence the validity of the EDD as calculated from the LMP, such as the following:
- Was the last period normal?
- What is the usual cycle length?
- Are the patient's periods usually regular or irregular?
- Was the patient using the oral contraceptive pill in the 3 months prior to conception? If so, calculations based on her LMP are unreliable.

Current pregnancy
Ask about the patient's general health and that of her fetus. If there is a presenting complaint, the details should be documented in full as on 📖 p. 33. Also ask about the following:
- Fetal movements
  - These are not usually noticed until 20 weeks' gestation in the first pregnancy and 18 weeks' in the second or subsequent pregnancies.
- Any important laboratory tests or ultrasound scans
  - This include dates and details of all the scans, especially the first scan (dating or nuchal translucency scan).

---

* Named after the German obstetrician Franz Naegele, following the rule's description in his *Lehrbuch der Geburtshuelfe*, published for midwives in 1830. The formula was actually developed by Harmanni Boerhaave. See Boerhaave H. (1744)*Praelectiones Academicae in Propias Institutiones Rei Medicae.* Von Haller A (ed). Göttingen: Vandehoeck. Vol. 5 (part 2), p. 437.

Box 14.15 Gravidity and parity

These terms can be confusing. Although it is worth knowing the definitions and how to use them, they should be supplemented with a detailed history and not relied on alone, as you may miss subtleties that alter your outlook on the case.

Gravidity (G)

- The number of pregnancies (including the present one) to *any* stage

Parity (P)

- The outcomes of the pregnancies. The notations after the *P* refer to full-term (F), premature (P), abortions (spontaneous or terminations) (A), and living children (L).

Examples

- A woman who is currently 20 weeks pregnant and has had two normal deliveries:
  - G 3 P 2002
- A woman who is not pregnant and has had a single live birth and one miscarriage at 17 weeks:
  - •G 2 P 1011
- A woman who is currently 25 weeks pregnant, has had three normal deliveries, one miscarriage at 9 weeks, and a termination at 7 weeks:
  - G 6 P 3023

Twins

- A woman who is not pregnant and had a delivery of twins at 34 weeks:
  - G 1 P 0202

Past obstetric history

Ask about all of her previous pregnancies, including miscarriages, terminations, and ectopic pregnancies.

For each pregnancy, note the following:
- Age of the mother when pregnant
- Antenatal complications
- Duration of pregnancy
- Details of induction of labor
- Duration of labor
- Presentation and method of delivery
- Birth weight and sex of infant

▶ Also ask about any complications of the puerperal period, which is the period from the end of the third stage of labor until involution of the uterus is complete (about 6 weeks).

Possible complications include the following:
- Postpartum hemorrhage
- Infections of the genital and urinary tracts
- Deep vein thrombosis (DVT)

- Perineal complications, such as breakdown of the episiotomy site or perineal wounds
- Psychological complications (e.g., postpartum depression)

Past gynecological history

- Record all previous gynecological problems with full details of how the diagnosis was made, treatments received, and the success or otherwise of that treatment.
- Record date of the last cervical smear and any previous abnormal results.
- Take a full contraceptive history.

Past medical history

Take a full PMH as on ⊞ p. 35. Note especially those conditions that may have an impact on the pregnancy:

- Diabetes
- Thyroid disorders
- Addison's disease
- Asthma
- Epilepsy
- Hypertension
- Heart disease
- Renal disease
- Infectious diseases, such as TB, HIV, syphilis, and hepatitis
  - Identification of such conditions allows early referral to a specialist for shared care as needed.
- All previous operative procedures
- Blood transfusions and receipt of other blood products
- Psychiatric history

Drug history

- Take a full drug history (⊞ p. 36), which should include all prescribed medications, OTC medicines, herbal treatments, vitamins, and illicit drugs.
- Record any drug allergies and their nature.
- If currently the patient is pregnant, ensure that she is taking 400 mcg of folic acid daily until 12 weeks' gestation to reduce the incidence of spina bifida.

Smoking and alcohol

A full history should be taken (⊞ p. 37).

Family history

Family history is an important aspect of the obstetric history and should not be overlooked.

- Ask about any pregnancy-related conditions, such as congenital abnormalities, problems following delivery (Box 14.16), etc.
- Ask also about a FH of diabetes.
▶ Ask especially if there are any known hereditary illnesses.
Appropriate counseling and investigations such as chorionic villus sampling or amniocentesis may need to be offered.

Box 14.16 A word about deliveries
The verb *to deliver* is often misused by students of obstetrics, as it is often misused by the public at large.

Babies are not delivered; the mothers are *delivered of* the child, as in being relieved of a burden.

Check your nearest dictionary!

Social history
A full standard SH (📖 p. 41) should be taken. Ask about the following:
- Her partner—age, occupation, health
- How stable the relationship is
- If she is not in a relationship, who will give her support during and after the pregnancy?
- Ask if the pregnancy was planned or not.
- If she works, ask about her job and if she has any plans to return to work.

ⓘ You may also use this opportunity to give advice on regular exercises and avoidance of certain foods, e.g., seafood (high mercury content), soft cheeses (risk of *Listeria*), and calf liver (high vitamin A content).

Presenting symptoms in obstetrics

Bleeding—during pregnancy

Treat as any symptom. In addition, you should build a clear picture of how much blood is being lost, and when and how it is affecting the current pregnancy (see also Box 14.17).

After establishing an exact timeline and other details about the symptom, ask about the following:

- Exact nature of the bleeding (fresh or old)
- Amount of blood lost
- Number of sanitary pads or tampons used daily
- Presence of clots (and, if present, size of those clots)
- Presence of pieces of tissue in the blood
- Presence of mucoid discharge
- Fetal movement

Box 14.17 Some causes of vaginal bleeding in early pregnancy

Ectopic pregnancy
- *Symptoms:* light bleeding, abdominal pain, fainting if pain and blood loss is severe
- *Signs:* closed cervix, uterus slightly larger and softer than normal, tender adnexal mass, cervical motion tenderness

Threatened miscarriage
- *Symptoms:* light bleeding; sometimes cramping, lower abdominal pain
- *Signs:* closed cervix, uterus corresponds to dates; sometimes uterus is softer than normal

Complete miscarriage
- *Symptoms:* light bleeding; sometimes light cramping, lower abdominal pain and history of expulsion of products of conception
- *Signs:* uterus smaller than dates and softer than normal; closed cervix

Incomplete miscarriage
- *Symptoms:* heavy bleeding; sometimes cramping lower abdominal pain, partial expulsion of products of conception
- *Signs:* uterus smaller than dates and cervix dilated

Molar pregnancy
- *Symptoms:* heavy bleeding, partial expulsion of products of conception that resemble grapes; sometimes nausea and vomiting, cramping lower abdominal pain, history of ovarian cysts
- *Signs:* dilated cervix, uterus larger than dates and softer than normal

Information adapted from World Health Organization, Department of Reproductive Health Research (2007). Vaginal bleeding in early pregnancy. In *Managing Complications in Pregnancy and Childbirth: A Guide for Midwives and Doctors.* Geneva: WHO.

Box 14.18 Some causes of bleeding in second and third trimesters (>24 weeks)

This is known as *antepartum hemorrhage* (APH).

Placenta previa

The placenta is positioned over the lower pole of the uterus, obscuring the cervix. Bleeding is usually after 28 weeks and often precipitated by intercourse. Findings may include a relaxed uterus, fetal presentation not in the pelvis, and normal fetal condition.

Placental abruption

This is detachment of a normally located placenta from the uterus before the fetus is delivered. Bleeding can occur at any stage of the pregnancy. Possible findings include a tense, tender uterus, ↓ or absent fetal movements, fetal distress, or absent fetal heart sounds.

- Associated symptoms, such as abdominal pain (associated with placental abruption; placenta previa is painless).
- Possible trigger factors—recent intercourse, injuries (see Box 14.18)
- Any history of cervical abnormalities and the result of the last smear

Abdominal pain

A full pain history should be taken as on 📖 p. 34, including site, radiation, character, severity, mode and rate of onset, duration, frequency, exacerbating factors, relieving factors, and associated symptoms.

Take a full obstetric history and systems review. Ask especially about a past history of preeclampsia, preterm labor, peptic ulcer disease, gallstones, appendectomy, and cholecystectomy.

🔵 Remember that the pain may be unrelated to pregnancy, so keep an open mind! Causes of abdominal pain in pregnancy include the following:
- **Obstetric:** preterm or term labor, placental abruption, ligament pain, symphysis pubis dysfunction, preeclampsia or HELLP (Hemolysis, Elevated Liver enzyme levels, Low Platelet count) syndrome, acute fatty liver of pregnancy
- **Gynecological:** ovarian cyst rupture, torsion, hemorrhage, uterine fibroid degeneration
- **Gastrointestinal:** constipation, appendicitis, gallstones, cholecystitis, pancreatitis, peptic ulceration
- **Genitourinary:** cystitis, pyelonephritis, renal stones, renal colic

Labor pain

This is usually intermittent and regular in frequency and associated with tightening of the abdominal wall.

Bleeding—after pregnancy

This is called *postpartum hemorrhage*, or PPH.
- **Primary PPH:** >500 mL blood loss within 24 hours following delivery
- **Secondary PPH:** any excess bleeding between 24 hours and 6 weeks post-delivery (No amount of blood is specified in the definition.)
▶ Take a full history as for bleeding during pregnancy, on 📖 p. 437. Ask

also about symptoms of infection, an important cause of secondary PPH (see Boxes 14.18 and 14.19).

Hypertension

Hypertension is a common and important problem in pregnancy. You should be alert to the possible symptoms that can result from it, such as headache, blurred vision, vomiting, and epigastric pain after 24 weeks, convulsions, or loss of consciousness.

Pregnancy-induced hypertension

- Two readings of diastolic blood pressure 90–110, systolic BP >140, 4 hours apart after 20 weeks gestation; no proteinuria

Mild proteinuric pregnancy-induced hypertension/preeclampsia

- Two readings of diastolic blood pressure 90–110, systolic BP >140, 4 hours apart after 20 weeks gestation, and proteinuria 1–2+

Severe proteinuric pregnancy-induced hypertension/preeclampsia

- Diastolic blood pressure 110 or greater after 20 weeks' gestation and proteinuria 3+.
- Other symptoms may include hyperreflexia, headache, clouding of vision, oligura, abdominal pain, pulmonary edema. There may be evidence of HELLP syndrome.

Eclampsia

- Convulsions associated with raised blood pressure and/or proteinuria beyond 20 weeks gestation. The patient may be unconscious.

Box 14.19 Some causes of postpartum hemorrhage

Primary
- Uterine atony (most frequent cause)
- Genital tract trauma
- Coagulation disorders
- Retained placenta
- Uterine inversion
- Uterine rupture

Secondary
- Retained products of conception
- Endometritis
- Infection

Box 14.20 Risk factors for postpartum hemorrhage
These include placental abnormalities, polyhydramnios, prolonged labor, very rapid labor, multiple gestation, previous PPH or APH, preeclampsia, coagulation abnormalities, genital tract lacerations, and small maternal stature.

Box 14.21 Minor symptoms of pregnancy
These so-called minor symptoms of pregnancy are often experienced by many women as normal, physiological changes occur. This is not to say that they should be ignored, as they may point to pathology.
- *Nausea and vomiting:* severity varies greatly and is more common in multiple pregnancies and molar pregnancies. Persistence of vomiting may suggest pathology such as infections, gastritis, biliary tract disease, or hepatitis.
- *Frequent urination:* An expected finding in pregnancy, it does not exclude the possibility of urinary tract infection.
- *Heartburn/gastroesophageal reflux:* Heartburn is a frequent complaint during pregnancy due partially to compression of the stomach by the gravid uterus. See 📖 p. 206.
- *Constipation:* often secondary to ↑ progesterone. It improves with gestation (📖 p. 212).
- *Shortness of breath:* due to dilatation of the bronchial tree secondary to ↑ progesterone. Peaks at 20–24 weeks. The growing uterus also has an impact. Other possible causes (such as PE) need to be considered. See 📖 p. 184.
- *Fatigue:* very common in early pregnancy, peaking at the end of the first trimester. Fatigue in late pregnancy may be due to anemia.
- *Insomnia:* due to anxiety, hormonal changes, and physical discomfort
- *Pruritus:* Generalized itching in the third trimester may resolve after delivery. Biliary problems should be excluded (📖 p. 216).
- *Hemorrhoids:* may resolve after delivery
- *Varicose veins:* especially at the feet and ankles
- *Vaginal discharge:* Exclude infection and spontaneous rupture of the membranes.
- *Pelvic pain:* Stretching of pelvic structures can cause ligament pain that resolves in the second half of the pregnancy. Symphysis-pubis dysfunction causes pain on abduction and rotation at the hips and on mobilization.
- *Backache:* often first develops during the fifth to seventh months of pregnancy
- *Peripheral paresthesias:* Fluid retention can lead to compression of peripheral nerves, such as carpal tunnel syndrome. Other nerves can be affected, e.g., lateral cutaneous nerve of the thigh.

Outline obstetric examination

Explain to the patient that you would like to examine her uterus and baby, and reassure her that the procedure will be quick and gentle. You should have a chaperone present, particularly if you are male.

As always, ensure that the room is warm and well lit, preferably with a moveable light source, and that you will not be disturbed.

As with the gynecological examination, you should follow an orderly routine. The authors' suggestion is shown in Box 14.22. It is standard practice to start with the cardiovascular and respiratory systems—this not only gives a measure of the general health of the patient but also establishes a physical rapport before you examine more sensitive areas.

General inspection

Always begin with a general examination of the patient (as in Chapter 3), including temperature, hydration, coloration, nutritional status, lymph nodes, and blood pressure. Note especially the following:

- Any brownish pigmentation over the forehead and cheeks, known as *chloasma*
- Distribution of facial and body hair, as hirsutism may be a presenting symptom of various endocrine disorders
- Height and weight, and calculate BMI (📖 p. 56)

▶ Blood pressure should be measured in the left lateral position at 45° to avoid compression of the IVC by the gravid uterus.

🔅 Anemia is a common complication of pregnancy, so examine the mucosal surfaces and conjunctivae carefully (📖 p. 51).

- Examine the cardiovascular and respiratory systems in turn(see Chapters 7 and 8).
  - Flow murmurs are common in pregnancy and, although usually of no clinical significance, must be recorded in detail.
- A routine breast examination is usually performed. Take note of inverted nipples, which may interfere with breast-feeding.

Box 14.22 Framework for obstetric examination

- General inspection
- Cardiorespiratory examination
- Breast examination
- Abdominal inspection
- Abdominal palpation
  - Uterine size
  - Fetal lie
  - Fetal presentation
  - Engagement
  - Amniotic fluid estimation
- Auscultation of the fetal heart
- Vaginal examination
▶ Perform urinalysis (particularly urine dipstick)

Abdominal examination

Inspection

Look for abdominal distension caused by the gravid uterus rising from the pelvis. Look also for the following:

- Asymmetry
- Fetal movements
- Surgical scars
  - Pubic hairline (transverse suprapubic Pfannenstiel incision)
  - Paraumbilical region (laparoscopic scars)
- Cutaneous signs of pregnancy
  - Linea nigra (black line), which stretches from the pubic symphysis upward in the midline
  - Red stretch marks of current pregnancy (striae gravidarum)
  - White stretch marks (striae albicans) from a previous pregnancy
  - Other areas that can undergo pigmentation in pregnancy include the nipples, vulva, umbilicus, and recent abdominal scars.
- Umbilical changes
  - Flattening as pregnancy advances
  - Eversion secondary to ↑ intra-abdominal pressure (e.g., caused by multiple pregnancies or polyhydraminios)

Palpation

Before palpating the abdomen, always ask about any areas of tenderness and examine those areas last. Palpation should start as for any standard abdominal examination (Chapter 9) before proceeding to more specific maneuvers in an obstetric examination.

Uterine size

This provides an estimation of gestational age in weeks (Fig. 14.7) and is objectively measured and expressed in centimeters as the *symphysial–fundal height* (distance from the symphysis pubis to the upper edge of the uterus) (Boxes 14.23 and 14.24).

🛈 You need a tape measure for this—don't start without it!

- Use the ulnar border of the left hand to press firmly into the abdomen just below the sternum.
- Move your hand down the abdomen in small steps until you can feel the fundus of the uterus.
- Locate the upper border of the bony pubic symphysis by palpating downward in the midline, starting from a few centimeters above the pubic hair margin.
- Measure the distance between the two points that you have found in centimeters, using a flexible tape measure.

Fetal lie

This describes the relationship between the long axis of the fetus and the long axis of the uterus (Fig. 14.8). In general, it can be the following:

- *Longitudinal:* The long axis of the fetus matches the long axis of the uterus. Either the head or breech will be palpable over the pelvic inlet.
- *Transverse:* The fetus lies at right angles to the uterus and the fetal poles are palpable in the flanks.

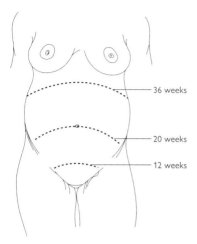

36 weeks

20 weeks

12 weeks

Fig. 14.7 The distance between the fundus (upper border of the uterus) and the pubic symphysis can be used as a guide to the number of weeks' gestation. You can also, therefore, judge whether the uterus is smaller or larger than expected, which may point to problems with the pregnancy.

Box 14.23 Symphysial–fundal height (cm) ≈ weeks gestation
At 16–36 weeks, there is a margin of error of ±2 cm, ±3 cm at 36–40 weeks, and ±4 cm at 40 weeks on.

Box 14.24 Uterine size—milestones
- The uterus first becomes palpable at 12 weeks' gestation.
- 20 weeks' gestation = at the level of the umbilicus
- 36 weeks' gestation = at the level of the xiphisternum

- *Oblique:* The long axis of the fetus lies at an angle of 45° to the long axis of the uterus; the presenting part will be palpable in one of the iliac fossae.

Examination technique
The best position is to stand at the mother's right side, facing her feet.
- Put your left hand along the left side of the uterus.
- Put your right hand on the right side of the uterus.
- Palpate systematically toward the midline with one hand and then the other hand—use dipping movements with flexion of the MCP joints to feel the fetus within the amniotic fluid.
- You should feel the fetal back as firm resistance or the irregular shape of the limbs.

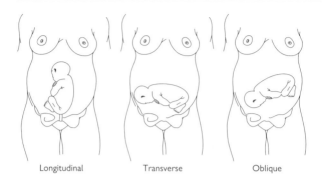

| Longitudinal | Transverse | Oblique |

Fig. 14.8 Some examples of fetal lie.

- Now palpate more widely, using the two-handed technique above to stabilize the uterus, and attempt to locate the head and the breech.
  - The head can be felt as a smooth, round object that is ballotable—that is, it can be bounced (gently) between your hands.
  - The breech is softer, less discrete, and not ballotable.

Fetal presentation

This is the part of the fetus that presents to the mother's pelvis. Possible presenting parts include the following:

- **Head:** cepahalic presentation. One option in a longitudinal lie
- **Breech:** podalic presentation. The other option in a longitudinal lie
- **Shoulder:** seen in a transverse lie

Examination technique

- Stand at the mother's right side, facing her feet.
- Place both hands on either side of the lower part of the uterus.
- Bring the hands together firmly but gently.
  - You should be able to feel either the head, breech, or other part as described under Fetal Lie.

It is also possible to use a one-handed technique (Paulik's grip) to feel for the presenting part—this is best left to obstetricians. In this technique, you use a cupped right hand to hold the lower pole of the uterus. This is possible in ~95% of pregnancies at about 40 weeks.

Engagement

When the widest part of the fetal skull is within the pelvic inlet, the fetal head is said to be *engaged*.

In a cephalic presentation, palpation of the head is assessed and expressed as the number of fifths of the skull palpable above the pelvic brim. A fifth of a fetal skull is roughly equal to a finger breath on an adult hand.

- The head is engaged when three or more fifths are within the pelvic inlet—that is when two or fewer fifths are palpable.
- When three or more fifths are palpable, the head is not engaged.

Number of fetuses

The number of fetuses present can be calculated by assessing the number of fetal poles (head or breech) present.

- If there is one fetus present, two poles should be palpable (unless the presenting part is deeply engaged).
- In a multiple pregnancy, you should be able to feel all the poles except one, as one is usually tucked away out of reach.

Amniotic fluid volume estimation

The ease with which fetal parts are palpable can give an indication of the possibility of ↓ or ↑ amniotic fluid volume.

- ↑ Volume will give a large-for-dates uterus that is smooth and rounded. The fetal parts may be almost impossible to palpate.
- ↓ Volume may give a small-for-dates uterus. The fetus will be easily palpable, giving an irregular, firm outline to the uterus.

Percussion

This is usually unhelpful in an obstetric examination, unless you suspect polyhydramnios (increased amniotic fluid volume). In this case, you may wish to attempt to elicit a fluid thrill (📖 p. 239).

Auscultation

Auscultation is used to listen to the fetal heart rate (FHR). This is usually performed using an electronic hand-held Doppler fetal heart rate monitor and can be used as early as 14 weeks.

Using Pinard's fetal stethoscope

With the prevalance and low cost of the modern fetal Doppler, a Pinard's fetal stethoscope is no longer likely to be seen or used. Fetascopes are not generally useful until 28 weeks' gestation. It is a simple-looking device that looks like an old-fashioned ear-trumpet (Fig. 14.9).

- Place the bell of the instrument over the anterior fetal shoulder, where the fetal heart sounds are best heard.
- Press your left ear against the stethoscope to hold it between your head and the mother's abdomen in a hands-free position, or hold the instrument lightly with one hand.
- Press against the opposite side of the mother's abdomen with your other hand to stabilize the uterus.
- It should sound like a distant ticking noise. The rate varies between 110 and 150/minute at term and should be regular.
▶ Record the rate and rhythm of the fetal heart.

Vaginal examination

Vaginal examination enables you to assess cervical status before induction of labor. You should attempt this only under adequate supervision if you are unsure of the procedure.

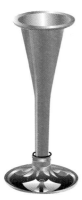

Fig. 14.9 A Pinard's stethoscope.

This examination allows you to assess the degree of cervical dilatation (in centimeters) using the examining fingers.

🜊 Examination of the vagina and cervix should be performed under aseptic conditions in the presence of ruptured membranes or in patients with abnormal vaginal discharge.

Technique

The examination should be performed as described on 🕮 p. 427. It takes experience to reliably determine the findings.

Findings

Assess the following:

• Degree of dilation
  • Full dilation of the cervix is equivalent to 10 cm.
  • Most obstetric departments will have plastic models of cervices in various stages of dilatation with which you can practice.
• Length of the cervix
  • Normal length is ~3 cm but shortens as the cervix effaces secondary to uterine contraction.
• Consistency of the cervix, which can be described as follows:
  • Firm
  • Mid-consistency
  • Soft (this consistency facilitates effacement and dilatation)
• Position
  • As the cervix undergoes effacement and dilatation it tends to be pulled from a posterior to an anterior position.
• Station of the presenting part
  • The level of the head above or below the ischial spines may be estimated in centimeters.

The elderly patient

It is easy to be seduced into thinking that the principal focus should be on very medical diagnoses, such as urinary tract infections, which contribute to significant morbidity (and mortality) in older people.

Continence issues are frequently overlooked in most clinical assessments. Large-scale surveys of prevalence have shown up to 20% of women over 40 reporting difficulties with continence. So while this is more common in older people, you should always be mindful of problems in younger adults as well.

Although continence issues are one of the geriatric giants of disease presentation, it is important to recall the physiology of postmenopausal changes, such as vaginal atrophy and loss of secretions, which can complicate urinary tract infections, continence, and uterovaginal prolapse in older patients.

Assessment

Tact and understanding

Although problems are common, patients may be reluctant to discuss them or have them discussed in front of others. Engaging in a discussion about bladder and/or sexual function can seem daunting, but if done empathetically, remembering not to appear judgmental or be embarrassed, you may reveal problems that have seriously affected your patient's quality of life.

Treating problems such as these, even with very simple interventions, can be of immeasurable value to the patient. Remember to consider STIs in your differential. "Elderly" does not mean sexual inactivity.

Holistic assessment of urinary problems

Learn to think when asking about bladder function, and work out a pattern of dysfunction—e.g., bladder instability or stress incontinence. Remember that bladder function may be disrupted by drugs, pain, or lack of privacy. Continence issues may reflect poor mobility or visual and cognitive decline.

Genital symptoms

Don't forget to consider vaginal or uterine pathology—view postmenopausal bleeding with suspicion. Discharges may represent active infection (if *Candida*, consider diabetes) or atrophic vaginitis (see Box 14.25).

Past medical history

Pregnancies and previous surgery in particular may help point to a diagnosis of stress incontinence. Are urinary tract infections recurrent—has bladder pathology been excluded?

Drugs

Many are obvious—diuretics and anticholinergics; some are more subtle—sedatives may provoke nocturnal loss of continence. Does your patient drink tea or coffee?

Tailored functional history

This is the cornerstone of these pages and of any assessment you perform. It largely relates to bladder function—is the bathroom located upstairs or down? How are the stairs? Does your patient already have continence aids, such as bottles, commodes, or pads, and do they manage well with them?

> **Box 14.25 A word on atrophic vaginitis**
>
> Up to 40% of postmenopausal women will have symptoms and signs of atrophic vaginitis. The vast majority will be elderly and may be reluctant to discuss this with their doctors. A result of estrogen decline, the subsequent ↑ vaginal pH and thinned endometrium lead to both genital and urinary symptoms and signs.
>
> An decrease in vaginal lubrication presents with dryness, pruritus, and discharges, accompanied by an ↑ rate of prolapse. Urinary complications can result in frequency, stress incontinence, and infections.
>
> Careful physical examination often makes the diagnosis clear with labial dryness, loss of skin turgidity, and smooth, shiny vaginal epithelium. A range of treatment options, including topical estrogens, simple lubricants, and continued sexual activity when appropriate, are all key interventions to manage this common condition.

Psychiatric assessment

Approach to psychiatric assessment

In taking a psychiatric history and assessing mental state, it is crucial to communicate to the patient with empathy, respect, competence, and interest, in a nonjudgmental fashion. This approach will create an atmosphere of trust that encourages the patient to talk honestly about their thoughts and feelings.

Central to the psychiatric interview process is the art of active listening to what is said and an awareness of any nonverbal communication between patient and assessor.

Be prepared to spend anywhere from 30 minutes to an hour, depending on the circumstances, conducting an interview. This might seem a daunting task in the early stages, particularly as patients rarely find a narrative. However, staying on track is often made easier by remembering to write out the headings for parts of the assessment in advance.

Preparation and preliminary considerations

The room

Before proceeding to questioning, adequate preparations should be made regarding the place where the assessment is to be carried out. An interview room should be a safe environment, especially when seeing a patient who is potentially violent. Your facility will normally have rooms specifically configured for the performance of psychiatric examinations.

- Inform your colleagues and departmental staff of your location.
- You should know where to locate, and how to use, the panic button.
- You should be accompanied by a colleague if you are seeing a patient with a history of violent behavior.
- Remove any objects that might pose a danger (i.e., those that can be used as a weapon).
- Know your nearest exit point and ensure that it is open or unblocked.
- Never allow the patient to come between you and the door.
- Ensure adequate privacy and lighting.
- Ideally, the patient should be sitting off-center, so that all of their body may be seen but without the situation appearing too threatening.
- The height of your seats should be equal or similar.

Conduct of interview

Begin by introducing yourself, explaining who you are and the purpose of your assessment. Use a handshake—a widespread sign of introduction and welcome. Establish whether or not the patient wishes a friend or relative to be present (and whether you feel it is appropriate).

The interview should generally start in an informal way to establish a friendly and concerned rapport. This might involve a short period of neutral conversation.

Try to avoid leading or direct questions. Use relatively broad, open, general questions and leave specific closed questions for further clarification later. Allow breaks and digressions within reason, especially with sensitive individuals. At appropriate intervals, clarify what the patient has said by repeating sentences and asking them to confirm this.

Examination

In psychiatry, you should be examining the patient's mental state; this is described later. However, don't overlook physical examination, as this is often an important part of the assessment. Conduct the physical examination is described in Chapters 2 and 3. A useful framework for psychiatric assessment is given in Box 15.1

Box 15.1 Framework for psychiatric assessment

History
- Name, age, marital status, occupation, ethnic origin, and religion
- Source, mode, and reason for referral
- Chief complaint
- History of present illness
- Risk assessment
- Past psychiatric history
- Past medical history
- Drug history
- Family history
- Personal history
  - Birth and early development
  - School
  - Occupational history
  - Psychosexual history
  - Marital history
  - Children
  - Forensic history
- Premorbid personality
- Social history

Mental state examination
- Appearance and behavior
- Speech
- Mood
- Thought content
- Perception
- Cognitive functioning
- Insight

Physical examination
- As appropriate

History

The psychiatric history is very similar in structure to the standard medical history described in Chapter 2. Symptoms and issues should be dealt with in the same way (see Box 15.2).

Patient profile

Start by making a note of the patient's name, age, marital status, occupation, ethnic origin, and religion.

Source, mode, and reason for referral

Record here all the information you have about the patient from other sources—relatives, caregivers, social workers, counselors, primary care team, and police, if relevant.

- Who has asked for the individual to be seen and why?
- What was the mode of referral—voluntary, or involuntary as a referral from other clinicians or law enforcement (as under the Baker Act)?

Chief complaint

Obtain a brief description of the principal complaint(s) and the time frame of the problem in the individual's own words.

This can be difficult if the patient is in a psychotic state and does not believe a problem exists. In these cases, try to comment on the presenting complaint as described by an informant.

Box 15.2 Factors asked about for a physical or mental symptom

The following is repeated from Chapter 2. Treat psychiatric symptoms in a similar way, but remember that the patient may not regard their issue as a symptom, so tailor your language carefully.

- Exact nature of the symptom
- Onset
  - Date it began
  - How it began (e.g., suddenly, gradually—over how long?)
  - If long-standing, why is the patient seeking help now?
- Periodicity and frequency
  - Is the symptom constant or intermittent?
  - How long does it last each time?
  - What is the exact manner in which it comes and goes?
- Change over time
  - Is it improving or deteriorating?
- Exacerbating factors
  - What makes the symptom worse?
- Relieving factors
  - What makes the symptom better?
- Associated symptoms

History of present illness

This is a detailed account of the presenting problems in chronological order (as for any other kind of symptom as in Chapter 2):

- Onset of illness (when was the patient last well?)
- How did the condition develop?
- Severity of the patient's symptoms
- Precipitating factors (including any significant life events preceding onset of the symptoms)
- Exacerbating factors (what makes the symptoms worse?)
- Relieving factors (what makes the symptoms better?)
- How has it affected the patient's daily life, pattern, or routine (effect on interpersonal relationships, working capacity, etc.)?
- Treatment history. Include treatment tried during the course of the present illness, previous drug treatments, electroconvulsive therapy, and psychosocial interventions.
- Associated symptoms
- Systematic inquiry. Similar to the standard medical history, run through other psychiatric symptoms and ask the patient if they have experienced them (see Box 15.3). Explore related symptoms; if the patient admits to a few depressive symptoms, ask about other symptoms of depression.

Risk assessment

This includes an assessment of not only self-harm but also the possibility of harm to others. This should be broached in a serious and sensitive way. Some useful questions in assessing suicide risk (Box 15.4) are as follows:

- How do you feel about the future?
- Does life seem worth living?
- Do you have thoughts of hurting or harming yourself?
- Have you had thoughts of harming others?
- Have you ever thought of ending it all?

If suicidal thoughts are present, ask how often they occur and if the patient has made a specific plan and what the plan is.

- Ask about the means, e.g., prescribed and over-the-counter drugs, guns, or knives.
- Explore for feelings of excessive guilt and loss of self-esteem.

Box 15.3 Tailoring the history

In the taking of a history in any specialty, you should formulate your questions according to what is said. Also, information may not be provided by the patient in the order you would like.

This is particularly true of psychiatry—if the patient is talking freely, you may find them providing information that comes under a number of different subheadings in your history. Be flexible, note the information in the appropriate places, and then fill in the gaps with direct questions.

Box 15.4 Risk factors for suicide

Biological
- Age >40 years
- Male gender

Medical and psychiatric history
- Previous suicide attempts
- Previous deliberate self-harm
- Psychiatric disorder (depression, substance misuse, schizophrenia, personality disorder, obsessive-compulsive disorder, panic disorder)
- Chronic physical illness
- History of trauma or abuse
- Substance misuse (including alcohol)

Personality
- Impulsivity, poor problem-solving skills, aggression, perfectionism, low self-esteem

Family history
- Family history of mental health, substance abuse, family violence, or suicide attempts among family members

Social
- Lack of social support, isolation
  - Unemployment or retired
  - Single, unmarried, divorced, or widowed
- Presence of firearms in the home
- History of previous incarceration
- Previous exposure to suicidal behaviors in others to whom they have had close exposure

Access to means
- Weapons in the home or through occupational or social activities

If thoughts involving harming others are present, ask about the specific persons and circumstances surrounding these thoughts.
- Ask about the means, e.g., presence of weapons such as guns or knives.

Previous history of self-harm
Ask about previous attempts—when, where, how, and why. Ask in detail about the most recent attempt:
- What events led up to the attempt (see Box 15.5)?
- Were there any specific precipitating factors?
- Was there concurrent use of drugs and alcohol?
- What were the methods used?
- Was it planned?
- Was there a suicide note?
- Were there any active attempts made to avoid being discovered?

Box 15.5 Factors that may precipitate suicide

The overriding theme here is loss—loss of occupation, independence, family member, friend, social supports, or freedom.
- Death, separation, or divorce
- Imprisonment, or threat thereof
- Humiliating event
- Job loss
- Reminder of a past loss
- Unwanted pregnancy

Box 15.6 Protective factors for suicide

- Strong family and social connections
- Hopefulness, good skills in problem solving
- Cultural or religious beliefs discouraging suicide
- Responsibility for children

- What is the meaning of the action (wanted to die, share distress)?
- Also ask about the circumstances surrounding discovery and how they were brought to medical attention (if at all).
- Was this what the patient expected?

Protective factors for suicide
These are factors that would stop a person from attempting suicide (Box 15.6). Record what social supports are available to the person (friends, church, doctor, counselor).

Assessing homicidal intent
If faced with a patient expressing homicidal intent, you should inform a senior colleague and law enforcement authorities immediately. Legal instruments such as the Baker Act should be used to prevent the patient's release in order to protect those individuals against whom they state this intent.

Some questions to assess a homicidal or violent patient are as follows:
- Are you upset with anyone?
- Do you have thoughts of hurting anyone?
- Have you made plans to harm someone?
- How would you harm them? (It is important to establish whether the patient has actually made plans for carrying out the action.)

Past psychiatric history
Explore in detail previous contact with psychiatry and other services for mental health problems. Include as far as possible:
- Dates of illness, symptoms, diagnoses, treatments, hospitalizations, previous outpatient treatment, and compulsory treatment under the Baker Act.

Past medical history
This should be evaluated in the same way as in the general medical history, but remember to ask in particular about obstetric complications, epilepsy, head injuries, and thyroid disorders.

Drug and alcohol history
- Ask about all current drug intake, including prescribed and over-the-counter medicines.
- Take a detailed history of substance abuse, if relevant, recording the type, quality, source, route of administration, and cost.
- Ask about alcohol, tobacco, and any allergic reactions. If necessary, use the CAGE questionnaire (📖 p. 221).

Family history
Explore family relationships in detail (parents, siblings, spouse, children). It is useful to draw a family tree and record age, health, occupation, personality, quality of relationship, family history of mental illness, including alcoholism, suicide, and deliberate self-harm, as well as any other serious family illnesses.

Also record the details and times of certain important family events, such as death, separation, or divorce, and their impact on the patient.

Personal history
The personal history is a chronological account of the individual's life from birth up to the present. This section, which is often lengthy, should be tackled under the following subheadings.

Birth and early development
- Begin with recording the place and date of birth, gestation at delivery, and any obstetric complications or birth injuries.
- Inquire about developmental milestones.
- Ask about neurotic traits in childhood (night terrors, sleep walking, bedwetting, temper tantrums, stammer, feeding difficulties).
- Ask about relationships with peers, siblings, parents, and relatives, particularly in adolescence.
- Record any adverse experiences (physical or emotional abuse).
- Note any significant life events, such as separations and bereavement.

School
- Explore how they did at school socially, academically, and athletically.
- Record the start and end of their education and qualifications.
- Ask about the type of school, relationships with peers, teachers, and extracurricular interests and whether there was a history of academic difficulty or truancy.

Occupational history
- Inquire about all previous jobs held, dates, and reason for change, level of satisfaction with employment, and ambitions.
- Include present job and economic circumstances.

Psychosexual history

This can be a difficult section of the history to elicit and is often dependent on how willing the patient is to volunteer such intimate details. However, try not to avoid it. It may have to be excluded if judged inappropriate or likely to cause distress.

- Record the onset of puberty (and menarche, if female).
- Sexual orientation (heterosexual, bisexual, gay, or lesbian)
- Gender identity (transsexual)
- First sexual encounter
- Current sexual practices (practice of safer sex?)
- Any of sexual abuse
- Record any history of sexual dysfunction.

Marital history

This includes a detailed account of number of marriages, duration, quality of relationships and personality, age and occupations of spouses, and reasons for breakup of relationship(s).

Children

- Ask about the sex, age, and mental and physical health of all children.

Forensic history

This may or may not be volunteered by the patient. Begin by asking non-threatening questions: "Have you ever been in trouble with the law?"

- Ask about criminal record and any previous episodes of violence or other acts of aggression.

Premorbid personality

This is the patient's personality before the onset of mental illness. An independent account is especially important for this part of the history.

- It may help to ask the patient how they would describe themselves and how they think others would describe them.
- Ask about social relationships and supports.
- Include interests and recreational activities.
- Inquire specifically about temperament—what's their mood like on most occasions?
- Ask the patient to describe the nature of their emotional reactions, coping mechanisms, and character (e.g., shy, suspicious, irritable, impulsive, lacking in confidence, history of obsession).
- What are their moral and religious beliefs?

Social history

Ask especially about finances, legal problems, occupation, dependants, and housing. If elderly, ask about social support, such as home care or attendance at a day center, and how they cope with activities of daily living (hygiene, mobility, domestic activity).

Mental status examination

The mental status examination is a vital part of the psychiatric assessment. It is your assessment of the patient's mental state based on your observations and interaction. It begins as soon as you see the patient. Mental state features prior to the interview, whether described by the patient or by other informants, are considered part of the history.

Appearance and behavior

This involves a brief descriptive note of your observations, both at first contact and through the interview process. It should include a description of the following:

- Dress and grooming
  - Patients with depression, dementia, and drug abuse may show evidence of self-neglect.
  - Flamboyant clothes with clashing colors may be worn by a manic patient.
  - Loose-fitting clothes may indicate an underlying anorexia or other eating disorder.*
- Facial appearance
- Eye contact
- Degree of cooperation
- Posture
- Mannerisms
- Motor activity
  - Excessive movement indicating agitation?
  - Very little movement (retardation) suggesting depression?
- Abnormal movements
  - E.g., tics, chorea, tremor, stereotypy—repetitive movements, such as rocking or rubbing hands
- Gait
- Any other physical characteristics worth noting

Speech

Describe in terms of the following:

- Rate
- Quantity (↑ = pressure of speech and is often associated with flight of ideas, ↓ = known as poverty of speech)
- Fluency
- Articulation (including stammering, stuttering, and dysarthria)
- Form: this is the way in which a person speaks, rather than actual content (see Box 15.7).

Mood and affect

Mood is a pervasive and sustained emotion that can color the patient's perception of the world over long periods. *Affect* is the patient's immediate emotional state, including the external expression of feeling.

---

* Loose-fitting clothing is usually not a sign of weight loss, contrary to popular belief. In fact, patients with anorexia tend to deliberately wear baggy clothes to hide their underlying skeletal appearance.

Box 15.7 Some examples of abnormal speech or thought form

The following are examples of abnormal speech; however, the speech is a manifestation of the underlying thought processes. One could argue, therefore, that the following are abnormalities of thought form.

- *Flight of ideas:* associated with mania. Ideas flow rapidly but remain connected although sometimes by unusual associations. The patient's train of thought tends to veer off on wild tangents.
- *Derailment:* loosening of association seen in formal thought disorders (e.g., schizophrenia) in which train of thought slips of the track. Things may be said in juxtaposition that lack a meaningful association or the patient may shift from one frame of reference to another.
- *Perseveration:* mainly seen in dementia and frontal lobe damage. The patient finds moving to the next topic difficult, resulting in an inappropriate repetition of a response.
- *Incoherence:* pattern of speech that is essentially incomprehensible at times
- *Echolalia:* feature of dementia. This is a repetitive pattern of speech in which a patient echoes words or phrases said by the interviewer.
- *Neologisms:* found mainly in schizophrenia and structural brain disease (see 🕮 p. 261). New words are invented that have no meaning.
- *Circumstantiality:* a long-winded pattern of speech loaded down with unnecessary detail and digression before finally getting to the point. The patient is, however, able to maintain their train of thought.

Examining mood and affect involves consideration of the patient's subjective emotional state and your objective evaluation.

Abnormalities of mood include depression, elation, euphoria, anxiety, and anger. You should note whether mood is consistent with thought and action or is incongruous.

Abnormalities of affect include the following:

- *Blunting:* the coarsening of emotions and insensitivity to social context. This is commonly used synonymously with affective "flattening."
- *Flattening of affect:* a reduction in range and depth of outward emotion
- *Lability:* superficially fluctuating and poorly controlled emotions. This may be found in delirium, dementias, frontal lobe damage, and intoxication.

Thought content

Preoccupations

These include phenomena such as *obsessive thoughts*, or ruminations characterized by an intrusive preoccupation with a topic. The patient cannot stop thinking about it even though they may realize that it is irrational.

Phobias represent a fear or anxiety that is out of proportion to the situation, cannot be reasoned or explained away, and leads to avoidance behavior.

Other types of ruminations particularly important to establish here include suicidal or homicidal thoughts, in addition to morbid ideation (e.g., ideas of guilt, unworthiness, burden, and blame).

Abnormal beliefs

Overvalued ideas

These are isolated beliefs that are not obsessive in nature and preoccupy an individual to the extent of dominating their life. That is, the patient is able to stop thinking about them, but they choose not to.

The core belief of anorexia nervosa—the belief that one is fat—is an example of an overvalued idea. Other examples include unusual sect or cult beliefs, forms of morbid jealousy, and hypochondriasis.

Delusions

These are fixed false beliefs based on an incorrect inference about reality, not consistent with a patient's intelligence and cultural background (see Box 15.8). Importantly, these cannot be corrected by reasoning. They can sometimes be difficult to differentiate from overvalued ideas. The difference is that the patient firmly believes the delusion to be true.

Box 15.8 Some examples of delusions and associated terminology

- *Mood-congruent delusion:* a delusion with content that has an association to mood. For example, a depressed person may believe that the world is ending.
- *Mood-incongruent delusion:* a delusion with content that has no association to mood. This is seen in schizophrenia.
- *Nihilistic delusion:* a false feeling that self, others, or the world is nonexistent or coming to an end
- *Paranoid delusion:* any delusion that is self-referential. In psychiatry, *paranoid* does not carry the lay meaning of *fearful* or *suspicious*.
- *Delusions of reference:* a false belief that others are talking about you or that events are somehow connected with you. For example, the patient may believe that people on TV or the radio are actually talking directly to them. The feelings and delusional messages received are usually negative in some way, but the fact that the patient alone is being spoken to has a grandiose quality.
- *Delusion of grandeur:* an exaggerated perception of one's importance, power, or identity. Usually, patients believe they have made an important achievement that has not been suitably recognized.
- *Delusions of control:* a false belief that a person's will, thoughts, or feeling are being controlled by external forces. These include disorders of the possession of thought.

Box 15.8 (Cont'd.)

- *Thought broadcasting:* the false belief that the patient's thoughts can be heard by others
- *Thought insertion:* the belief that an outside force, person, or persons are putting thoughts in the patient's mind. *Thought withdrawal* is the belief that thoughts are being removed.
- *Thought echo:* thoughts being heard spoken aloud
- *Thought blocking:* the experience of having one's train of thought halted
- **Passivity feelings:** examples of delusions of control. They may include *made acts and impulses*, where the individual feels they are being made to do something by another, *made movements*, where patients believe their limbs are controlled by someone else, *made emotions*, where they are experiencing someone else's emotions.
- **Erotomania:** a belief that another person is in love with the patient. Patients often believe that innocent glances from another person have a deeper, sexual meaning.
- **Capgras delusion[1]:** belief that those around you (often loved ones) have been removed and replaced with exact replicas. Patients exist in a world of impersonators. The delusion may extend to animals and objects. Patients may believe that they are their own double.
- **Religious delusions:** any delusions with a religious or spiritual content.
  ⓘ Be careful here! Beliefs considered normal for a person's religious or cultural background (e.g., a Christian believing that God has cured their illness) are not classed as delusions.

[1] Capgras JMJ, Reboul-Lachaux J (1923). L'illusion des 'sosies' dans un délire systématisé chronique. *Bulletin de la Société clinique de médecine mentale* 11:6–16.

Delusions may be *primary* with no discernable connection with any previous experience or mood (characteristic of schizophrenia) or *secondary* to an abnormal mood state or perception. In this way, the content of the delusions can give a clue to the nature of the mental illness.

Perception
Alteration in normal perception consists of changes to our normal, familiar awareness or ordinary experiences. These include sensory distortions (heightened or dulled perception), sensory deceptions (illusions and hallucinations), and disorder of self-awareness (depersonalization, derealization).

Disorders of self-awareness
- *Depersonalization* is the feeling that the body is strange and unreal.
- *Derealization* is the perception of objects in the external world as being strange end unreal.

Both of these phenomena commonly occur in stressful situations, with drug intoxication, anxiety, depressive disorders, and in schizophrenia. Many psychologically normal people can experience an element of derealization or depersonalization if sleep deprived.

Illusions

An *illusion* is a misperception or misinterpretation of real sensory stimuli. It may affect any sensory modality. Inquire as to when they occur and what significance they have.

Illusions frequently arise from a sensory impairment, such as partial sightedness or deafness, and represent an understandable attempt at filling in the gap. Most people have experienced some form of visual illusions—for example, mistaking a distant object for a person, particularly in poor lighting (e.g., at night).

Hallucinations

Hallucination is a false perception that is not based on a real external stimulus. It is experienced as true and coming from the outside world.

They may occur in any sensory modality, although visual and auditory hallucinations are most common (Box 15.9).

Importantly, not all hallucinations point to psychiatric disease. For example, some hallucinations occur in normal people when falling asleep (hypnagogic) or on waking (hypnopompic), and although the nature of dreams is heavily debated, it could be said that they are hallucinations. Note also the Charles Bonnet syndrome (Box 15.10).

Box 15.9 Some examples of hallucinations

- **Auditory hallucinations:** false perception of sounds, usually voices, but also other noises such as music. The hallucination of voices may be classed as *second person,* where the voice is speaking to the patient ("you should do this") or *third person,* where the voice or voices are talking about the patient ("he should do this").
- **Visual hallucinations:** false perceptions involving both formed (e.g., faces, people) and unformed (e.g., lights, shadows) images
- **Scenic or panoramic hallucinations:** a form of visual hallucination involving whole scenes, such as battles
- **Olfactory hallucinations:** the false perception of odors
- **Gustatory hallucinations:** the false perception of taste
- **Tactile hallucinations:** the false perception of touch or surface sensation (e.g., phantom limb; crawling sensation in or under skin in delirium tremens—formication)
- **Somatic hallucination:** the false sensation of things occurring in or to the body, most often visceral in origin. Somatic hallucinations include *haptic* (touch, tickling, pricking), *thermic* (heat/cold), and *kinathetic* (movement and joint position).
- **Pseudohallucinations:** These are recognized as not being real by the patient, acquiring an as-if quality, and have some degree of voluntary control.

Box 15.10 Charles Bonnet syndrome

This is a good example of hallucinations in a psychiatrically normal patient. In this syndrome, patients with some kind of visual impairment (usually older people) see visual hallucinations within the area of impaired vision. The hallucinations are often cartoon-like characters or faces. For example, the authors once came across a patient with a visual scotoma due to retinal injury. The voice of our Irish consultant would trigger the hallucination of a leprechaun dancing and cavorting within their blind spot.

The syndrome is also an example of pseudohallucination, as often the patient realizes that the visions are not real.

It was first described by the Swiss philosopher Charles Bonnet in 1760, whose 87-year-old grandfather admitted seeing visions of buildings and people after developing severe cataracts in both eyes.

Charles Bonnet syndrome is likely much more common than most medical people realize. Older sufferers are often afraid to admit to it, for fear of being diagnosed with a psychiatric disorder or being labeled "insane."

Sensory distortions

This includes heightened perception with especially vivid sensations (e.g., hyperacusis), dulled perception, and changed perception. For example, patients may experience objects as having a changed shape, size, or color.

Cognitive function

Cognition can be described as the mental processes of appraisal, judgment, memory, and reasoning. Evaluation of cognitive functioning is important for detecting impairment, following the course of an illness, and monitoring improvement or response to treatment.

The Mini-Mental State Examination (MMSE)

The MMSE provides a brief quantitative measure of cognitive functioning and can be used in both a psychiatric or general medical setting. It tests attention, orientation, immediate and short-term recall, language, and the ability to follow verbal and written commands (see Box 15.11).

Notes on conducting the MMSE

It is important to remember that there are no half marks in this test—be strict and rigorous. The maximum total score is 30.

- *Orientation:* Rather than asking for each part of the date in turn, ask the patient for today's date and then ask specifically for those parts omitted. Do the same for place ("where are we now?").
- *Registration:* Say the name of the objects clearly and slowly, allowing about 1 second to say each. The first repetition determines the patient's score, but keep repeating the names of the object until the patient has got all three, to enable testing of recall later.

Box 15.11 Mini-Mental State Examination (MMSE) Sample Items

Orientation to time
"What is the date?"

Registration
"Listen carefully. I am going to say three words. You say them back after I stop. Ready? Here they are...
APPLE (pause), PENNY (pause), TABLE (pause). Now repeat those words back to me." [Repeat up to 5 times, but score only the first trial.]

Naming
"What is this?" [Point to a pencil or pen.]

Reading
"Please read this and do what it says." [Show examinee the words on the stimulus form.]
CLOSE YOUR EYES

- *Attention and calculation:* If the patient can't perform this mathematical task, ask them to spell the word *WORLD* backward. The score is the number of letters in the correct order (e.g., dlrow = 5, dlorw = 3).
- *Repetition:* Allow one trial. Score 1 only if the repetition is completely correct. Make sure you say it slowly and clearly so that the patient can hear!
- *Three-stage command:* Say all three stages of the command before giving the piece of paper to the patient. Do not prompt the patient as you go. Score 1 point for each part conducted correctly.
- *Reading:* Say "read this sentence and do what it says." Score 1 point if the patient closes their eyes, no points if they simply read the sentence out loud.
- *Writing:* Be sure not to dictate a sentence or give any examples. The sentence must make sense and contain a subject and a verb. Correct grammar, punctuation, and spelling are not necessary.
- *Copying:* All 10 angles must be present, and 2 must intersect. Ignore mistakes from tremor and ignore rotation of the diagram.

Interpreting the final score

The MMSE score will vary within the normal population by age and number of years in education (decreasing with advancing age and increasing with advanced schooling). The median score is 29 for people with 9 years of education, 26 for 5–8 years of education, and 22 for 0–4 years.[1]

As a rule of thumb, scores of <23 are taken to indicate mild, <17 moderate, and <10 severe cognitive impairment. This is a nonlinear scale, however. For more information, see Crum et al. (1993).[1]

Insight

This is how well the patient is able to understand or explain their condition. When assessing insight, ask the following questions:

- Do they recognize and accept that they are suffering from a mental or physical illness?
- Are they willing to accept treatment and agree to a management plan?

Note also whether an individual's attitudes are constructive or unconstructive, realistic or unrealistic.

If not accepting of a psychiatric diagnosis, to what does the patient attribute their difficulties or abnormal experiences?

[1] Crum RM, Anthony JC, Bassett SS, Folstein MF (1993). Population-based norms for the Mini-Mental State Examination by age and educational level. *JAMA* 18:2386–2391.

Summary

At the end of the assessment, a summary should be made of history and mental state examination, which should encompass a statement of diagnosis or differential diagnosis, etiolgical factors, and a plan for further investigations and management.

Physical examination

A full physical examination, particularly that of the neurological system should be seen as an integral part of the assessment of a psychiatric patient.

You may want to tailor an examination to look for, or exclude, physical conditions that give rise to the psychiatric symptoms and signs that you have discovered. See the end of this chapter for details.

Important presenting patterns

Schizophrenia

The term *schizophrenia** is often described as a single disease, but the diagnostic category includes a group of disorders, probably with heterogeneous causes, but with somewhat similar behavioral symptoms and signs (Box 15.12). It is a psychosis, characterized by splitting of normal links between perception, mood, thinking, behavior, and contact with reality.

The prevalence of schizophrenia is ~0.5% worldwide, with equal incidence in both sexes. The onset is usually in adolescence or early adulthood. Symptoms tend to remit, although a return to baseline is unusual.

Clinical features

Schizophrenia is characterized by delusions and hallucinations with no insight. These symptoms are often followed by a decline in social functioning. Historically, several different diagnostic classifications have been developed. For the latest diagnostic criteria, see the ICD-10 or DSM-IV or DSM-V (due in 2012).

Bleuler's four A's

In 1910, Bleuler coined the term *schizophrenia*. He went on to characterize the key features, summarized as the four A's.

- Associative loosening (disconnected, incoherent thought process)
- Ambivalence (the ability to experience two opposing emotions at the same time—e.g., loving and hating a person)
- Affective incongruity (affect disassociated with thought)
- Autism (self-absorption and withdrawal into a fantasy world)

Box 15.12 Subtypes of schizophrenia

- **Simple:** Negative symptoms tend to predominate.
- **Paranoid:** Delusions and hallucinations are prominent and tend to include religious, grandiose, and persecutory ideas.
- **Hebephrenic:** Affective incongruity predominates, with shallow range of mood. Delusions and hallucinations tend to lack an organized theme.
- **Catatonic:** Anhedonia, avolition, alogia, and poverty of movement are the key features. This may lead to a "waxy flexibility," where the patient's limbs can be moved into, and stay in, certain positions.

---

* *Schizophrenia* comes through Latin from the Greek *skhizein*, "to split" and *phren*, "mind." The term *phrenic* refers also to the diaphragm. This is because in ancient Greece, the mind was thought to lie in the diaphragm.

Crow's positive and negative symptoms

In 1980, Crow[1] suggested that the symptoms of schizophrenia could be divided into two distinct groups—those that are positive and those that are negative. This remains a useful way to think of the symptoms.

Crow went on to suggest that schizophrenia could be split into two syndromes, comprising mostly positive or negative symptoms, respectively.

Positive symptoms
- Delusions (including ideas of reference)
- Hallucinations
- Thought disorder

Negative symptoms
- Blunted affect
- Anhedonia (lack of enjoyment)
- Avolition (lack of motivation)
- Alogia (poverty of speech)
- Social withdrawal
- Self-neglect

Schneider's first-rank symptoms

Kurt Schneider listed his first-rank symptoms of schizophrenia in 1959[2]. One of these, Schneider said, is diagnostic of schizophrenia in the absence of organic brain disease or drug intoxication.
- Third-person auditory hallucinations (running commentary, arguments, or discussions about the patient)
- Thought echo, or "echo de la pensée"
- Disorders of thought control (withdrawal, insertion, broadcast)
- Passivity phenomena
- Delusional perception
- Somatic passivity

Schneider's criteria have been criticized for being too narrow, providing a snapshot of a patient at only one time, and for not taking into account the long-term negative symptoms.

For information on etiology, treatment, and prognosis, see appropriate other Handbooks in this series.

Delirium

Delirium, or acute confusional state, is a transient global disorder of cognition that is characterized by an acute onset and a fluctuating course. It represents one of the most important and misdiagnosed problems in medicine and surgery (see Box 15.13 for assessment).

Delirium may occur in as many as 10–20% of hospital inpatients, with elderly patients being the most vulnerable. Approximately 60% of patients suffer delirium following hip fracture.

[1] Crow TJ (1980). Molecular pathology of schizophrenia: more than one disease process? *BMJ* 280:66–68.
[2] Schneider K (1959). *Clinical Psychopathology*. New York: Grune and Stratton.

Box 15.13 Confusion assessment method (CAM)

This is method is commonly used to assess delirium in the clinical set-ting.[1] The patient must display both features 1 and 2 *plus* either 3 or 4.

- 1 *Acute onset and fluctuating course:* often best obtained from a relative or member of the ward staff. Onset is hours to days, lucid periods are often in the morning.
- 2 *Inattention:* easily distracted, attention wanders in conversation
- 3 *Disorganized thinking:* rambling or irrelevant conversation, illogical flow of ideas, unable to maintain a coherent stream of thought
- 4 *Altered level of consciousness:* drowsy or over active, may fluctuate. May experience nightmares and hallucinations.

[1] Inouye S, van Dyck C, Alessi C, et al. (1990). Clarifying confusion: the confusion assessment method. *Ann Intern Med* 113(12):941–948

Following is a brief summary of the main features and causes. You should bear all the possible causes in mind and tailor your physical examination and investigations accordingly (see Chapter 10).

Predisposing factors (risk factors)

- Increasing age
- Pre-existing cognitive defect
- Psychiatric illness
- Severe physical comorbidity
- Previous episode of delirium
- Deficits in hearing or vision
- Anticholinergic drug use
- New environment or stress

Causes (precipitants)

Delirium is usually multifactorial, with a single cause being difficult or impossible to identify. Some factors include the following:

Intracranial factors

- Trauma
- Vascular disease (e.g., stroke)
- Epilepsy and postictal states
- Tumor
- Infection (meningitis, encephalitis, tuberculosis, neurosyphilis)

Extracranial factors

- Drugs—both prescribed and recreational, intoxication, and withdrawal
- Electrolyte imbalances
- Infection (e.g., urinary tract, chest, septicemia)
- Endocrine (e.g., thyroid dysfunction, hypo- and hyperglycemia)
- Organ failure (heart, lung, liver, kidney)
- Hypoxia
- Acid–base disturbance

- Nutritional deficiencies
- Postoperative or postanesthetic states
- Miscellaneous
  - Sensory deprivation
  - Sleep deprivation
  - Fecal impaction
  - Change of environment

Symptoms
- Fluctuating level of consciousness
- Difficulty maintaining, or frequently shifting, attention
- Disorientation (often worse at night)
- Illusions
- Hallucinations (often simple, visual)
- Apathy
- Emotional lability
- Depression
- Disturbance of the normal sleep–wake cycle

Differential diagnosis
- Dementia (often coexists with delirium and ↑ risk of delirium 2- to 3-fold), depression, psychosis, AIDS-related complex

Anxiety disorders*

Generalized anxiety disorder (GAD)
The main feature is excessive anxiety and worry about events or activities that the patient finds difficult to control, such as work or school performance. The symptoms must be present for more than 6 months and include three or more of the following:
- Restlessness or feeling on edge
- Easily fatigued
- Difficulty concentrating or mind goes blank
- Irritability
- Muscle tension
- Sleep disturbance (insomnia and fatigue on waking)

Panic disorder
This involves spontaneous occurrence of severe panic attacks (periods of fear that peak within 10 minutes).

These should be accompanied by four or more of the following: tachycardia, sweating, trembling or shaking, shortness of breath, a feeling of choking, chest pain, dizziness, lightheadedness or presyncope, paresthesia, depersonalization or derealization, nausea, abdominal pain, fear of dying, fear of losing control, and hot flushes.

Phobic disorders
A *phobia* is an irrational fear that produces an avoidance of the subject of the fear (an object, person, activity, or situation). A phobia is perceived by the patient as excessive (i.e., they have insight).

---

* Based on DSM-IV criteria.

Agoraphobia

Agoraphobia† is not fear of wide open spaces per se, as is commonly thought, but is anxiety caused by being in places or situations from which escape may be difficult or in which help might not be available in the event of a panic attack. These situations may include being outside, being home alone, being in a crowded place, or traveling on a bus or train.

Social phobia

This is a fear of social situations in which the person is exposed to unfamiliar people or to possible scrutiny by others. The fear is of the resulting humiliation caused by a poor performance.

Avoidance behavior, anticipation, or distress at the time of the social encounter leads to impairment in functioning at work or in school and can have a significant impact on the patient's life.

Other specific phobias

These are marked and persistent fears cued by the presence or anticipation of specific objects or situations. The list is manifold. Our favorites, from which no medic can suffer, include bromidrosiphobia (the fear of body odor), spermophobia (the fear of germs), belonephobia (the fear of needles), phronemophobia (the fear of thinking), iatrophobia (the fear of doctors), and, of course, pinaciphobia (the fear of lists).

Obsessive-compulsive disorder (OCD)

This is characterized by time-consuming obsessions or compulsions that cause social impairment or mental distress.

Obsessions are intrusive thoughts, feelings, ideas, or sensations. They are recognized by the patient as their own (compare with thought insertion)—the patient usually tries to ignore or suppress them.

Compulsions are conscious, purposeful behaviors through which the person attempts to neutralize or prevent a discomfort or dreaded event. Examples include repeated hand-washing, checking, and counting.

The key here is that the obsessions and compulsions are recognized as coming from within the patient, and the patient feels powerless to stop and is distressed by their presence. Severe obsessions and compulsions can occur in depression, schizophrenia, generalized anxiety disorder, panic disorder, and other disorders.

Dementia

Dementia is usually a disease of older people and refers to a global deterioration of higher mental functioning, without impairment in consciousness, that is progressive and usually irreversible.

Dementia usually presents with a history of chronic, steady decline in short- and long-term memory and is associated with difficulties in social relationships, work, and activities of daily living. Important manifestations include disruption of language and intelligence as well as changes in personality and behavior. Apathy, depression, and anxiety are frequently found, and psychotic phenomena may be seen in a third of patients.

† *Agoraphobia* comes from the Greek *agora*, meaning "the marketplace."

A diagnosis of dementia is based on MMSE results and information from other sources, such as the patient's family, friends, and employers.

Dementia may be primary or secondary to diseases:

- *Chronic CNS infection:* HIV, syphilis, meningitis, encephalitis
- *CNS trauma:* anoxia, diffuse axonal injury, dementia pugilistica (repeated head injury—seen in boxers), chronic subdural hematoma
- ↑ *Intracranial pressure:* neoplasia, hydrocephalus
- *Toxins:* heavy metals, organic chemicals, chronic substance abuse
- *Vitamin deficiencies:* B$_{12}$, folate
- *Autoimmune disease:* SLE, temporal arteritis, sarcoidosis

Other possible causes include endocrinopathies, Wilson's disease, and lipid storage diseases.

Alzheimer's disease

The key pathological changes in Alzheimer's disease (AD) are decreased brain mass and increased size of the ventricles. There is neuronal loss and occurrence of amyloid plaques and neurofibrillary tangles. AD makes up ~50% of all cases of dementia and ~90% of all primary dementias. The main features are memory impairment and at least one of the following:

- Aphasia (📖 p. 260)
- Apraxia (📖 p. 328)
- Agnosia (📖 p. 327)
- Abnormal executive functioning (planning, organizing, abstracting, sequencing)

Vascular dementia/multi-infarct dementia

This makes up about 20–30% of all cases of dementia. Onset may be abrupt and/or with a stepwise decline. Vascular dementia is associated with more patchy cognitive impairment then AD, often with focal neurological signs and symptoms such as hyperreflexia, extensor plantar responses, pseudobulbar, bulbar, or other cranial nerve palsies, gait abnormalities, and focal weakness.

The primary pathology is multiple small areas of infarction (cortex and underlying white matter). It is important to note vascular risk factors such as previous stroke, hypertension, heart disease, diabetes, and smoking.

Lewy body dementia

Lewy body dementia accounts for up to 20% of all cases. Patients with this disorder show features similar to AD but also often have recurrent visual hallucinations, fluctuating cognitive impairment, parkinsonian features, and extrapyramidal signs.

Frontotemporal dementia

This accounts for 5% of all dementia. Pick's disease is a form of frontotemporal dementia characterized by the presence of neuronal Pick's bodies (masses of cytoskeletal elements).

The predominance of frontal lobe involvement is evidenced by profound personality changes, social impairment, and stereotyped behavior. However, visuospacial skills are usually preserved. The patient may also show primitive reflexes (📖 p. 307).

Huntington's disease

Huntington's is an autosomal dominant disease presenting as early as the third decade and is associated with a subcortical type of dementia. Apart from the movement disorder showing involuntary choreiform movements of the face, shoulders, upper limbs, and gait, the symptoms of the dementia include psychomotor slowing and personality alteration with apathy or depression.

Parkinson's disease

Patients with Parkinson's disease have cognitive slowing along with the signs described earlier (📖 p. 325). Dementia is seen in later stages of disease.

Creutzfeldt–Jakob disease (CJD)

Contrary to common perception, this is not a new disease or one that affects young people. The most frequently seen of this family of diseases is sporadic CJD, which has no known cause. Onset is usually between the forth and sixth decades of life and is associated with a very rapid progression of dementia, in addition to signs such as myoclonus, seizures, and ataxia—the time to death is typically a few months.

Variant CJD (vCJD) is a disease mainly confined to the UK, first reported in 1996, and is thought to have resulted from transmission of infection from cattle suffering from bovine spongeiform encephalopathy (BSE). The average age of onset is 27 years, presenting initially with behavioral symptoms. The duration is of a year or more.

Affective disorders

Bipolar disorder

Bipolar disorder, previously known as manic-depression, is usually characterized by periods of deep, prolonged depression with periods of excessively elevated and irritable mood, known as *mania*.

It is important to note that patients presenting only with mania, and no evident depression, are said to have bipolar disorder. There are three main patterns of disease:

- *Bipolar I disorder*: one or more episodes of major depression with episodes of mania
- *Bipolar II disorder:* milder bipolar disorder consisting of recurrent periods of depression and hypomania but no manic episodes
- *Cyclothymic disorder:* characterized by frequently occurring hypomanic and depressive symptoms that do not meet the diagnostic criteria of manic episodes or major depression

Mania

Manic episodes are characterized by profound mood disturbance, consisting of an elevated, expansive, or irritable mood that causes impairment at work or danger to others (Box 15.14). These patients may suffer delusions and hallucinations, the former usually involving power, prestige, position, self-worth, and glory. The key feature is disinhibition.

Box 15.14 Typical mental state examination in affective disorders

Mania
- *Appearance:* bright, colorful, or garish clothing, hyperactivity, hypervigilance, restlessness
- *Speech:* fast, pressured, flight of ideas
- *Mood and affect:* joy, elation, jubilance, euphoria, annoyance, irritability
- *Thought content:* expansive and optimistic thinking, excessively self-confident or grandiose, distractible, rapid production of ideas and thoughts
- *Perception:* mood-congruent and mood-incongruent delusions. Fleeting auditory or, more rarely, visual hallucinations. Delusions of wealth, power, influence, or religious significance
- *Cognitive functioning:* usually unaffected
- *Insight:* seriously impaired judgment and no insight

Depression
- *Appearance:* reduced eye contact, poor grooming and hygiene, change in weight, psychomotor agitation, or retardation
- *Speech:* slow, monotonous, or lacking in spontaneity
- *Mood and affect:* sadness, numbness, irritability, anhedonia, reduced concentration, loss of energy, and motivation
- *Thought content:* preoccupied with negative ideas and nihilistic concerns, overwhelmed or inadequate, helpless, worthless, hopeless, suicidal
- *Perception:* delusions and hallucinations (usually mood congruent), especially second-person auditory hallucinations. For example, auditory hallucinations of voices call the patient worthless.
- *Cognitive functioning:* poor memory and concentration but level of consciousness is normal. Depressed patients may score falsely low on an MMSE if they are not willing to answer the questions ("I don't know")—pseudodementia.
- *Insight:* diminished judgment and insight

There may be several of the following:
- Inflated self-esteem or grandiosity
- Reduced need for sleep
- Racing thought, flight of ideas, and distractibility
- Excessive talking or pressured speech
- ↑ Level of goal-focused activity at home, at work, or sexually
- Psychomotor agitation
- Excessive involvement in pleasurable activities, often with unfortunate consequences (especially sexual indiscretions, unrestrained spending)

Depression

Depressive disorders can be classified as bipolar or unipolar and as mild, moderate, or severe. They may include somatic symptoms and psychotic symptoms (delusions and hallucinations that are usually mood-congruent) in the case of severe depression.

The diagnostic criteria, treatment, and prognosis can be found in the *Oxford Handbook of Psychiatry*. Depression can cause significant social impairment and distress.

In general terms, features of major depression include the following:

- Depressed mood with feelings of worthlessness
- Diminished interest or pleasure (anhedonia)
- Significant weight loss or gain
- Insomnia or hypersomnia
- Psychomotor agitation or retardation
- Fatigue or loss of energy
- Diminished ability to think or concentrate; indecisiveness
- Recurrent thoughts of death, suicide, suicide attempts, or specific plans for suicide

Hypomania

Hypomanic episodes are characterized by a persistently elevated, expansive, or irritable mood with features similar to mania. However, the episode is not severe enough to cause marked impairment in social or occupational functioning, and delusions and hallucinations do not occur.

Medical conditions with psychiatric symptoms and signs

There are many medical conditions that can produce psychiatric clinical features. This can sometimes lead to failure of the underlying medical condition to be recognized and treated appropriately. It is important in psychiatry to consider possible organic causes for the symptoms and signs before starting psychiatric treatment. Further, many medical disorders are associated with psychiatric diagnoses.

The following is a sample of such situations, aimed at illustrating the above points, rather than providing an exhaustive list.

Neurological disorders

Seizure disorder

- Ictal events, including status epilepticus, may mimic psychosis.
- Automatisms are seen in some temporal lobe seizures.
- The preictal prodrome can involve changes in mood, particularly irritability, and auras (including auditory and olfactory hallucinations) can be seen in temporal lobe epilepsy. These may also include epigastric sensations, *déja vu* or *jamais vu*.
- The postictal state often involves confusion and disorientation.

Parkinson's disease

- Patients may suffer from major depression, anxiety syndromes, hallucinations, and delusions.

Brain tumors and cerebrovascular events (depend on location)

- *Frontal:* personality change, cognitive impairment, motor and language disturbance
- *Dominant temporal lobe:* memory and speech impairment, Korsakoff psychosis in bilateral lesions
- *Occipital lesions:* visual agnosis, visual hallucinations
- *Limbic and hypothalamic:* affective symptoms, rage, mania

Multiple sclerosis (MS)

- Cognitive deficits, dementia, bipolar disorder, major depression

Infectious diseases

- **Neurosyphilis:** primarily affects the frontal lobe (irritability, poor self-care, mania, progressive dementia)
- **Meningitis:** especially with indwelling shunts, can cause acute confusion, memory impairment
- **Herpes simplex encephalitis:** bizarre and inconsistent behavior, seizures, anosmia, hallucinations (olfactory and gustatory), psychosis
- **HIV encephalitis:** progressive subcortical dementia, major depression, suicidal behavior, anxiety disorders, abnormal psychological reactions

Endocrine disorders

- **Hyperparathyroidism:** delirium, sudden stupor and coma. Visual hallucinations with associated hypomagnesaemia

- *Hypoparathyroidism:* psychosis, depression, anxiety
- *Hyperthyroidism:* depression, anxiety, hypomania, psychosis
- *Hypothyroidism:* depression, apathy, psychomotor retardation, poor memory, delirium and psychosis myxoedema madness

Rheumatological disorders

- *Systemic lupus erythematosus (SLE):* delirium, psychosis, severe depression

Metabolic disorders

- *Hyponatraemia:* confusion, depression, delusions, hallucinations, seizures, stupor, coma
- *Hypernatremia:* acute changes of mental state
- *Encephalopathy*
- *Uremia encephalopathy:* memory impairment, depression, apathy, social withdrawal

Vitamin deficiencies

- B_1 *(thiamine):* asthenia, fatigue, weakness, depression
- B_{12} *(cyanocobalamin):* impaired cognitive function

Pediatric assessment

History-taking

Children and providers

The specialty of pediatrics is very different from adult medicine. Children grow, change, and mature. Your style and approach to history-taking and examination will depend greatly on the child's age, independence, and understanding, so flexibility is essential. The most important thing to remember during your time as a provider is that pediatrics should be pleasurable.

An approach to the child patient

The child needs to be put at ease and made to feel welcome.

- Make a complimentary remark, or show them an interesting toy. The fascination of how to turn on a tuning fork can amaze many children.
- Tell the child your name, and ask theirs.
- Make friends with them by asking what their favorite class is at school or what they had for breakfast.
- Shake hands with children—even toddlers may enjoy this formality.

History

A structured approach to history-taking is important to keep from forgetting things, but avoid excessive rigidity, as it is sometimes necessary to pursue a different line of questioning to gain essential information. Box 16.1 is a list of useful headings in pediatric history-taking that should be memorized to avoid missing essential information.

Talking to the child

Ask the child to give their account of events with parental corroboration. Children under 5 years old may lack the vocabulary to describe their symptoms but will be able to point to parts that hurt. Sometimes it is important to quiet the eager parent to hear from the patient!

Talking to parents

Most of the history is likely to be gained from the parents or guardians. First confirm the relationship of the history provider.

- Ask if they have an infant medical record book—this contains information about height and weight percentiles, immunizations, development, and illnesses in the first few years of life.
- Ask if they have any views on what the cause of the child's trouble is. Listen carefully to the parents; they are the observer of their child.
- Ensure that all terms used are appropriately defined—you should be gleaning information from the parents' observations and *not* their interpretation of the symptoms.

For example, the word *wheeze* is often used incorrectly; sometimes a demonstration can be helpful. Further, the parent may interpret a baby's cries as pain, when, in fact, it is your task to establish the circumstances of the cries and thus the cause.

As children get older, parents may have a hazy memory for early events. Establishing symptoms in relation to easily remembered events (e.g. first walked) may clarify the timeline.

Box 16.1 Outline of pediatric history

- Presenting complaint and history of presenting complaint
- Birth history
  - Place of birth
  - Gestation and pregnancy
  - Birth weight
  - Delivery
  - Perinatal events and subsequent hospital course
- Feeding methods and weaning
  - If the child is bottle fed, note how the formula is mixed (how many scoops or number of ounces).
- PMH, including hospital admissions, infections, injuries
- Developmental history
- School progress
- Immunizations
- Drugs
- Allergies
- Family tree with sibling's ages, including deaths, miscarriages, and stillbirths
- Parental age and occupation
- Family illnesses and allergies
- Housing
  - Include a discussion about the child's bedroom, with furnishings, as they may spend 12 hours of each day there.
- Travel
- Systems review

"You can do anything with children if you only play with them."
—Otto von Bismarck, 19th century

Examination: an approach

Examination of children varies depending on the age and cooperation of the child (see also Box 16.2). School-age children and babies may be examined on an exam table with a parent nearby, whereas toddlers may be best examined on the parent's lap (Box 16.3). If the child is asleep on the parent's lap, much of the examination should be completed before waking them.

Undressing

Let the parent undress the child, and only expose the part of the body you will be examining.

Positioning

Some children may prefer to be examined standing up. Only lay the child down when you have to, as this can be very threatening.

Putting the child at ease

Slowly introduce yourself into the child's space during the examination by exchanging toys, for example.

Explain what you are going to do and be repeatedly reassuring, children can be embarrassed by silence after a provider's question but will be comforted by endless rambling. And remember—don't ask permission, as this will often be refused!

Examination

First, use a hands-off approach. Allow the child to look at you, and let them play in your presence. Watch the child. How do they interact with their parents? Do they look well or ill? Do they look clean, well nourished, and well cared for?

Kneel on the floor so that you are at the child's level. Use a style and language appropriate to the age of the child—a toddler will understand the word *tummy* better than the word *abdomen*.

Box 16.2 Some distraction techniques to help examination

- Playing peek-a-boo
- Letting toddlers play with your reflex hammer or tuning fork
- Giving infants something to hold
- Asking mom or dad to wave a bright toy in front of the child

---

Box 16.3 The mother's lap

1. Be cautious about taking any baby or young child to an exam table. It is often better to leave them on their mother's knee for most of the examination.
2. Avoid taking a baby off their mother's knee if they are beyond 7–8 months of age—this will invariably result in screaming.

Be opportunistic

Do not adhere to a rigid examination protocol—e.g., you may have to listen to the heart first while the child is quiet, then look at the hands later. Never examine the presenting part only. Be thorough and train yourself to be a generalist (Box 16.4).

Sometimes, demonstrating with a cooperative older sibling, parent, or a stuffed toy may put a child more at ease about what is to be done.

Leave unpleasant procedures, such as examination of the ears and throat, for last.

Presenting your findings

When presenting your findings, translate what you see into appropriate terminology. Informing a colleague that a child "looks funny" is not very helpful, but the saying that the child is dysmorphic, followed by a detailed description is acceptable. Describe in simple terms the relevant features that make the child look unusual, e.g., low-set ears, wide-set eyes.

▶ There is no substitute for examining lots of normal children.

> "Pediatrics is a specialty bound by age and not by system."
> —Apley

Box 16.4 Using this chapter

The examination routines in this chapter describe the techniques to employ and the signs to look for in each body system. For more detailed information about how to perform certain aspects, the reader should refer to the relevant organ system chapter elsewhere in this book (e.g., how to perform accurate percussion, where to listen to heart sounds, and so on).

Respiratory system

Key points from the history

- Is the child short of breath or wheezy (remember to define terms)?
- Is there stridor or croup?
- Is there a cough? Does it disturb sleep?
- Does anything trigger the symptoms—sports, cold weather, pets?
- Has the child expectorated or vomited any sputum?
- Is the infant short of breath during breast or bottle feeding?
- Is there a possibility the child could have inhaled a foreign body?
- Is there a FH of respiratory problems, such as asthma or cystic fibrosis?
- Does the child have a fever—suggestive of infection?
- Has anyone else been ill? Any contacts with tuberculosis?
- What's happening at the child-care facility?
- Has the child traveled abroad recently?
- How does the respiratory problem limit the child's life—how much school is missed, can they participate in sports, how far can they run, is sleep disturbed?

Examination

Inspection

Look around for any clues—is the patient on oxygen? Are there inhalers or nebulizers at the bedside? Remember if mom or dad's clothing smells of tobacco, the child is breathing smoke too.

General inspection

- Is the child comfortable or in respiratory distress (Box 16.5)? Look for the following:
  - Nasal flaring
  - Use of accessory muscles of respiration
  - Intercostal retractions (sucking in of the muscles between the ribs) and subcostal retractions (drawing in of the abdomen)
  - Grunting (a noise at the end of expiration, which is the infant's attempt to maintain a positive end expiratory pressure)
- Is the child running around or just sitting on the parent's knee?
- Are they restless or drowsy?
- Count the respiratory rate (see Table 16.1).
- Listen for wheeze or stridor (a harsh inspiratory sound caused by upper airways obstruction).
- What type of cough does the child have (Box 16.6)?

Box 16.5 Pain

Children may complain of pain when they wish to indicate distress or discomfort that their vocabulary will not allow. Remember also that diseases may present differently in children than in adults. For example, children may describe chest pain with chest tightness and asthma.

Pneumonia often produces abdominal pain in children.

- Has the child coughed up any sputum? (Children under 5 years will swallow sputum, which is often vomited after a bout of coughing.)

Hands
- Clubbing (cystic fibrosis, bronchiectasis)
- Measure the radial pulse—pulsus paradoxus (Chapter 7, 📖 p. 159) is an important feature of acute, severe asthma in children.

Face
- Check the conjunctiva for anemia.
- Look for central cyanosis in the tongue.
- Look for petechiae (nonblanching spots from small burst blood vessels) around the eyes from a prolonged bout of coughing.

Chest
- Look for chest movement. Is it symmetrical? Is the child splinting (failing to move) one side of the chest?
  - Children who splint their chest as a consequence of pneumonia often also have a slight spinal scoliosis.
- Look at the chest shape. Is there any chest wall deformity?
  - *Harrison's sulcus:* permanent groove in the chest wall at the insertion of the diaphragm in long-standing asthma
  - *Barrel chest:* air trapping in asthma
  - *Pectus carinatum:* "pigeon chest" seen in long-standing asthma *Pectus excavatum:* normal variant

Table 16.1 Normal respiratory *and heart rates*, by age

Age (years)	Heart rate (bpm)	Respiratory rate
<1	120–160	30–60
1–3	90–140	24–40
3–5	75–110	18–30
5–12	75–100	18–30
12–16	60–90	12–16

Box 16.6 Some childhood coughs

The following factors may give important clues to origin of the cough:
- *Productive:* cystic fibrosis, bronchiectasis, pneumonia
- *Nocturnal:* asthma, cystic fibrosis
- *Worse on wakening:* cystic fibrosis
- *Brassy:* tracheitis
- *Barking:* croup (laryngotracheobronchitis)
- *Paroxysmal:* pertussis, foreign body
- *Worse during exercise:* asthma
- *Disappears when sleeping:* habitual cough
- *During or after feeding:* aspiration

Palpation
- Feel the neck for enlarged cervical lymph nodes.
- Palpate the trachea to ensure that it is midline.
- Then move onto the chest.
  - Feel for the apex beat. This may be displaced in effusion, collapse, or tension pneumothorax.
  - Assess expansion (see 📖 Chapter 8, p. 194), commenting on extent and symmetry.
  - In young children, you may be able to feel crackles.

Percussion
Percussion is rarely useful in infants and toddlers. Remember to also percuss for the normal cardiac dullness as well as the upper and lower borders of the liver.
- Dull = consolidation
- Hyperresonant = air-trapping or pneumothorax
- Stony dull = pleural effusion

Auscultation
🔔 Before using a stethoscope on the child, pretend to auscultate the parent's or an older sibling's chest or a less vulnerable part of the child's body (e.g., their leg).

▶ Remember to listen under the axillae as well as the anterior and posterior chest wall.

▶ Especially in young children, upper airway noises may be transmitted to the chest, so if they are old enough, ask them to cough to clear them.

Listen for the following:
- Breath sounds
  - Are they vesicular (normal), absent, or bronchial?
- Added sounds (e.g., wheeze or crackles—see 📖 Chapter 8, p. 198, for more details) (see Table 16.2 for some associated conditions)
- Absent breath sounds in one area suggests a pleural effusion, pneumothorax, or dense consolidation.

▶ ↑ Respiratory rate and work of breathing are the most important signs of a lower respiratory tract infection in infancy, as sometimes palpation, percussion, and auscultation will be normal.

Table 16.2 Some common respiratory conditions and signs

Condition	Age	Inspection	Auscultation
Bronchiolitis	<1 year	Pale, coryza, cough, retractions, tachypnea	Wheezes and crackles throughout chest
Croup (laryngo-tracheobronchitis)	1–2 years	Stridor, hoarse voice, barking cough	Clear
Asthma	>1 year	Tachypnea, retractions ± audible wheeze and use of accessory muscles	Wheeze, variable air entry throughout chest. Crackles in young children
Pneumonia	Infant	Tachypnea, retractions, flushing due to fever, grunting	May be clear, reduced breath sounds over affected area, crackles
Pneumonia	Child	Tachypnea, retractions, flushed, generally ill	Abdominal pain (may be the only symptom), crackles and bronchial breathing over affected area

Ear, nose, and throat

Ear, nose, and throat (ENT) conditions are a common reason for children to present to the provider.

❶ Examination of this system should be left until last, as many children find it unpleasant.

Key points from the history

- Does the child pull at their ears (suggests infection)?
- Does the child complain of an earache or a sore throat?
- Is there coryza (runny nose)?
- Does the child have a fever?
- Does the infant drool more than normal (suggests sore throat)?

Examination

Ears

- Sit the child on the parent's lap, facing to the side.
- Ask the parent to hold the child's head against their chest with one hand, and to firmly hold the child's arms and upper body with the other hand (see Box 16.7).
- With an infant, gently pull the pinna back before inserting the otoscope. When examining an older child, pull the pinna up.
- Use the otoscope as in adults—see Chapter 6, 🕮 p. 132.

See Table 16.3 for common conditions of the eardrum.

Box 16.7 More on ear examination

While asking the parent to hold the child's head during the ear examination is the usually taught method, this often leads to a struggle.

It is equally appropriate to allow the child free movement of the head, providing you splint the hand holding the otoscope against the child's face so that your hand (and otoscope) will move as the child's head moves. This can lead to a less distressing examination.

❶ In infancy, the pinna should be pulled forward (not back) to straighten the auditory canal.

Table 16.3 Some common findings when examining the eardrum

Appearance of drum	Condition
Translucent, clear light reflex	Normal
Red, bulging, loss of light reflex	Acute otitis media
Retracted, loss of light reflex, dull	Glue ear (chronic otitis media with effusion)

Nose

- Examine the nose externally for discharge.
- The nose may be examined very gently, using an otoscope.
  - Polyps are a common finding in asthma and cystic fibrosis.
  - Pale, boggy nasal mucosa suggests allergic rhinitis.

Throat

- Sit the child upright on the parents lap facing toward you.
- Ask the parent to hold the child's forehead with one hand, with the back of the child's head against their chest.
  - The parent should firmly hold the child's arms with the other hand.
- The difficulty now is encouraging the child to open their mouth!
  - Ask the child to open their mouth "as wide as a lion's."
  - Tempt an infant to open their mouth with the pacifier.
  - Sometimes children will be more inclined to open their mouth if you promise not to use a tongue depressor.
- When the child's mouth is open, gently depress the tongue with the tongue depressor if it is obstructing view of the tonsils.
- Decide whether the tonsils are
  - Normal: pink and small
  - Acutely inflamed: red, enlarged, with purulent areas
  - Chronically hypertrophied: enlarged and pitted, but not inflamed

Lymph nodes

- Always feel for cervical and supraclavicular lymphadenopathy.

Cardiovascular system

Key points from the history

- Does the child ever have blue spells (cyanosis)?
- Does the child become tired, pale, or sweaty (indicating heart failure)?
- If the patient is an infant, ask how long the child takes to feed from a bottle. Breathlessness may inhibit feeding.
- Is the child growing normally? Plot on a percentile chart.
- Does the child suffer from recurrent chest infections?
- Does the child suffer from abdominal pain (caused by organomegaly)?
- Is there a history of fainting or collapse?
- Has the child ever complained of their heart racing (would imply an arrhythmia such as supraventricular tachycardia)?
- Is there a FH of congenital heart disease?

Examination

Inspection

Search for evidence of heart failure: pallor, cyanosis, sweating, respiratory distress, and tachypnea.

Hands

- Clubbing is seen in cyanotic congenital heart disease.
- Search for signs of endocarditis, including splinter hemorrhages, Janeway lesions, and Osler's nodes.

Face

- Anemia in the conjunctiva
- Central cyanosis ("stick your tongue out!")

Neck

The jugular venous pulse and pressure are difficult to appreciate in young children, given the relative shortness of the neck.

Peripheral pulses

Palpate the radial, brachial, and femoral pulses.

❶ The femoral pulse, although sometimes awkward to feel, must always be sought to ensure coarctation of the aorta is not missed. Assess:

- *Volume:* Is it full or thready? (You need to practice feeling many pulses to appreciate the difference.) A thready, weak, or small volume pulse indicates hypovolemia. Look for pulsus paradoxus (📖 Chapter 7, p. 159).
- *Rate:* Heart rate varies with age, activity, distress, excitement, and fever (pulse rate will ↑ by 10 bpm with every temperature rise of 1°C).
- *Rhythm*
  - Sinus arrhythmia: an ↑ in pulse rate on inspiration, with slowing on expiration. This is very common in children.
  - Occasional ventricular ectopic beats are normal in children.
- *Character*
  - Collapsing pulse in children is most commonly due to a patent ductus arteriosus.
  - Slow rising pulse suggests ventricular outflow obstruction.

Blood pressure

Blood pressure readings in children are not easy, but they are important, so remember to perform this test. The use of the correct cuff size is vital to prevent inaccurate readings.

Anxiety and poor technique are the most common causes for raised blood pressure in children, so it should be measured several times.

Chest

Note the presence of the following:

- Precordial bulge: causes the sternum and ribs to bow forward
- Visible ventricular impulse: right ventricular (RV) impulse may be visible under xiphoid process. The left ventricular (LV) impulse (PMI) is often visible in thin children and in children with true LV hypertrophy.
- Scars: indicative of previous heart surgery

Palpation

- Feel the PMI to determine its location and character. It is usually situated in the fourth intercostal space in the mid-clavicular line in infants or toddlers (often difficult to localize if they are plump), and in the fourth or fifth intercostal space in older children.
  - LV hypertrophy results in a diffuse, forceful, and displaced apex beat, felt as a heave.
  - If the apex is impalpable, consider dextrocardia (inverted heart with apex pointing to the right) or pericardial effusion. *Levocardia* is the normal orientation of the heart to the left.
- *Right ventricular heave:* Place your fingertips along the left sternal border (LSB). If the child has RV hypertrophy, you will feel your fingers lift up with each impulse.
- Palpate in *the four valve areas* (aortic, pulmonary, tricuspid, and mitral) for thrills.
- *Palpate the abdomen* for hepatomegaly, which suggests heart failure (percuss the upper border of the liver—a normal-sized liver may be displaced downward by lung disease such as bronchiolitis.) Raised JVP, pulmonary, and peripheral edema are rarely seen in children.

Auscultation

Listen to the heart sounds in the four valve areas with the diaphragm and bell of the stethoscope (preferably pediatric size).

First heart sound (S1) is best heard at the apex with the bell.

- Loud S_1 is heard with high cardiac output states (e.g., anxiety, exercise, fever).
- Soft S_1 is heard with emphysema and impaired LV function.

Second heart sound (aortic = A2 and pulmonary = P2) is best heard at the base with the diaphragm. It is normally split in children.

- Soft P_2 is heard with stenotic pulmonary valve (e.g., tetralogy of Fallot).
- Loud P_2 is heard with pulmonary hypertension.
- Wide fixed splitting is caused by atrial septal defect.

Third heart sound is due to rapid ventricular filling.
- Causes include ↑ LV stroke volume (aortic or mitral regurgitation) and restricted ventricular filling (constrictive pericarditis, restrictive cardiomyopathy). It may be normal in children.

Fourth heart sound is due to forceful atrial contraction.
- Causes include hypertrophic cardiomyopathy and severe hypertension.

Murmurs

Auscultate for murmurs (Table 16.4) over the four valve areas and at the back. About 30% of children have innocent murmurs.

Innocent murmurs

The patient is asymptomatic. These are systolic (except venous hum), with no radiation or thrill. Change occurs with altering patient posture.
- *Venous hum:* due to turbulent flow in the head and neck veins. A continuous murmur in diastole and systole is heard below the clavicles, which disappears when the child lies flat.
- *Ejection murmur:* due to turbulent flow in the outflow tracts of the heart. It is heard in the second to fourth left intercostals spaces.

Pathological murmurs

These are systolic or diastolic and may radiate. The patient may have a thrill and may be symptomatic.
- *Atrial septal defect:* soft ejection systolic murmur at the upper LSE due to ↑ RV outflow. Fixed wide splitting of the second heart sound may first be detected at school entry.
- *Ventricular septal defect:* parasternal thrill. Loud pansystolic murmur occurs at the lower left sternal border (LSB). It radiates throughout the precordium. Signs of heart failure may be present.
- *Coarctation of the aorta:* ejection systolic murmur is heard between the shoulder blades. Femoral pulses are weak or absent.
- *Patent ductus arteriosus:* collapsing pulse. A continuous "machinery murmur" is heard below the left clavicle.
- Also see 📖 Chapter 7, p. 171.

Table 16.4 Quick guide to common pediatric murmurs

Symptom	Cause
Cyanosis + murmur	Usually tetralogy of Fallot
Cyanosis + murmur + operation	Possibly tetralogy of Fallot or transposition of the great arteries
Pink + loud systolic murmur	Probable ventricular septal defect (most common form of CHD)
Pink + murmur + impalpable femorals	Coarctation of the aorta
Continuous low-pitched murmur	Probable patent ductus arteriosus

Abdomen and gastrointestinal system

Key points from the history

Determine whether the child takes in sufficient calories for growth and has a well-balanced diet. Ask about height and weight gain.
▶ This may be an appropriate time for dietary teaching.

When taking a history, start at the head and work down to avoid missing things.

- Does the child have a good appetite?
- Does the child vomit?
  - How much?
  - Are they hungry afterward?
  - Is it forceful (projectile) or effortless (regurgitation)?
  - Is it related to eating?
  - What does it contain? Ask about coffee grounds or other appearances of the vomit. (Bile-stained vomiting in an infant always indicates obstruction and must be considered pathological.)
- Does the child suffer from abdominal pain?
- Does the child ever have a bloated abdomen?
- Are there any urinary symptoms?
- Ask about bowel habit—is the child constipated?
- Have there been any frequent or loose stools? Are the stools particularly offensive (suggests malabsorption)?
- Is there a relevant FH (e.g., celiac or inflammatory bowel disease)?

Examination

Inspection

Start with a general inspection of the patient, looking especially for the following:

- Visible liver edge or spleen
- Peristalsis (important in diagnosing pyloric stenosis during a test feed)
- Jaundice
- Observe for signs of liver disease (see 📖 Chapter 9, p. 246), including spider nevi, xanthomata, and purpura.
- Edema over the tibia and sacrum
- Whether the child is under- or overweight
- Wasted buttocks (suggesting weight loss—typical of celiac disease)

Hands

- Clubbing, palmar erythema

Face

- Check the conjunctiva for anemia.
- Periorbital edema (e.g., in nephrotic syndrome)

Abdomen

- Abdominal distension (see Boxes 16.8 and 16.9)
- Gross ascites may be evident—the abdomen will be distended and the umbilicus everted.
- Caput medusae (cutaneous collateral veins with blood flowing away from the umbilicus due to ↑ portal venous pressure; see Chapter 9, 📖 p. 229).

Box 16.8 Causes of abdominal distension in a child

- Fat
- Fluid
- Flatus
- Feces
- Organomegaly
- Muscle hypotonia
- Exaggerated lordosis (normal in young children)

Box 16.9 Detecting peritoneal inflammation

A further useful technique is to ask the patient to make their belly "as fat as possible" and "as thin as possible." Also ask them to cough. If peritonitis is present, any of these maneuvers may result in pain.

Palpation

ℹ Young children may resist abdominal examination. First try distraction techniques. If these fail, use the child's hand to guide yours around the abdomen. If there is doubt as to the significance of tenderness in a child's abdomen, listen with your stethoscope and gently apply more pressure. Often, quite firm pressure can be tolerated in this way where there was previously tenderness.

The aims of palpation are to
- Determine the presence of normal abdominal organs.
- Detect enlargement of the abdominal organs.
- Detect the presence of abnormal masses or fluid.

Procedure
- Ensure the child is relaxed and that your hands are warm.
- Inquire about pain before you begin.
- Palpate for tenderness (light palpation first, then deep palpation).
  - Feel for guarding (tensing of the abdominal muscles, which may indicate underlying tenderness).
- Palpate the spleen. This is normally felt 1–2 cm below the costal margin in infancy. It is soft and can be tipped on inspiration. Begin palpation in the right iliac fossa and move toward the left upper quadrant, to avoid missing a very large spleen. It may help to turn the child onto their right side.
- To palpate the liver, start in the right iliac fossa and move upward in time with the child's respiratory movements until the liver edge meets your fingers. A liver edge 1–2 cm below the costal margin is normal up to the age of 2 or 3 years. See Box 16.10 regarding hepatomegaly.
- Kidneys are not easy to palpate in children (they are easier to palpate in newborns), so if you can feel them, they are probably enlarged. They are best palpated bimanually. The kidneys move with respiration and have a smooth outline, and one can get above them (unlike the liver and spleen).
- Palpate for other masses and check for constipation (usually felt as a hard, indentable, nontender mass in the left iliac fossa).

Box 16.10 Confirming hepatomegaly

If in doubt, confirmation of liver enlargement can be made by
- Placing the stethoscope over the xiphoid process.
- Gently rubbing the abdomen, progressing up from the right iliac fossa.
  - When the rubbing hand is over the liver, the sound will be heard through the stethoscope.

Percussion

- Ascites. Test for shifting dullness (described in 📖 Chapter 9, p. 240) as a sign of ascites.
- Gaseous distension
- Percuss to determine the size of the liver and spleen

Auscultation

- Bowel sounds

Rectal examination

This is rarely indicated in children. However, it is often useful to inspect the perianal region for fissures, tags, soiling, and pinworms.

Male genitalia

Penis

- Note the state of hygiene.
- True micropenis is rare. If the penis looks small, it is probably because it is buried in suprapubic fat.
- Check the urethral orifice is at the tip of the glans. If not, is there epispadius (dorsal opening, very rare) or hypospadias (ventral opening)?

Scrotum

The child should be standing up.
- Inspect for normal rugosity of the scrotum.
- Palpate for the testes.
  - If they are not present in the scrotum, feel at the inguinal canal and, if found, try to milk the testis down.
  - Many undescended testes are subsequently found on re-examination as retractile testes, so be gentle in your approach to avoid provoking a cremasteric reflex!

Female genitalia

Inspect the female external genitalia if there are urinary symptoms.

Nervous system

Key points from the history
- Detailed birth and perinatal history, including maternal drugs or illness
- Careful history of developmental milestones
- Hearing or visual concerns. Did the child pass the newborn hearing screen?
- Any change in school performance, personality or behavior (e.g., aggression)?
- Ask about symptoms of raised intracranial pressure (e.g., headache, vomiting).
- Any change in gait or frank ataxia?
- Does the child have limited function—what can they do? What do they need help with?
- Obtain relevant FH of learning difficulties or genetic conditions.

Examination

Examination of the nervous system in school-age children should be performed as in adults. Young children cannot cooperate with a formal neurological examination, so assessment is opportunistic—observation becomes important. The assessment of a young child is described below.

Young children—where to start
Palpate the anterior fontanel when the child is quiet to
- Determine the presence of raised intracranial pressure (felt as fullness or bulging).
- Determine the degree of dehydration (felt as a sunken fontanel).
▶ It is impossible to assess fontanel tension in crying babies.
▶ Pulsation of the fontanel is normal.
- Measure the maximum occipitofrontal head circumference and plot this on a percentile chart.

Cranial nerves
It is not possible to systematically examine cranial nerves in infants or young children; below is a rough guide (see 📖 Chapter 10).
- *I (olfactory):* very difficult
- *II (optic):* Ask the parents—can the child see?
- *III, IV, VI (eye movements):* Gain the infant's visual attention with an object and move it back and forth. Watch for the range of ocular movements as the child tracks the object. Pendular nystagmus may indicate a visual defect. See Box 16.11 for assessment of strabismus.
- *V (trigeminal):* rooting reflex
- *VII (facial):* Facial palsy will become apparent when the child cries. Asymmetry will be more obvious. Does the child close both eyes?
- *VIII (vestibulocochlear):* Formal hearing tests are performed at birth.
- *IX, X:* swallowing
- *XI (accessory):* neck and shoulder movements
- *XII (hypoglossal):* tongue movement

Box 16.11 Assessment of strabismus

Any strabismus persisting beyond the age of 6 weeks needs specialist assessment, as strabismus may lead to amblyopia (cortical blindness).
- Ask when the strabismus is most apparent—latent strabismus may only be present when the child is tired.

Examination
- *Corneal light reflection test:* shine a penlight at a spot directly between the patient's eyes to produce a reflection in the cornea. The reflected light that you see should be at the same spot on each eye. If the reflection from the corneas is asymmetrical, strabismus is probably present.
- *Eye movements:* to detect a paralytic strabismus (rare)
- *Cover test:* encourage the child to fix on a toy, and cover the normal eye with a card or occluder. If the fixing eye is covered, the affected eye moves to take up fixation.
  - *Manifest (constant) strabismus:* on removal of the cover, the eyes move again as the fixing eye takes up fixation.

- *Pupils:* Check for size, shape, and reaction to light.
- *Fundi* should be examined but should be left to the end of the examination, as it is unpleasant (and sometimes impossible).

Tone
- Observe the child's response to gravity.
  - *Hypotonic infant:* slips through in ventral suspension (holding them up with a hand in each axilla), droops over your hand during ventral suspension, head lags when pulled to sit, frog legs posture.
  - *Hypertonic infant:* scissoring of lower limbs when the baby is picked up. Resistance to movement of limbs. The baby will seem to move in one piece.

Move limbs through their range of movements. Important areas to examine include the following:
- Arm flexors and extensors
- Arm supinators and pronators (most sensitive for ↑ tone)
- Hip adductors
- Leg extensors
- Leg flexors
- Ankle extension

Power
Observe for the following:
- Symmetry
- Spontaneous movements (Reduced movement is indicative of muscle weakness.)

Sensation
This is difficult to assess. Only response to pain can be confidently elicited in young children, but please don't try this!

Table 16.5 Some primitive reflexes and age of extinction

Reflex	Age of extinction
Stepping reflex	2 months
Palmar grasp	3–4 months
Moro reflex	4–5 months
Asymmetric tonic neck reflex	6 months

Reflexes
- *Tendon reflexes* can be elicited by tapping the tendon with a finger for babies, and using a reflex hammer for children.
  - The examiner should know the nerve roots responsible for the reflexes (see 📖 Chapter 10, p. 330).
- ▶ Remember that the plantar response is upward until age 8 months.
- *Primitive reflexes:* The presence of primitive reflexes beyond 6 months of age is abnormal and will inhibit normal development.
  - Persistence is indicative of a UMN lesion (e.g., cerebral palsy). See Table 16.5.

Coordination (assess in older children)
Ask the child to do the following:
- Stand on one leg and then hop.
- Walk on tiptoes.
- Walk on heels. This is a good test for coordination and overall neurological integrity. Patients with any kind of spasticity, for example, will be unable to do this.
- Do the finger-to-nose test and heel-to-shin test if child is old enough.

Gait (assess in older children)
- *Spastic gait:* Spasticity of extensor muscles causes a stiff gait on a narrow base. Toes catch the ground first (e.g., cerebral palsy).
- *Hemiplegic gait:* If the spasticity is unilateral, the affected leg drags stiffly and is circumducted as it is brought forward.
- *Ataxic gait:* broad based, unsteady, with frequent falls
- *Lower limb weakness (distal):* The affected leg is lifted over obstacles, then the foot returns to the ground with a slap.
- *Lower limb weakness (proximal):* There is a waddling gait as the pelvis is thrown side to side, being poorly supported by lower limbs (e.g., muscular dystrophy)
- *Limp* has several causes, but always rule out dislocation of the hip.

Developmental assessment

Development is a continuous process, the rate of which varies considerably among normal children.

Development is divided into four areas:
- Gross motor
- Fine motor and vision
- Speech and hearing
- Social

Delay in all four areas is usually abnormal, but delay in one area may not be (Table 16.6). For example, some children become expert at bottom shuffling or scooting. Thus having learned an effective means of traveling, the need to walk becomes less important.

Performing a developmental assessment

- Observation is key. Young children will often not cooperate. Take a history from the parents about milestones the child has achieved (Table 16.7).
- Be systematic and evaluate each of the four developmental areas.
- Learn a few essential milestones, as it is difficult to remember them all.
▶ If an infant was born prematurely, allow for this by calculating their corrected age from their expected due date.
- Limit distractions and present one task at a time.

Equipment for developmental assessment

- Wooden blocks: for assessing palmar grasp and building towers
- Coins or Cheerios: for testing pincer grip
- Pencil and paper: for assessing fine motor skills
- Different-colored cards or colorful book

Table 16.6 Developmental warning signs

Age	Warning sign
Any	Regression in previously acquired skills or a halt in developmental progress
8 weeks	No smiling
6 months	Persistent primitive reflexes. Hand preference (this should not appear until 18 months)
12 months	No sitting. No pincer grip. No double babble
18 months	Not walking. No words
4 years	No words

Table 16.7 Developmental milestones

Age	Gross motor	Fine motor	Language	Social
3 months	Head control, pushes up with arms	Opens hand	Laughs	Smiles (6 weeks)
6 months	Sits	Palmar grasp, reaches, transfers	Babbles (monosyllabic: ba, ka, da)	Eats solid food
9 months	Crawls, pulls to stand	Pincer grip begins to develop	Double babble (dada, mama, baba)	Stranger awareness, waves bye-bye
12 months	Walks	Developed pincer grip	Mommy, daddy, specifically	Peek-a-boo
18 months	Walks upstairs, jumps	Scribbles, 3-block tower	2-word phrases	Mimics
2 years	Kicks, runs	Draws straight line, 6–8 block tower	Begins to use clauses (including verbs)	Uses spoon skillfully, undresses, symbolic play
3 years	Hops, walks upstairs adult-style	Draws a circle, builds a bridge with blocks	Says name, knows colors	Dresses, has a friend, dry diapers by day
4 years	Stands on one leg, hops	Draws a cross, makes 3 steps with blocks	Sentences of 5+ words	Does up buttons
5 years	Can ride a bicycle	Draws a triangle		Ties shoelaces, dry all night

The newborn

The vast majority of newborns have a normal intrauterine life and normal birth and are physically normal. However, because there is wide variation in the spectrum of normal, it is important to stress the value of examining a large number of neonates to appreciate the normal spectrum.

In the delivery room

All newborns should have a brief examination at birth to determine whether resuscitation is needed and to rule out any major abnormalities.

The APGAR score is used to gauge the need for resuscitation (Table 16.8).

In the nursery

A more thorough examination is carried out prior to discharge. At this stage, the baby is unrecognizable from the one you met in the delivery room—they will be pink, vigorous, and feeding well.

Ask briefly about whether the baby has passed urine and meconium (the first, black sticky stool), and inquire about the progress of feeding as well as a FH of congenital anomalies. Of particular importance is a FH of dislocated hips, renal abnormalities, and deafness.

• Examination should start at the top and work down, to ensure nothing is missed.
• Undress the baby yourself as the examination proceeds, to get a feel for how the baby handles.

General observation

First observe the baby without disturbing him or her.

• *Color:* pink, pale, cyanosed, or jaundiced? Acrocyanosis (cyanosis of the hands and feet) is normal, provided the lips and tongue are pink.
• *Rash:* a blotchy erythematous rash occurs in about half of all neonates; this is usually harmless and is called *erythema toxicum*.
• Peeling of skin is common, especially in post-dates babies.

Table 16.8 APGAR score

Sign	0	1	2
Appearance	White/blue	Blue extremities, pink trunk	Pink
Pulse	Absent	<100bpm	>100 bpm
Grimace on stimulation of foot	None	Frown/grimace	Cry
Activity, tone	Floppy	Some limb flexion	Active movement
Respiratory effort	Absent	Irregular, slow	Loud cry

Hand and face

- *Shape of the head* can vary widely in the first week.
- *Fontanels* should be soft and flat. The size of the anterior fontanel also varies widely, from 1 to 4 cm in diameter. The posterior fontanel may accept a little fingertip.
- *Cranial sutures:* Are they fused?
- *Look for trauma from the birth,* such as caput succedaneum (edema caused by pressure over the presenting part) and molding (head changing shape as it passes through the birth canal), forceps marks, and subconjunctival hemorrhages. In general, these conditions will resolve within the first week.
  - A *cephalhematoma* is a localized, fluctuant swelling, usually over the parietal bone, caused by subperiosteal bleeding. This will resolve over a few months.
- *Ears* can be of different shape and size. Look for preauricular sinuses and ear tags, and observe their position.

Mouth

- *Palate:* Look at it when the infant cries, then palpate it for a cleft with a clean finger.
  - *Epstein's pearls* are small, white cysts in the midline of the hard palate. They are normal and resolve spontaneously.
- *Jaw:* A small jaw (micrognathia) may be part of the Pierre Robin sequence (midline cleft, small jaw, posterior displacement of the tongue, which can cause upper airway obstruction).
- *Tongue:* Note the size. If it is large and protruding, this may indicate a number of syndromes (e.g., Down syndrome).

Eyes

- Note the position and size.
- Look for the red reflex with an ophthalmoscope to exclude a cataract, which would be seen as a white reflection.
  - To encourage the baby to open their eyes, wrap them in a blanket (a crying baby will not open their eyes) and sit them upright.
  - If this fails, give the baby something to suck on, or startle with the Moro reflex.
- Sticky eyes can be the result of ophthalmia neonatorum (purulent conjunctivitis in the first 3 weeks of life), usually due to accumulation of lacrimal fluid due to incomplete drainage of the nasolacrimal duct.

Respiratory system and chest

- *Observe:* This is best done with a quiet baby (either sleeping or with the aid of a pacifier).
- *Chest:* Comment on size, symmetry, and shape.
- *Respiratory rate* should be <60/minute. Note the work of breathing. Are there any subcostal or intercostal retractions? Is the baby grunting?
  - Normal newborn respiration should be quiet, effortless, and predominantly diaphragmatic (abdomen moves more than the chest).
- *Auscultate* the lung fields to ensure symmetrical air entry. Crepitations may be normal in the first few hours of life.
- *Breasts:* Engorgement is common in male and female infants.

Cardiovascular system
- *Observe:* Note color, respiratory effort, and precordial heave.
- *Apex beat:* Palpate and feel for any thrills (common in neonates).
- *Femoral pulse:* This is extremely important; its absence may imply coarctation of the aorta. This requires a relaxed, still baby and lots of patience.
- ℹ Remember that too much pressure may obliterate it. A collapsing pulse (water hammer) suggests patent ductus arteriosus.
- *Heart rate* should be between 100 and 160 bpm.
- *Auscultate* for the heart sounds and murmurs. Systolic murmurs are common and usually best heard along the left sternal edge.

Abdomen
- *Observe:* Distension could be bowel obstruction or abdominal mass.
- *Umbilical stump:* Count the three vessels. Note any signs of infection, such as an unpleasant smell, discharge, or periumbilical erythema.
  - The cord will spontaneously separate around the fourth or fifth day.
- *Palpate:* Gently feel the abdomen for intra-abdominal organs and exclude organomegaly. Use warm hands and a pacifier, if necessary.
- ℹ The liver edge is soft and easily missed.
- *Kidneys:* Determine presence and size by balloting.
  - It is possible to palpate the lower poles of the kidneys in normal neonates.
- *Bladder:* Palpate suprapubically. If felt, this suggests outlet obstruction.
- *Anus:* Infants with an imperforate anus may still pass meconium via a fistula, so check that the anus is patent and in the correct position.

Male genitalia
- *Urethra:* Identify the urethral orifice and exclude hypospadias.
- *Testes:* Palpate gently. If they cannot be found in the scrotum, commence in the inguinal area and palpate downward.
  - If a testis appears larger than normal, transilluminate the scrotum (📖 Chapter 12, p. 384) to check for the common condition hydrocele.
- *Inguinal hernia:* These are more common in preterm infants.
- ℹ Put the diaper back on quickly, for obvious reasons. In the event of failure to quickly cover the genitalia, note the urinary stream, as a weak stream may indicate posterior urethral valves.

Female genitalia
- *Labia minora* may not be fully covered, especially in preterm infants.
- *Vaginal tags* are common and resolve spontaneously in the first week.
- *Vaginal discharge* and occasionally bleeding can occur, and is normal.
- Note ↑ pigmentation and clitoromegaly.

Limbs
- Ensure that all joints have full range of movement, to exclude any congenital contractures.
- Examine fingers and toes for syndactyly (fused digits) or polydactyly (extra digits).

Examination of the hips
This is to detect congenital dislocation and instability of the hips, and should be left until last, as it will make the baby cry.
- Observe for unequal leg length and asymmetry of skin creases.

Hip examination is in two parts:
- Lay the infant supine on a flat surface with hips and knees at 90*.
- Stabilize pelvis with one hand and with the other, grasp the knee between thumb and palm, with the fingertips over the greater trochanter.
  - *Barlow test* assesses whether the hip *can be* dislocated. Pull the hip up and then push down and laterally.
  - *Ortolani test* assesses whether the hip *is* dislocated. Pull the hip up into the acetabulum (producing a "clunk"); then the hip can be abducted (Ortolani = out).

Feet
- *Talipes equino varus:* primary clubfoot. This is usually a fixed structural deformity requiring early manipulation and fixation.
- *Calcaneo valgus:* common. Dorsum of the foot is in a position close to the shin. It resolves after about 2 months with ↑ calf muscle tone.
- *Positional talipes* is extremely common and involves no bony deformity. It is easily corrected by movement and treated with physiotherapy.

Spine
Lay the infant prone in one hand and with the other, palpate the spine, checking for spina bifida occulta or a dermal sinus.

Neurological examination
Because infants with little or no cerebral cortex can show normal reflexes and tone, you should observe the baby's state of consciousness through-out the examination. This should vary from quiet sleep to semi-wakeful-ness to an alert state.
   A normal infant will be consolable when they cry, whereas it is very difficult to settle a neurologically abnormal infant.

Inspection of the spine
Any midline lesion over the spine needs immediate investigation. A single hair might indicate communication with the spinal column (spina bifida).

Posture
Posture is generally flexor, although abnormal intrauterine positions can distort this, such as extended breech position.

Movements
Watch spontaneous limb movements, noting the presence of jitteriness.

Tone
Assess and compare the flexor recoil of the limbs.
   Evaluate tone in response to gravity:
- Pull-to-sit test. Let the baby grasp your fingers and pull the baby up to sit. The head should flex and follow the traction to an upright position and hold momentarily. Also observe the tone in the baby's arms.

- Ventral suspension is assessed by grasping the infant under each axilla. A normal infant will support themselves in this position by extending their back and hips, lifting their head, and flexing their arms and legs.

Primitive reflexes (see Box 16.12)
These are used to assess asymmetry of function, gestational age, and neurological function.

Vision
Assessment of vision should be carried out with the infant in an alert state. The baby will fix on an interesting object 8 inches away and will follow the target.

Hearing
This can be assessed by sounding a loud rattle outside of the infant's vision. The baby should look toward the noise.

Head circumference and weight
Finally, measurement and plotting of head circumference and birthweight on a growth chart is of utmost importance.

Box 16.12 Primitive reflexes

- *Palmar grasp:* Fingers close to hold an object placed in the palm.
- *Rooting:* When pressure is applied to the cheek, the head turns toward the pressure and the mouth opens.
- *Sucking:* When a finger is placed in the mouth, the infant will suck vigorously.
- *Stepping:* Hold the infant with both hands and lower the feet onto a surface. The legs will move in a stepping fashion.
- *Moro reflex:* Lay the infant supine on your hand and forearm. When the head is dropped a couple inches, the upper limbs abduct, extend, and flex in a symmetrical flowing movement. A unilateral response indicates damage (usually transient) to the fifth and sixth cervical roots, producing Erb's palsy.

Examination under special circumstances

Overview

This chapter provides an overview and Web URLs for some special considerations that medical personnel should address within the topics of natural disasters, terrorism events, public health emergencies, and sexual assault. Detailed information is beyond the scope of this text.

In many communities, there are specific laws that address and define the working relationship among health and law enforcement officials. Healthcare providers should be aware of these laws and incorporate a working knowledge of all appropriate regulations (or at least where to locate the information) before it is needed.

Often in these situations, support personnel, such as social workers, may have left for the day, and providing timely and appropriate care can be challenging without basic knowledge and skills.

Disasters, terrorism, and public health emergencies

The need for increased opportunities for health-profession students and providers to learn about emergency preparedness is a direct outcome of horrific natural disasters (Hurricane Katrina, the Haiti earthquake), terrorism events (Oklahoma City, New York City), and concerns about pandemic influenza.

The U.S. Centers for Disease Control and Prevention (CDC) has extensive training opportunities and information on its Web site (www.bt.cdc. gov). A readiness assessment survey for health-care facilities can be found at http://www.ahrq.gov/prep/cbrne. Personal readiness information can be found at http://www.fema.gov/areyouready

Skills such as good communication and teamwork are essential in dealing with emergencies. An understanding of the role of primary providers in the Public Health Surveillance systems is critical, as they may be the first to see the effects of widespread biological or radiation exposures. Early identification will lead to appropriate treatment and has the potential of saving lives.

Beyond participating in surveillance activities and having a high index of suspicion, providers should acquire competencies in patient care that prepares them to assist in disasters, terrorism events, or public health emergencies. They should be knowledgeable about reporting sentinel events to the appropriate public health authorities.

Providers should be able to determine the absence or presence of symptoms characteristic of exposure to chemical, biological, radiological, nuclear, or explosive agents (CBRNE). They should also know to assess for evidence of psychological trauma. This could be a result of the event or triggered by experiences of previous events. Providers should watch for delayed stress reactions in responders or community members.

Physical assessment and evaluation need to be appropriate to the exposure or trauma. It is essential to know how to access information in the event of a local emergency. The Internet may not always be accessible in an emergency, so a reliable backup plan should be in place.

Care will be both acute (trauma, antibiotics, vaccines, antidotes) and chronic (burn and wound long-term care, physical therapy) and should address physical and emotional aspects of healing. There may be a need to collect and preserve evidence for forensic purposes; this should be done once life-threatening injuries are attended to.

Appropriate precautions must be taken to avoid exposures spreading to other patients, care providers, and the wider population. As such, providers should be familiar with and have access to personal protective equipment, isolation levels, isolation rooms, and decontamination areas.[1]

---

[1] Markenson D, DiMaggio C, Redlener I (2005). Preparing health professions students for terrorism, disaster, and public health emergencies: core competencies, *Acad Med* 80(6):517–526.

Sexual assault

Sexual assault victims have suffered an extreme trauma and need to be treated with respect and understanding. Many localities will have a victim advocacy program, through which advocates can come to the clinic or emergency room to support the victim and help arrange for aftercare counseling.

Providers should be aware of state laws and the proper procedure for collecting forensic evidence (often there are evidence collection kits with all the materials needed for collecting evidence and maintaining the integrity of the evidence chain).

In addition to the physical trauma, providers should also address the psychological effects of the assault. It is essential that the necessary exam and specimen/culture collection not retraumatize the patient. Allowing patients to control the pace of the exam and ensuring that they know what is going to happen to them each step of the way is paramount.

If the victim was assaulted by an intimate partner, the provider may have to notify law enforcement authorities, regardless of whether the victim wants to do this. If the victim is a minor, child protective services may need to be called in.

Appropriate cultures and monitoring for STIs and pregnancy should be initiated. Patients will need long-term follow-up, which should be arranged at the initial visit. Providers should remember that victims can be of either gender; providers need to make an extra effort to remain nonjudgmental in their approach.

Since the 1970s, programs to educate sexual assault nurse examiners (SANE) have been developed. A comprehensive development and operation guide is available online from the U.S. Department of Justice, Office of Justice Programs, Office for Victims of Crime, at: www.ojp.usdoj.gov/ovc/publications/infores/sane/saneguide.pdf.

These programs have allowed specialized services for assault victims to become available nationwide.

Other thoughts

Hints

Consider keeping an inexpensive disposable or digital camera in the patient care area for photodocumentation.

Practical procedures

Using this chapter

This chapter describes those practical procedures that the primary care provider may be expected to perform.

Obviously, some of these are more complicated than others, and some should only be performed once you have been trained specifically in the correct technique.

Each procedure has a difficulty icon as follows:

⚠   Requires no specific further training and primary care providers should be competent to perform.

▶   Requires some skill. Experienced providers should be able to perform with ease.

▶▶   More complex procedures that you may only come across in specialty jobs and will not be required to perform without specific guidance from specialists or highly experienced clinicians.

Rules are made to be broken

Many procedures and practical skills do not have a "correct" method but have an accepted method. These methods should, therefore, be abided by, although deviation from the routine by a competent practitioner, when circumstances demand, is acceptable.

Many procedures have local variations—if in doubt, check the standard method used in your hospital or facility.

Infiltrating anesthetic agents

A large number of procedures involve the infiltration of local anesthetic agents. The importance of this procedure cannot be overlooked. Injection of a large amount of anesthetic into a vein could lead to potentially fatal cardiac arrhythmias. It is also important, of course, to ensure that you do not damage any vessels.

Advance and withdraw

Whenever you inject anything, you should advance the needle and attempt to withdraw the plunger at each step. If you do not aspirate blood, you may *then* go ahead and infiltrate the anesthetic.

Making a surface bleb

- Take the syringe of anesthetic (e.g., 1% lidocaine) and a small needle.
- Pinch a portion of skin, insert the needle horizontally into the surface.
- Withdraw the plunger to ensure no blood is aspirated then inject a small amount of the anesthetic—you should see a wheal of fluid rise.
- The area of skin will now be sufficiently anesthetized to allow you to infiltrate deeper.
- *Remember*—no epinephrine-containing anesthetic agents for infiltration into the digits!

Sterility and preparation

Most equipment will come in prepacked sterile wrapping. When performing a procedure in which sterility is important, all packaging should be opened using a no-touch technique.

Large packs of equipment

Some equipment is available in pre-prepared sterile packs. For example, a catheterization pack may contain gauze, cotton balls, a cleansing agent, lubricant, and a sterile vessel. These come wrapped in plastic and then internally wrapped with material for the placement of a sterile field while opening the pack.

Any such packs should be placed on a stand that has first been appropriately cleaned. You should then carefully open the pack, touching the corners only, and using sterile gloved hands.

The opened pack can then be used as a sterile surface on which to place additional sterile equipment.

Smaller pieces of equipment

Most equipment (e.g., needles, syringes) comes sterilized and wrapped in paper or plastic. These should also be opened using a no-touch technique if absolute sterility is needed.

For example, unwrap a needle by peeling back the packaging as if peeling a banana and allow the needle to drop onto the pre-prepared sterile field.

⚠ **Hand-washing**

Theory

Hand-washing is the single-most important procedure for preventing the spread of infections. It is underperformed in frequency and quality.

Hands should be washed before every episode of care that involves direct contact with a patient's skin, their food, invasive devices, or dressings, and after any activity or contact that could result in hands becoming contaminated, such as using community computers to enter data.

Alcohol sanitizers can also be regularly used when entering or leaving a patient care area and before and after examining patients.

Equipment

- Soap and alcohol gel
- Disposable paper towels
- Moisturizer (if required)

Procedure

If hands are not visibly soiled, hand-sanitizing with alcohol-cleansing agents may be as if not more effective than hand-washing.

When required to wash our hands, we should use soap and warm water. Those parts often missed are the tips of fingers, thumbs, and between the fingers.

The following routine is advised (Fig. 18.1):

- First, rub hands palm to palm (Fig. 18.1a).
- Rub right palm over the left dorsum.
- Rub left palm over the right dorsum.
- Wash palm to palm with the fingers interlaced (Fig. 18.1b).
- Wash the backs of the fingers with opposing palms, with fingers interlocked (Fig. 18.1c).
- Perform rotational rubbing of the right thumb clasped with the left fist (Fig. 18.1d).
- Perform rotational rubbing of the left thumb clasped with the right fist.
- Wash the right palm with rotational rubbing using fingers of left hand.
- Wash the left palm with rotational rubbing using the finger of the right hand (Fig. 18.1e).
- Wash the space between the thumbs and first fingers by interlocking them and rubbing together (Fig. 18.1f).
- Rinse away all soap and pat dry using disposable paper towels.
- Apply moisturizer to protect the skin from the drying effects of regular washing.

▶ Hints

- Keep nails short, clean, and polish free.
- Avoid wearing wristwatches and jewelry, especially rings with ridges or stones.
- Any cuts or abrasions should be covered with waterproof dressing.

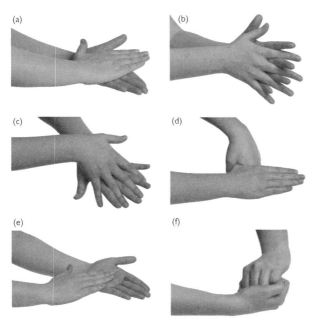

Fig. 18.1 The correct stages of hand-washing as described on previous page.

⚠ Injections

Theory

This is an important and routine procedure that is often carried out by nursing staff, although providers may be asked to administer medication at times. Good injection technique can make the experience for the patient relatively painless. Three commonly used routes of administration are sub-cutaneous (SC), intramuscular (IM), and intradermal (ID).

▶ Before gloving for any procedure, confirm the absence of latex allergy.

▶ Before attempting an injection, familiarize yourself with the operation of any syringe cover or guard device.

Equipment

- Syringe (size depends on injection)
- Needles: 25-gauge (G) for SC route; 21–23G for IM route
- Extra 21G needle for drawing up dose
- Alcohol swab
- Gloves
- Cotton
- Sharps container
- Medication for injecting
- Band-aid for covering injection site

Procedures

Subcutaneous injections

The SC route is used for a slow absorption of medication and is ideal for drugs such as insulin.

- Introduce yourself, confirm the identity of the patient, explain the procedure, and obtain verbal consent.
- Wash your hands and put on a pair of gloves.
▶ Always check that you have the correct drug and correct dose and that it is within the expiration date before injecting it.
- Draw up the medication using a 21G needle and double check the medication, dose, and expiration date.
- Expel any air in the syringe and replace with a 25G needle or other needle appropriate for the medication being injected.
- Clean the injection site with the alcohol swab.
- Pinch a fold of skin so as to lift the adipose tissue away from the underlying muscle.
- Insert the needle horizontally into the fold and draw back to ensure you are not in a vein.
- Inject the medication.
- Withdraw needle and apply cotton to the site to absorb any bleeding.
Suitable SC sites include the forearm, triceps area, and abdomen.

Intramuscular injections

IM injections are administered through the epidermis, dermis, and SC tissue into the muscle. They provide rapid systemic action and allow relatively large doses to be absorbed.

Suitable IM sites typically include the deltoid muscle, dorsogluteal site, ventrogluteal site, and lateral thigh or vastus lateralis muscle, depending on available muscle mass. A related method of IM injection, the Z-track method, is used for "sealing" the injection site to prevent staining from medications such is iron.

❶ Remember to avoid sites of inflammation, swelling, infection, or skin lesions.

- Introduce yourself, confirm the identity of the patient, explain the procedure, and obtain verbal consent.
- Wash your hands and put on a pair of gloves.
▶ Always check that you have the correct drug and correct dose and that it is within the expiration date before injecting it.
- Draw up the medication using a 21G needle and have a colleague double check the medication, dose, and expiration date.
- Expel any air in the syringe and replace with a 25G needle or other needle appropriate for the medication being injected.
- Inspect the proposed site for adequate muscle mass.
- Clean the injection site with the alcohol swab.
- IM injections should be given at a 90^0 angle to ensure the needle reaches the muscle and to reduce pain.
- A good way to ensure accuracy and avoid a needle-stick injury is to rest the heel of the palm on the thumb of the nondominant hand.
- Pull the skin down or to one side at the intended site.
- Hold the syringe between the thumb and forefinger and insert the needle at full depth.
- Draw back on the syringe to ensure the needle is not in a vein.
- Slowly inject the medication.
- After needle insertion and injection, allow 10 seconds before removing the needle, to facilitate diffusion of the medication into the muscle.
- Withdraw the needle and wipe the area clean with cotton.

Intradermal injections

The ID route provides a local, rather than systemic, effect and is used primarily for diagnostic purposes, such as allergy or tuberculin testing.

This involves the same preliminary procedures as for IM injection except a 25G needle is inserted at a $10–15^0$ angle, bevel up, just under the epidermis.

Up to 0.5 mL is injected until a wheal appears on the skin surface—just as when creating a bleb of local anesthetic.

⚠ **Venipuncture**

Two methods exist: the common method of collecting blood directly into the tubes by Vacutainer®, and the traditional needle-and-syringe method.

Equipment

- Gloves
- Alcohol swabs
- Tourniquet
- Sticky tape
- Gauze or cotton ball
- Needle (try 21G first), a syringe, and blood collection bottle or:
- Vacutainer® tube, holder, and blood collection needle
- Don't forget a band-aid!

Procedure

Using a needle and syringe

- Introduce yourself, confirm the patient's identity, explain the procedure, and obtain verbal consent.
- The patient should be lying or sitting comfortably with the arm from which blood is to be taken resting on a pillow.
- Select a vein site—usually the antecubital fossa (see Fig. 18.2).
- Apply tourniquet proximal to the puncture site and recheck vein.
- Put on gloves and ask the patient to clench their fist a few times.
- Cleanse the area with an alcohol swab in spirals, inside to out.*
- Attach the needle to a syringe and unsheathe it.
- Use the thumb of your nondominant hand to gently anchor the skin just below the puncture site.
- ❶ Warn patient to expect a sharp scratch and to not move their arm.
- Insert the needle firmly through the skin, bevel up, at an angle of 20–40° over the vein.
- With experience, you will feel a slight give as the vein is entered. Blood will visibly enter the hub (plastic portion) of the needle (flashback).
- Carefully holding the needle in position, pull back on the plunger.
  - There are several ways of doing this. The authors favor holding the needle and syringe in the nondominant hand, once in place, and pulling back with the dominant hand.
- When enough blood is taken, release the tourniquet *before* removing the needle from the vein.
- Apply a clean cotton ball or folded gauze to the puncture site as the needle is withdrawn. Pressure should be applied for >1 minute. (Ask the patient to do this for you, if they are able.)
- Apply a band-aid to the site, and thank the patient.
- Vacuum blood tubes are filled by puncturing the rubber top with the needle and allowing the blood to enter the tube.
- Remember to label the tubes correctly, ideally at the patient's bedside, and dispose of sharps in a sharps bin.

---

* There is no solid evidence for benefit in using alcohol wipes unless there is *visible* dirt at the venipuncture site. However, their use is policy in most facilities and should be used accordingly.

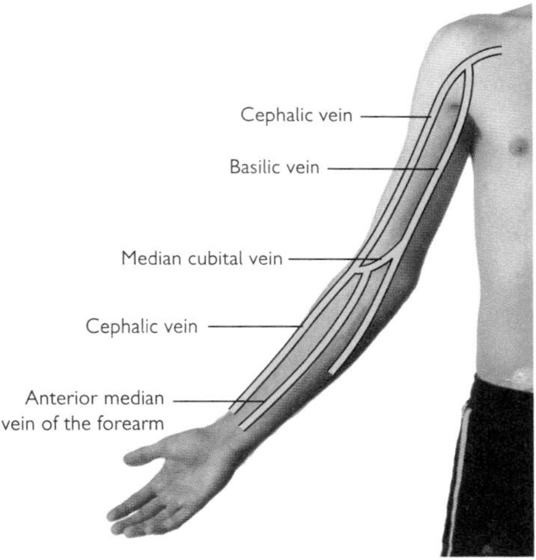
Cephalic vein
Basilic vein
Median cubital vein
Cephalic vein
Anterior median
vein of the forearm

Fig. 18.2 Representation of peripheral veins of the upper limb.

Using a Vacutainer® system

Much of the procedure is the same as for using a needle and syringe.

- Vacutainer® needles are double-ended, one standard needle and one needle covered by a rubber sleeve.
- Attach a Vacutainer® holder over the covered needle (see Fig. 18.3).
- The needle is inserted into the vein as with a syringe, but no flashback will be visible.
- Once in place, the Vacutainer® tubes are attached to the needle directly by pushing them onto the covered needle using the tube holder.
- Allow enough blood to enter the tube (some tubes must be filled—check local laboratory guidance).
- Multiple tubes may be filled by removing and replacing tubes while carefully holding the needle in position.

Inappropriate sites for venipuncture

- Edematous areas
- Cellulitic areas
- Hematomas
- Phlebitis or thrombophlebitis
- Scarred areas
- Arm in which there is a transfusion or infusion
- Arm on the side of previous mastectomy
- Arms with AV fistulae or vascular grafts

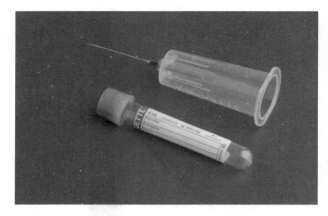

Fig. 18.3 Vacutainer® blood collection system, ready for use.

Hints
- If extraction of blood with the Vacutainer® proves difficult, it may be easier to switch to the needle-and-syringe technique, as this gives you more control over the flow of blood.
- Venipuncture can be performed at *any* peripheral vein. Inpatients from whom it is difficult to draw blood often have the blood taken from the back of their hands, feet, or legs.
- In difficult to reach places, it is often easier to use a butterfly needle. This is a smaller needle attached to a length of tubing that can be used with either technique. It allows for greater control of the needle.

Box 18.1 Taking blood from a central venous catheter

Theory
Central lines should only be used for taking blood if it is not possible to obtain a sample via the peripheral route. Do not risk catheter sepsis or a clotted line unless there are no alternatives!

Practicality
Central lines are frequently used for taking blood for assorted reasons. Avoidance of additional needle-sticks for patient comfort is a primary concern.

Blood culture requirements may preclude use of the central line for obtaining a sample. However, blood may need to be obtained from the central line and a peripheral site simultaneously to assist in differentiation of a source of sepsis.

In any case, caution must be observed to appropriately obtain a specimen from a port that may have been salinized or heparinized, and proper care of the port must be exercised after use of the port. Proper caution will decrease risk of catheter sepsis or a clotted line.

Facility policy will dictate what is done.

Equipment
- 3 x 10 mL syringes
- 0.9% isotonic or heparinized saline
- Chlorhexidine, povidone-iodine, or other recommended agent
- Gauze
- Sterile gloves
- Drape

Procedure
- Introduce yourself, confirm the identity of the patient, explain the procedure, and obtain verbal consent.
- Stop any infusions for at least 1 minute before sampling.
- Place the patient in a supine position.
- Ask the patient to turn their head away from the line site during the procedure.
- Drape the site in case of splash, and put on a pair of sterile gloves.
- Spray or paint the line with the chosen sanitizing agent.
- Clamp the line before removing the cap.
- Connect a 10 mL syringe to the line before unclamping.
- Withdraw 5–10 mL of blood, clamp the line, and remove syringe.
- Discard the blood.
- Connect a new 10 mL syringe to the line, unclamp it, and withdraw another 10 mL of blood.
- Clamp the line and remove the syringe (keep this sample).
- Fill a further syringe with saline and attach to the line.
- Unclamp the line, instill the saline, and clamp the line again.
- Remove the syringe and replace the cap.

⚠ **Peripheral IV catheterization**

Theory

Peripheral IV catheterization is a generic skill that most students should have learned early in their education. A thin tube line is inserted into a vein, allowing easy venous access that is used in many situations, including the administration of fluids and IV medication.

Equipment

- Gloves
- Alcohol swabs
- Tourniquet
- Saline for injection
- Sticky tape
- Gauze or cotton ball
- Catheter of appropriate size (see Box 18.2, Fig. 18.4)
- 5 mL syringe

Procedure

- Introduce yourself, confirm the patient's identity, explain the procedure, and obtain verbal consent.
- The patient should be lying or sitting comfortably with the arm in which the catheter is to be inserted resting on a pillow.
- Apply the tourniquet to the arm and identify a suitable vein.
- ❶ Often those veins that can be *felt* are more reliable than those that are *seen*. The vein should be superficial and have a straight course for a few centimeters.
- Put on gloves and clean the overlying skin with the alcohol swab.
- Remove the catheter from its packaging.
- Ensure that the catheter is functioning properly by slightly withdrawing the needle and replacing it. Fold down the wings and open and close the port on the top.
- ❶ Warn patient to expect a sharp scratch and to not move their arm.
- Insert the catheter firmly through the skin, bevel up, at an angle of 20–40° over the vein.
- With experience, you will feel a slight give as the vein is entered. Blood will visibly enter the hub (plastic portion) of the catheter (flashback).
- Once the flashback is seen, hold the needle in place with one hand and slide the catheter off the needle—into the vein—with the other. Once the catheter is fully inserted, the needle should be sitting just within it, preventing blood from spilling.
- Release the tourniquet.
- Press over the vein at the tip of the catheter, remove the needle, and dispose of it safely in a sharps bin.
- Put the cap on the catheter and fix it in place with tape and the appropriate dressing.
- Draw up saline into the syringe and flush it through the catheter using the port on the top. Watch the vein—if the catheter is misplaced, the saline will enter the subcutaneous tissues, causing swelling.
- ▶ Don't forget to do this—it confirms that the catheter is working and clears it of blood that would form a clot.

Hints

- Try to avoid the antecubital fossa. Although this is often the easiest place to see and feel a vein, catheters at that site can become

Box 18.2 Sizing catheters

Like needles, catheters are color-coded according to size. Each is given a gauge (G), which has an inverse correlation to the external diameter. Color-coding is standardized across manufacturers.

The standard-size catheter is green, or 18G, but for most hospital patients, a pink, or 20G, cannula will suffice. Even blue catheters are adequate in most circumstances unless fast flows of fluid are required.

Gauge	External diameter (mm)	Length (mm)	Approximate maximum flow rate (mL/min)	Color
14G	2.1	45	290	Orange
16G	1.7	45	172	Gray
18G	1.3	45	76	Green
20G	1.0	33	54	Pink
22G	0.8	25	25	Blue

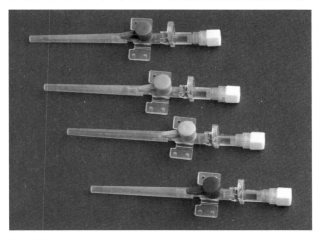

Fig. 18.4 A selection of standard IV catheters.

kinked and blocked as well as cause pain for the patient on bending the arm.
- Avoid an arm with a fistula or AV shunt.
- Bring a selection of different-sized catheters to the bedside, allowing you to choose a smaller gauge if you experience problems.
- Don't be afraid to ask for assistance from nursing or auxiliary staff if the patient is likely to move their arm during the procedure.

⚠ **Setting up an infusion**

Theory

Fluid therapy is one of the core skills for nurses. While it is usually the nursing staff that sets up an IV infusion, providers should nevertheless be competent at this technique.

Equipment

- Gloves
- An appropriate fluid bag
- Tubing (infusion) set
- IV (standard) pole
- Infusion pump, if required

Procedure

❶ IV infusions require IV access—see 📖 p. 522. Check the fluid in the bag and fluid prescription chart.

- Ask a colleague to double-check the prescription and the fluid and sign their name on the chart.
- Open the fluid bag and tubing set, which come in sterile packaging.
- Unwind the tubing set and close the adjustable valve.
- Remove the sterile cover from the bag outlet and from the sharp end of the tubing set (see Fig. 18.5).
- Using a lot of force, push the tubing set end into the bag outlet.
- Invert the bag and hang it on a stand.
- Squeeze the drip chamber to half fill it with fluid.
- Partially open the valve to allow the drip to run, and watch fluid run through to the end (it might be best to hold the free end over a sink in case of spills).
- If bubbles appear, try tapping or flicking the tube.
- Once the tubing is filled with liquid, connect it to the catheter.
- Adjust the valve and watch the drips in the chamber.
- Adjust the drip rate according to the prescription (see Box 18.3).

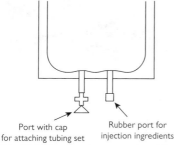

Port with cap   Rubber port for
for attaching tubing set   injection ingredients

Fig. 18.5 Diagrammatic representation of the base of a fluid bag and the port in which the tubing set should be inserted.

Box 18.3 Drip rate

Most infusions tend to be given with electronic devices that pump the fluid in at the prescribed rate. However, it is still important that health-care professionals be able to set up a drip at the correct flow rate manually.

Using a standard tubing set, clear fluids will form drips of about 0.05 mL—that is, there will be approximately 20 drips/mL. You can then calculate the number of drips per minute for a given infusion rate.

Infusion and drip rates

Prescription number of hours per liter of fluid	Infusion rate (mL/hr)	Infusion rate (mL/min)	Drip rate (drips/min)
1	1000	16	320
2	500	8	160
4	250	4	80
6	166	3	60
8	125	2	40
10	100	1.6	32
12	83	1.4	28
24	42	0.7	14

▶ External jugular vein catheterization

Theory

The external jugular vein lies superficially in the neck, running down from the angle of the jaw and across the sternocleidomastoid muscle before passing deep to drain into the subclavian vein. It is sometimes used to provide essential venous access in cardiac arrest and other emergency situations in which no peripheral access is obtainable.

See Fig. 18.6 for the surface anatomy of the external jugular vein.

Equipment

- Antiseptic solution or antiseptic wipe
- 2 x 5 mL syringes
- 1 25G orange needle
- 1 21G green needle
- 1% lidocaine
- 14G or 16G catheter
- 0.9% saline flush
- Dressing
- Gloves
- Sharps bin

Procedure

- Introduce yourself, confirm the identity of the patient, explain the procedure, and obtain verbal consent, if possible.
- Wash your hands and put on a pair of gloves.
- Tilt the patient to 10–15° head-down to facilitate venous filling.
- Once the external jugular vein is visible, clean the area with antiseptic solution.
- Reconfirm the patient's identity, the procedure, and the site.
- Attach a 25G (orange) needle to a 5 mL syringe and make a SC bleb of 1–2 mL of 1% lidocaine and infiltrate around the insertion site.
- ⊕ Be careful not to insert any anesthetic into the vein.
- Position yourself at the head of the bed.
- Remove the cap from the catheter and attach a clean 5 mL syringe.
- Turn the patient's head away from the side of insertion.
- Catheterize using the same technique as for peripheral venous access.
- ▶ Remember to aspirate as you advance the catheter. Correct placement will be confirmed once you are able to aspirate venous blood.
- Fix the catheter in place, using a suitable dressing.
- Flush the catheter with 5 mL of 0.9% saline solution.
- Dispose of all sharps in a sharps bin, wash your hands, and help the patient to a comfortable position.
- Document details of the procedure in patient record.

Hints

In an emergency situation, you may forgo the anesthetic, as venous access may be needed swiftly.

▶▶ Central venous catheterization

Theory

Central venous access is the placement of a catheter in a vein that leads directly to the heart. There are a number of central veins, including the internal jugular, external jugular, subclavian, femoral, and antecubital.

For each of these, the basic equipment and preparation are the same. Central venous catheterization is performed for vascular access, total parenteral nutrition (TPN), infusion of irritant, vasoactive, and inotropic drugs, measurement of central venous pressure (CVP), cardiac catheterization, pulmonary artery catheterization, transvenous cardiac pacing, and hemodialysis or plasmaphoresis.

Single- and multi-lumen catheters are available; the type to be used should be decided on prior to insertion according to the anticipated use (e.g., concurrent CVP monitoring and multiple-drug infusion). Frequently, quad-lumen catheters are used because of their versatility. Decisions on catheter selection are also contingent on length of the catheter needed relative to the size of the patient.

For the inexperienced, a CVP kit it can be overwhelming, given the variety of materials included for performing the procedure.

Equipment

- Appropriate instrument stand
- Sterile pack including sterile drapes
- Sterile gown and gloves
- Suture material e.g., 2/0 silk on a curved needle
- Antiseptic solution
- Local anesthetic—approximately 5 mL of 1% lidocaine
- Central venous line kit
- 21G green and 25G orange needles
- Saline or heparinized saline to prime and flush the line prior to and after insertion
- Sterile dressing
- Ultrasound machine

Procedure—internal jugular vein

- Introduce yourself, confirm the identity of the patient, explain the procedure, and obtain verbal consent.
- Remember, this can be a potentially frightening procedure. Explanations and reassurance must be given before and during the procedure.
- Put on a sterile gown and gloves.
- Unwrap all equipment.
- Check that the wire passes through the needle freely. Attach 3-way taps to all catheter ports. Flush all lumens with heparinized saline.
- Place the patient in a supine position, at least 15^0 head-down.
  - This is usually quite easy on a tilting bed and is performed to distend the neck veins and reduce the risk of air embolism.
- Turn the head away from the venipuncture site.
- Cleanse the skin with antiseptic solution and drape the area.
- Stand at the head of the bed.

- Locate the cricoid cartilage and palpate the carotid artery lateral to it.
- The site for insertion is approximately 1/3 of the way up the sternocleidomastoid, just between its two heads.
- Reconfirm the patient's identity, the procedure, and the site.
- Use local anesthetic to numb the venipuncture site once located.
- Infiltrate the skin and deeper tissues with a smaller orange needle and then replace with a green needle.
- Introduce the large-caliber introducer needle, attached to an empty syringe, into the center of a triangle formed by the two lower heads of the sternocleidomastoid muscle and clavicle.
- Keep your finger on the carotid artery and ensure that the needle enters the skin *lateral* to the artery.
- Direct the needle caudally at an angle of 30–40⁰ to the skin, toward the ipsilateral nipple. The vein is usually within 2–3 cm of the skin.
- Aspirate as the needle is advanced. Once you see blood, catheterize the vein using the Seldinger technique.
- Remove the syringe and occlude the needle lumen with a thumb.
- Straighten the J tip of the spring guide wire and advance into the vessel through the needle.
- Holding the spring-wire in place, remove the needle while maintaining a firm grip on the wire at all times.
- Enlarge the cutaneous puncture site with the cutting edge of the scalpel positioned away from the spring-wire guide.
- Use the dilator provided to enlarge the site and thread the tip of the catheter into the vessel using the spring-wire guide.
- Grasp the catheter near the skin and, using a slight twisting motion, advance into the vein.
- Make sure before you push the catheter forward that the wire is visible at the proximal end. *Hold the wire at all times* to prevent it from getting lost inside the patient.
- Hold the catheter and remove the spring-wire guide.
- Check lumen placement by aspirating through the pigtails and flush with saline.
- Lock off the 3-way taps. The patient can now be leveled.
- Secure the catheter in place with a suture and cover with an adhesive sterile dressing. (Do not forget to anesthetize suture sites as well.)
- Request a chest X-ray to verify correct catheter position and to exclude a pneumothorax.
- Catheters have a radio-opaque strip for this purpose.
- The catheter tip should lie in the SVC at the level of the carina.
- Dispose of your sharps and clear the instrument stand.
- Document the details of the procedure in the patient record.

Complications of internal jugular vein catheterization

- Pneumothorax
- Hemothorax
- Chylothorax
- Air embolism
- Arrhythmais
- Carotid artery puncture

- Infection
- Thrombosis of vessel
- Neural injury
- Cardiac tamponade
- AV fistula
- Patient discomfort

Procedure: femoral vein

The femoral vein lies medial to the femoral artery immediately beneath the inguinal ligament. It is commonly used in an ICU setting for placement of a double-lumen hemofiltration line and when central access is not feasible by other routes. This is impractical for mobile patients and raises concerns regarding the sterility of the groin area.

- Introduce yourself, confirm the identity of the patient, explain the procedure, and obtain consent.
- Extend the patient's leg and abduct slightly at the hip.
- Use full aseptic technique.
- Before initiating the procedure, reconfirm the patient's identity, the procedure, and the site.
- Locate the femoral artery, keep a finger on the artery, and introduce a needle attached to a 10 mL syringe at 45^0, 1.5 cm medial to the femoral artery pulsation, 2 cm below the inguinal ligament.
- Slowly advance the needle cephalad and posteriorly while gently withdrawing the plunger.
- When a free flow of blood appears, follow the Seldinger approach as detailed for the internal jugular vein.
- Ultrasound can be used to identify the vessels and ensure that the vein is punctured near the inguinal ligament where the artery and vein lie side by side.[*]

Procedure: subclavian vein

The subclavian vein is preferred for central venous access if the patient has a cervical spine injury and is best for long-term parenteral nutrition, pacing wires, or Hickman lines. It is, however, associated with a higher incidence of incorrect line placement than internal jugular catheterization. Given the local anatomy, pressure cannot be exerted on the subclavian artery if it is accidentally punctured.

The subclavian vein is a continuation of the axillary vein and runs from the apex of the axilla, behind the posterior border of the clavicle and across the first rib to join the internal jugular vein, forming the brachio-cephalic vein behind the sternoclavicular joint (Fig. 18.6).

- Introduce yourself, confirm the identity of the patient, explain the procedure, and obtain verbal consent.
- Place the patient in a supine position, head-down.
- Turn the head to the contralateral side.
- Reconfirm the patient's identity, procedure, and site prior to starting.
- Using full sterile technique, introduce a needle attached to a 10 mL syringe, 1 cm below the junction of the medial 1/3 and outer 2/3 of the clavicle.

---

[*] U.K. Guidelines produced by the National Institute for Clinical Excellence (NICE) in September 2002 encourage the routine use of 2-D (B-mode) ultrasound guidance for CVC insertion into the internal jugular vein in adults and children in elective and emergency situations. There is, however, limited evidence supporting ultrasound use for subclavian and femoral vein catheterization based on anatomy. Ultrasonography enables direct visualization of the anatomy before and during catheterization. Portable ultrasound machines can be used at the bedside. An additional review of this issue can be viewed in McGee DC, Gould MK (2003). Preventing complications of central venous catheterization. *N Engl J Med* 348;1123–1133.

Assorted U.S. procedural guidelines can be seen at http://www.guidelines.gov

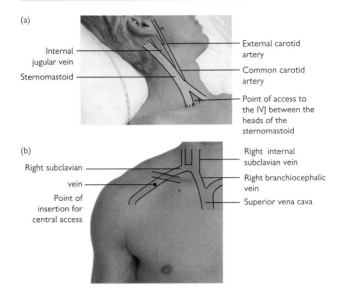

Fig. 18.6 Surface anatomy of the internal jugular vein (a) and subclavian vein (b).

- Direct the needle medially, slightly cephalad, and posteriorly behind the clavicle toward the suprasternal notch.
- Slowly advance the needle while gently withdrawing the plunger.
- When a free flow of blood appears, follow the Seldinger approach as detailed for internal jugular vein catheterization.
- The catheter tip should lie in the SVC above the pericardial reflection.
- Perform a chest X-ray to confirm position and exclude pneumothorax.
- As before, ultrasound can be used to guide puncture of the vein, using a more lateral approach.

Removing internal jugular venous catheters
- Remove any dressing and suture material.
- Ensure that all drugs and infusions have been stopped.
- Lay the patient down to reduce the risk of air embolism.
- Ask the patient to take a deep breath and fully exhale.
- Remove the line smoothly with a steady pull, while the patient is breath-holding, and apply firm pressure to the puncture site for at least 5 minutes to stop bleeding.
- Sit the patient up.
- If infection is suspected, send the tip of the line in a sterile dry specimen container for culture.

⚠ Blood pressure measurement

Theory

BP is measured with a sphygmomanometer, usually at the brachial artery.

Machines, operated by nurses or health-care assistants usually measure BP, but these are not fool-proof and a good working knowledge of the "old-fashioned," manual method of BP measuring is still essential.

A cuff is applied to the upper arm and inflated to cut off the arterial supply. The pressure is released slowly and a stethoscope used to listen for the blood flow.

When the pressure in the cuff equals the systolic blood pressure, blood will audibly pulse through the artery. When the cuff pressure falls below the diastolic blood pressure, the blood will flow continuously and the sound of intermittent blood flow will disappear.

Equipment

- A (functioning) sphygmomanometer with:
- An appropriately sized cuff (see Table 18.1)
- Stethoscope

Procedure

- Introduce yourself, explain the procedure, and obtain verbal consent.
- ▶ Check that the sphygmomanometer is working and is within the calibration box or that the dial reads "0."
- The patient should be sitting, relaxed for 5 minutes beforehand.
- Apply the cuff to the upper arm with the air bladder anteriorly (indicator over the brachial artery).
- Using your left arm, support the patient's arm so that it is held horizontally at the level of mid-sternum (avoid hyperextension of elbow).
- Close the valve (may be a screw or lever), monitor the patient's radial artery, and inflate the cuff until the radial pulse is no longer palpable.
- Listen over the brachial artery at the antecubital fossa, using the diaphragm or the bell of the stethoscope, while deflating the cuff at a rate of 2–3 mmHg/second.
- Note the point at which the pulsation is audible (Korotkoff* phase I—the systolic BP)

Table 18.1 National Guideline Clearinghouse guidelines for choice of BP cuff*

Arm circumference (cm)	Cuff size	Bladder dimensions (cm)
22–26	Small adult/child	12 × 22
27–34	Adult	16 × 30
35–44	Large adult	16 × 36
45–52	Adult thigh cuff	16 × 42

*Available at: www.guideline.gov

- And the point at which the sounds disappear (Korotkoff phase V—the diastolic BP).
- Record the BP as "systolic/diastolic" to the nearest 2 mmHg.

▶ **Hints**

- In some people with normal blood pressure, the sounds may not disappear completely. In this case, a distinct muffling of the noise (Korotkoff phase IV) should be used to indicate the diastolic BP.
- BP recording may be particularly difficult in a noisy environment or at the time of an emergency (which is when providers are most often asked to record the BP) or when the BP is very low. In this case, a rough estimation of the systolic BP may be made by feeling for the return of the radial pulse as the cuff is deflated.

⚠ **Recording a 12-lead ECG**

Theory

The ECG is a recording of the electrical activity of the heart. Electrodes are placed on the limbs and chest for a 12-lead recording. The term *12-lead* relates to the number of directions that the electrical activity is recorded from and is *not* the number of electrical wires attached to the patient!

Equipment

- ECG machine capable of recording 12 leads
- 10 ECG leads (4 limb leads, 6 chest leads)—should be attached to machine
- Conducting sticky pads (ECG electrodes)

Procedure

- Introduce yourself, confirm the identity of the patient, explain the procedure, and obtain verbal consent.
- Position the patient so that they are sitting or lying comfortably with their upper body, wrists, and ankles exposed.
- Each electrode is attached by clipping it to the sticky pads and sticking them to the patient's skin.
- The leads are usually labeled. The limb leads are often color-coded:
  - Right arm—red
  - Left arm—yellow
  - Right leg—green
  - Left leg—black
- The arm leads are of medium length and should be attached to a hairless part of the patient's wrists.
- The leg leads are the longest and should be attached to the patient's ankles (the hairless part just superior to the lateral malleolus is ideal).
- Position the chest leads as follows (see Fig. 18.7):
  - V1—fourth intercostal space at the right sternal border
  - V2—fourth intercostal space at the left sternal border
  - V3—midway between V2 and V4
  - V4—fifth intercostal space in the mid-clavicular line on the left
  - V5—left anterior axillary line, level with V4
  - V6—left mid-axillary line, level with V4
- Turn on the ECG machine. These are usually self-explanatory and require just one button to be pressed—marked *analyze* or *record*.
- Check the calibration and paper speed:
  - 1 mV should cause a vertical deflection of 10mm.
  - Paper speed should be 25 mm/sec (5 large squares per second).
- Ensure that the patient's name, DOB, as well as date and time of the recording are clearly recorded on the trace.
- Remove the leads and discard the sticky electrode pads.

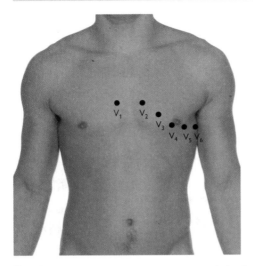

Fig. 18.7 Correct positioning of electrodes for a standard 12-lead ECG.

▶ Hints
- Encourage patient to relax, as muscle contraction causes interference.
- Ensure that you cleanse the area gently with an alcohol swab before attaching an electrode, to ensure a good connection.
- AC electrical lines and fluorescent lights may cause 60-cycle interference. If this is the case, try turning off the fluorescent lights.

⚠ Arterial blood gas sampling

Theory
An arterial sample is obtained to assess pH, PO_2, PCO_2, HCO_3^-, and base excess or deficit. It is also sometimes used for rapid assessment of electrolytes.

Equipment
- ABG kit (usually contains heparin-filled syringe, needle and vented cap)
- Gauze or cotton ball
- Tape
- Sterile gloves

Procedure
- Wash your hands and put on gloves.
- Verify patient identity, explain the procedure, and obtain verbal consent. Be sure to warn the patient of potential pain, and ask them to keep as still as possible.
- Note the patient's temperature and oxygen support.
- Chose a site for arterial puncture.

Radial
Because there are no adjacent nerves or vessels, this is the most commonly used site.
- Assess for adequate ulnar arterial circulation by performing the Allen's Test.
- Obstruct the radial artery with fingertip pressure.
- Ask the patient to make a tight fist to expel blood from the hand and maintain pressure on the radial artery.
- Ask them to open their hand and watch for flushing of the palm; this indicates adequate perfusion.
- Take the blood gas syringe, ensuring that the heparin has coated the inside by withdrawing and advancing plunger.
- Attach the needle and expel the excess heparin.
- Position the wrist in extension.
- Palpate the radial arterial pulse along its length using your middle and index fingers.
- Clean the skin.
- Having chosen a suitable spot, insert the needle with the bevel facing toward the direction of blood flow, using an appropriate angle.
- Advance the needle until arterial pressure fills the syringe.
- Obtain a sample of 1–3 mL and withdraw the needle.
- Apply pressure to the puncture site with gauze or a cotton ball until bleeding has stopped (minimum 2 minutes).
- Remove and discard the needle with care and place a vented cap on the syringe. Holding vertically, expel any air through the vent.
- Mix sample gently and take it to a blood gas analyzer.

Femoral
- Position patient with the hip extended and slightly internally rotated.
- Note that the femoral nerve is just lateral to the artery, so maintain a medial approach.
- Use the same procedure as above but use a 21G needle, aiming at the pulsation positioned between your index and middle finger.

Brachial
- Position the elbow in extension.
- Watch for adjacent nerves (see Fig. 18.8).

Appropriate angles for needle insertion
- Radial artery—45°
- Brachial artery—60°
- Femoral artery—90°

Hints
- The key to success is carefully lining up the needle over a palpable pulsation—take your time!
- If there is no flashback, withdraw the needle slightly, change the angle, and advance. Note that most pain is from puncturing the skin, so do not remove the needle fully when repositioning.
- If there will be some delay in analyzing the sample, store the blood-filled syringe on ice.
- Sources of blood gas result errors are as follows:
  • Air in the sample
  • Delay in analyzing sample or delay in icing
  • Excess heparin in the syringe
  • Accidentally obtaining a venous or mixed AV sample
  • Alterations in temperature

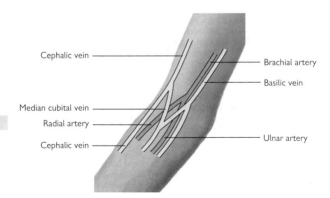

Fig. 18.8 Position of the brachial artery and surrounding structures at the antecubital fossa. The right arm is pictured.

⚠ Peak flow measurement

Theory
Peak expiratory flow rate (PEFR) is a measure of the maximum *speed* of expiration. Expressed in liters/minute, this simple and easy-to-administer test is a useful indicator of airway caliber and may be performed before and after administration of a bronchodilator to assess reversible airway obstruction.

Normal values are based on gender, age, and height.

Equipment
- Peak flow meter (see Fig. 18.9)
- Clean disposable mouthpiece

Procedure
- Introduce yourself, explain the procedure, and obtain verbal consent.
- The patient should be standing or sitting upright.
- Ensure that the meter is set to 0.
- Ask the patient to take a deep breath in, hold the mouthpiece in their mouth, and seal their lips tightly around it.
- The patient should blow out as hard and as fast as possible.

▶The PEFR needs a *hard* and *short* maximal blow-out. The patient does *not* have to blow out completely.
- Make note of the reading achieved.
- The procedure should be repeated and the best of 3 efforts recorded.
- The result should be compared to the normal value on the Nunn-Greggs nomogram.
- If the patient is to keep a record, be sure to explain how to record the readings appropriately. (Sometimes a 2-week diary is kept by the patient to assess diurnal variation.)

▶ Hints
- If the patient is having difficulty performing the test correctly, a brief demonstration often proves useful.
- If a patient has very variable flow measurements, repeat your demonstration and go on asking for flows until three consistent readings have been recorded.

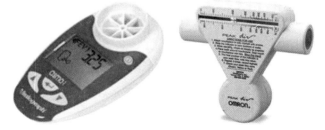

Fig. 18.9 Electronic and mechanical peak flow meters.

⚠ Inhaler technique

A person new to respiratory medicine may be surprised by the sheer number of different inhaler devices on the market. Each has its advantages and disadvantages and a different set of drugs that it can deliver.

Here we outline the inhaler devices currently available and the instructions for use, written as you would explain them to a patient. We suggest that providers become familiar with the different devices by asking your pharmacist if you can see placebo versions.

Instructions for use of devices are typically available from the manufacturer's Web site. Full video demonstrations illustrating appropriate use of devices are often available at manufacturer's Web sites, so these sites should not be overlooked.

Devices are constantly changing. Many devices are currently used, some of which have gone out of production. Some common devices include Clickhaler, Spinhaler, Aerohaler, Diskhaler, Rotahaler, Foradil inhaler, and Pulvinal. Included here is Handihaler, which is in current use.

Metered-dose inhaler (MDI)

This is the first device developed and the one people think of as a typical inhaler (Fig. 18.10). It is small and cheap and has many different drugs and doses. However, there is no dose counter and it requires much coordination to use correctly, making it unsuitable for the very young or elderly or those with arthritis or other ailments affecting the hands.

Instructions for use
- Take one dose at a time.
- Remove the cap and shake the inhaler several times.
- Sit upright, hold the head up, and breathe out.
- Place the inhaler in the mouth and seal lips around the mouthpiece.

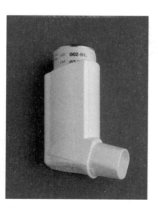

Fig. 18.10 A metered-dose inhaler (MDI).

- Breathe in, press the canister down to release drug, and continue to take a deep breath in. (The canister should be pressed *just after* the start of inhalation, not before.)
- Remove inhaler and hold breath for as long as possible, up to 10 sec.
- Recover before taking the next dose, and replace the cap.

Autohaler

This is one of the breath-actuated inhalers, releasing a dose of the drug when a breath is taken (Fig. 18.11). This eliminates the need for hand coordination and can reassure patients that a dose has been successfully administered.

Some people, however, may still find the priming lever hard to use or may have difficulty remembering to prime the device for each dose. Also, the puff and click during inhalation can be distracting.

Instructions for use

- Remove the cap and shake the inhaler several times.
- Prime the device—push the lever right up, keeping the inhaler upright.
- Sit upright, hold the head up and breathe out.
- Seal lips around the mouthpiece.
- Inhale *slowly* and *deeply*—don't stop when the inhaler clicks, and continue taking a really deep breath.
- Remove the inhaler and hold breath for as long as possible, up to 10 seconds.
- Push lever down and replace the cap.
- Recover before taking the next dose.
- Advise the patient that they won't feel the spray hitting the back of the throat, although there may be a slight taste disturbance.

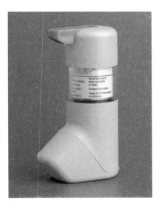 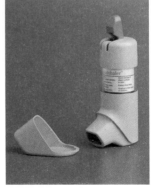

Fig. 18.11 Autohaler. Note the lever on the top. The inhaler must be primed for each dose.

▶ **Hints**
- Patients unable to push the lever up by hand can sometimes use the edge of a table to push it against.
- Patients should breathe in steadily, not as fast as possible.

Diskus

This is one of the dry-powder devices (Fig. 18.12) and has superseded the Diskhaler. Like most of the other inhalers, it is preloaded and has an integral cap. It also has a dose counter. However, it is more expensive than some of the other devices and has a several-step priming mechanism that some patients may not be able to cope with.

Instructions for use
- Hold the outer casing and push the thumb grip away from you, exposing the mouthpiece, until you hear a click.
- Holding the mouthpiece toward you, slide the lever back until it clicks (the device is now primed and the dose counter moves on 1).
- Sit upright, hold the head up, and breathe out.
- Holding the Diskus lever, seal lips around the mouthpiece.
- Inhale deeply and steadily.
- Remove the inhaler and hold breath for as long as possible, up to 10 seconds.
- To close, slide the thumbgrip toward you, so that the cover moves over the mouthpiece, until you hear a "click."
- Recover before taking the next dose.
- Advise the patient that they won't feel the spray hitting the back of the throat, although there may be a slight taste disturbance.

Turbohaler

This is another dry-powder device with preloaded drug (Fig. 18.13). There is no dose counter, but a window that turns red after 20 doses—the device is empty when there is red at the bottom of the window. Some

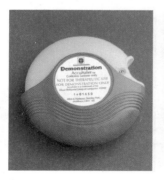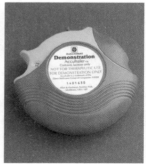

Fig. 18.12 Accuhaler (Diskus) closed and open. Note the thumbgrip, lever, and mouthpiece.

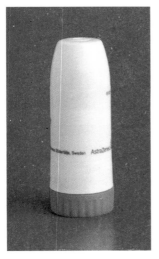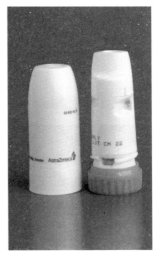

Fig. 18.13 Turbohaler. Note the tiny dose-indicating window.

people find the lack of taste disadvantageous (they like to be sure the dose has been given). Again, those with hand problems or deformities may find it difficult to use.

Instructions for use
- Unscrew and remove the white cover.
- Hold the inhaler upright.
- Twist the grip clockwise then counterclockwise as far as it will go until a "click" is heard.
- Sit upright, hold the head up, and breathe out.
- Seal lips around the mouthpiece.
- Inhale slowly and as deeply as possible.
- Remove the inhaler and hold breath for 10 seconds.
- Replace cover.
- Recover before taking the next dose.
- Advise the patient that they won't feel the spray hitting the back of the throat, although there may be a slight taste disturbance.

There are devices available that can calculate whether a person has a sufficient inspiratory flow rate to deliver the drug into the airways.

Handihaler
At the time of this writing, this is relatively new to the market and only available for tiotropium. It is a dry-powder device with an integrated cap and requires a lower inspiratory flow rate than other devices (Fig. 18.14).

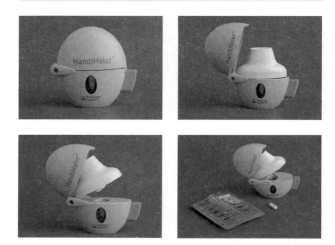

Fig. 18.14 Handihaler. Note the button at the side for piercing the capsule and the small window at the front.

However, it is not preloaded, thus a dose needs to be inserted via capsule at each use. This task requires some dexterity. Some people also find the cap hard to open, as a moderate amount of strength is needed to get it right.

Instructions for use
- Open cap by pulling upward, exposing the mouthpiece.
- Open the mouthpiece by pulling upwards exposing the chamber.
- Take a capsule from the blister-pack and insert it into the chamber.
- Replace the mouthpiece (make sure it clicks) and leave the cap open.
- Press the side button in a few times to pierce the capsule (you can watch through the small window).
- Sit upright, hold the head up, and breathe out.
- Seal lips around the mouthpiece.
- Breathe in deeply to a full breath (you should hear the capsule vibrate).
- Remove inhaler and hold breath for as long as is comfortable.
- Breathe out slowly.
- Remove the use capsule and replace the cap.

Spacer devices
These are used with a standard MDI and allow the drug to be puffed into a chamber before it is inhaled. This reduces deposition of the drug in the upper airways (and the local side effects) and increases peripheral lung deposition. This also means that no coordination is required and the

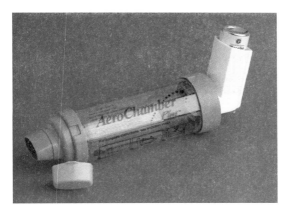

Fig. 18.15 Aerochamber with MDI inserted in the end.

patient has more time to inhale the drug. These are particularly useful for the very young or elderly, or those with severe breathlessness.

These devices are, however, bulky, which patients may find embarrassing. They also require a certain amount of dexterity to put together.

There are a number of spacer devices available, but only the Aerochamber (Fig. 18.15)is discussed here.

Instructions for use (Aerochamber)
- Remove cap of the MDI, shake the inhaler, and insert into the back of the Aerochamber.
- Breathe out.
- Seal lips around the mouthpiece.
- Press down the canister once to release the drug.
- Breathe in slowly and deeply—the Aerochamber will whistle if you breathe too quickly.
- Hold breath for 10 seconds.
- Breathe out through mouthpiece and breathe in again (do not press the canister a second time). This may be repeated up to 4 or 5 breaths.
- If a second dose is required, relax for a minute and repeat steps 3–5.
- Remover the inhaler and replace the cap.

Cleaning the Aerochamber
- The device must be rinsed daily in soapy water.
- Allow to air-dry on a drainer—do not rub (creates static electricity).
- Aerochambers should be replaced by a new model every 6 months.

⚠ Oxygen administration

Theory

This is the administration of supplementary oxygen when tissue oxygenation is impaired.

The aim is to achieve adequate tissue oxygenation (without causing a significant ↓ in ventilation and consequent hypercapnia or oxygen toxicity) while minimizing cardiopulmonary workload.

▶ Oxygen is a drug with a correct dosage and side effects, which, when administered correctly, may be life saving.

The primary responsibility for oxygen prescription lies with the hospital medical staff. It is good practice to record the following:

- Whether delivery is continuous or intermittent
- Flow rate/percentage used
- What SaO_2 should be

When to treat

- Tissue hypoxia is difficult to recognize, as clinical features are nonspecific. They include altered mental state, dyspnea, cyanosis, tachypnea, arrhythmias, and coma.
- Treatment of tissue hypoxia should correct any arterial hypoxemia (cardiopulmonary defect or shunt, e.g., PE, pneumonia, asthma), any transport deficit (anemia, low cardiac output), and the underlying causes.

▶ Remember, SaO_2/PaO_2 can be normal when tissue hypoxia is caused by low cardiac-output states.

Equipment

See 📖 p. 546.

Procedure

- Explain what is happening to the patient and ask their permission.
- Choose an appropriate oxygen delivery device (see next page).
- Choose an initial dose:
  - Cardiac or respiratory arrest: 100%
  - Hypoxemia with $PaCO_2$ <40 mmHg: 40–60%
  - Hypoxemia with $PaCO_2$ >40 mmHg: 24% initially
- Decide on the acceptable level of SaO_2 or PaO_2 and titrate oxygen accordingly.
- If possible, try to measure a PaO_2 in room air prior to giving supplementary oxygen. (This is not absolutely necessary, especially if the patient is in severe respiratory distress or is hypoxic.)
- Work with nursing staff, respiratory therapist, or outreach services for support in setting up equipment.
- Apply the oxygen and monitor via oximetry (SaO_2) and/or repeat ABGs (PaO_2) in 30 minutes.
- If hypoxemia continues, the patient may require respiratory support either invasively or noninvasively—consult with a respiratory specialist.
- Stop supplementary oxygen when tissue hypoxia or arterial hypoxemia has resolved.

Hints

- Only 10% of patients with COPD are susceptible to CO_2 retention with oxygen therapy. Use Venturi-style masks and monitor closely.
- Think about what is normal for the individual.

Oxygen administration equipment

The method of delivery will depend on the type and severity of respiratory failure, breathing pattern, respiratory rate, risk of CO_2 retention, need for humidification, and patient compliance.

Each oxygen delivery device (Fig. 18.16) comprises an oxygen supply, flow rate, tubing, interface 9 humidification. (Humidification should be used for patient comfort, presence of thick tenacious secretions, or flows >4 L/min.)

Nasal cannulas

These direct oxygen via two short prongs up the nasal passage They
- Can be used for long periods of time.
- Prevent rebreathing.
- Can be used during eating and talking.

Local irritation, dermatitis, and nose bleeding may occur, and rates of above 4 L/min should not be used routinely.

Low-flow oxygen masks

These deliver oxygen concentrations that vary depending on the patient's minute volume. At these low flow rates there may be some rebreathing of exhaled gases (they are not sufficiently expelled from the mask).

Fixed performance masks

These achieve a constant concentration of oxygen independent of the patient's minute volume.

The masks contain Venturi barrels where relatively low rates of oxygen are forced through a narrow orifice, producing a greater flow rate that draws in a constant proportion of room air through several gaps.

Partial and non-rebreather masks

Masks such as these have a reservoir bag that is filled with pure oxygen and depend on a system of one-way valves that prevent mixing of exhaled gases with the incoming oxygen.

The concentration of oxygen delivered is set by the oxygen flow rate.

High-flow oxygen masks

Masks or nasal prongs generate flows of 50–120 L/min using a high-flow regulator to mix air and oxygen at specific concentrations.

These masks are highly accurate, as delivered flow rates will match a high respiratory rate in patients with respiratory distress. It should always be used with humidification.

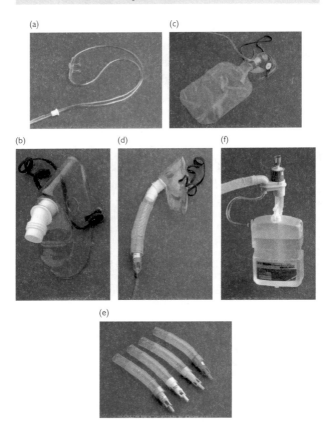

Fig. 18.16 (a) Nasal cannula. (b) Low-flow/variable-concentration mask. (c) Non-rebreather mask. (d) Mask with Venturi valve attached. (e) Selection of Venturi valves. (f) Humidification circuit.

▶ Basic airway management

Theory

An inadequate airway (Box 18.4) leads rapidly to hypoxemia and, if uncorrected, brain damage and death. Endotracheal intubation remains the gold standard for securing an airway and protecting the patient from aspiration (Box 18.5).

Airway management without intubation is an important skill to master and consists of the use of one or more of the following: triple maneuver, face masks, oropharyngeal and nasopharyngeal airways, laryngeal masks, and other supraglottic devices, e.g., Combitube. It may be carried out when intubation equipment or skills are unavailable, if intubation is difficult, or on a patient with a partially obstructed airway.

Urgency is an important factor in planning and securing an airway in the most appropriate manner. This will depend on risk of vocal cord injury, degree of patient cooperation, anatomy of airway, equipment at hand, and your own experience.

Before you start

▶ Think about simple positioning and the recovery position of the patient, especially for airway protection alone.

Assess for airway obstruction:
- LOOK (into mouth and for chest or abdominal movement)
- LISTEN (snoring, gurgling, wheezing)
- FEEL (expired air)

▶ Complete airway obstruction is *silent*.

Make sure that you have the following:
- Oxygen tubing
- Suction equipment
- Ambu-bag
- Rebreather bag

Hints

- A fully conscious, talking patient is able to maintain his or her own airway and needs no further assessment.

🛈 Do not use a head tilt or chin lift in suspected cervical spine injury, except as a last resort.

Airway maneuvers

The following techniques are performed with the patient lying supine, and all aim to open the airway with simple physical maneuvers. These are

Box 18.4 Common causes of airway obstruction

- Tongue (due to unconciousness)
- Soft tissue swelling (trauma, tumor)
- Foreign material (blood, vomit)
- Direct injury
  - Secretions
  - Bronchospasm

Box 18.5 Secure airways

A secure airway may be necessary in patients with the following:
- Apnea
- Glasgow Coma Scale <9/15
- High aspiration risk
- Respiratory failure
- Unstable mid-face trauma
- Airway injuries

useful as a first step in managing a patient with a compromised airway and are used in conjunction with an oxygen mask. They are also useful in situations where no airway devices are available.

If unsuccessful, you should go on to use additional equipment.

Head tilt
Place your hands around the patient's forehead and tilt backward to achieve upper cervical extension (Fig. 18.17).

Chin lift
- This is usually used with the head tilt.
- Place the tips of the index and middle fingers of your right hand under the front of the patient's mandible.
- Lift up, pulling the mandible anteriorly (Fig. 18.18).

Jaw thrust
- Use this maneuver if there is suspicion of an injury to the cervical spine. This is a two-handed technique.
- Holding the patient from behind, place the fingers of both hands behind the angle of the mandible.
- Lift the mandible with these fingers while using your thumbs to displace the chin downward, opening the mouth (Fig. 18.19).

▶ **Hint**
❶ Do not use a head tilt or chin lift in a patient with (or suspected to have) cervical spine injuries.

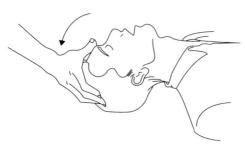

Fig. 18.17 Performing a head tilt.

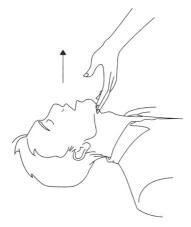

Fig. 18.18 Performing a chin lift.

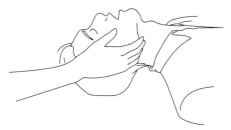

Fig. 18.19 Performing a jaw thrust.

Airway devices

Face masks

▶ Use the smallest-fitting mask to fit over the mouth and nose.
  This is a simple mask that is fitted over the nose and mouth. You may use an airway to aid ventilation or to clear any obstruction.

One-hand technique
- Place your thumb and index finger on the mask in a C shape (see Fig. 18.20).
- Grasp the jaw with the remaining fingers, pulling face into the mask.

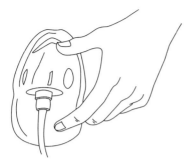

Fig. 18.20 Use of a face mask, one-handed technique.

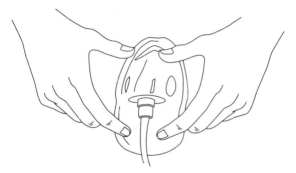

Fig. 18.21 Use of a face mask, two-handed technique.

Two-hand technique
- Place your thumbs on either side of the nasal portion of the mask.
- Use your index fingers to support the body of the mask.
- Use your other fingers to lift the jaw and extend the neck (Fig. 18.21).

Oropharyngeal airway

▶ Use this when the patient is semiconscious.

This device consists of a flange (limits depth of insertion), bite portion (teeth of patient rest against this), and curved body (follows curvature of the tongue), which has a lumen allowing passage of air and suction.

Different sizes are available and are color coded. The correct size is determined by measuring the airway against the distance between the corner of the mouth and the angle of the jaw (Figs. 18.22 and 18.23).

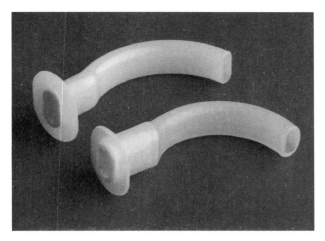

Fig. 18.22 Oropharyngeal airways.

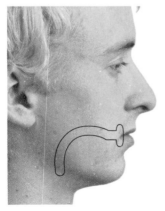

Fig. 18.23 Chose size of the oropharyngeal airway by measuring from the patient's teeth to the angle of the mandible.

Technique
- Lubricate and insert the airway upside down.
- Once it is well into the mouth rotate 180° and advance to full position.
  - Alternatively, hold the tongue down and forward with a tongue depressor until the airway is in place.

• Check for no gagging, snoring, or vomiting and that air is moving in and out.
• Use a size 10/12/14 catheter for suction, if required.

Nasopharyngeal airway

▶ This is tolerated better than the oropharyngeal airway in alert patients. This device consists of a flange (limits depth of insertion). The pharyngeal end has a bevel to facilitate nontraumatic insertion and a curved body with lumen allowing passage of air and suction. Some airways come without an adequate flange, so a safety pin is used at the nasal end to prevent the airway from falling back into the nose (see Fig. 18.24).

Different sizes are available. Determine the correct size by comparing with the distance between the nostril and the tragus (see Fig. 18.25).

Technique
• The wider nostril is traditionally chosen, but most airways are beveled for introduction into the left nostril.
• Lubricate airway and pass directly into the nasal passage, passing along the floor of the nose or aiming for the back of the opposite eyeball.
• Use a size 10/12 catheter for suction, if required.

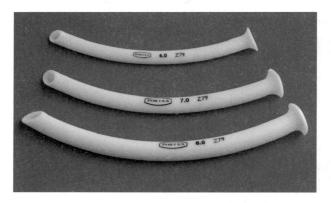

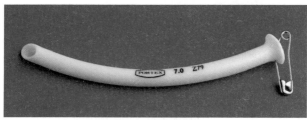

Fig. 18.24 Nasopharyngeal airways.

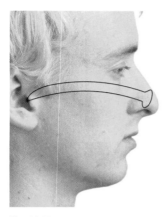

Fig. 18.25 Chose size of the nasopharyngeal airway by measuring from the patient's nostril to the tragus.

Laryngeal mask airway (LMA)

This consists of a tube with an inflatable cuff designed to seal around the laryngeal opening (Fig. 18.26). The patient must be deeply unconscious.

Technique
- Maintain oxygenation by bag and mask.
- Deflate the cuff of the LMA using a 20 mL syringe.
- Lubricate the outer cuff with aqueous gel. This part will not be in contact with the larynx.
- The patient should be in a supine position with head and neck in alignment.
- Stand behind the patient or, if this is not possible, from the front.
- Hold the tube like a pen and pass it into the mouth with the distal aperture facing the feet of the patient.
- Push back over the tongue while applying the tip to the surface of the palate until it reaches the posterior pharyngeal wall.
- The mask is then pressed backward and down until it reaches the back of the hypopharynx and resistance is felt.
- The black line on the tube should be aligned with the nasal septum.
- Inflate the cuff with usually 20–30 mL of air.
- The tube should lift out of the mouth slightly; the larynx is pushed forward if it is in the correct position.
- Attach breathing circuit and gently ventilate patient with 100% oxygen.
- Confirm correct placement by auscultating the chest in the axillary regions and observe for bilateral chest movement.
- Insert a bite block or oropharyngeal airway alongside the tube and secure the airway with the tape or tie provided.

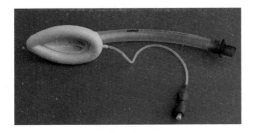

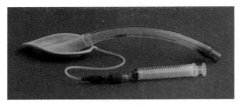

Fig. 18.26 A laryngeal mask airway.

▶▶ Tracheostomy management

Theory

A *tracheostomy* is an opening in the anterior wall of the trachea below the larynx that can facilitate ventilation and respiration.

A *mini-tracheostomy* is a narrow-diameter, cuffless tube inserted into the trachea, through which a catheter can be passed to stimulate a cough and/or suction. This is not a method for protecting the airway or delivering any kind of ventilatory support except emergency oxygen therapy.

Tracheostomy may be performed if the need for an endotracheal tube is prolonged, to facilitate weaning, to identify an inability to maintain or protect an airway, and to secure and clear an airway.

Patients may have a permanent tracheostomy in place or even a stoma. These often do not need humidification or suction unless the patient is acutely ill.

Equipment

Tracheostomy tube

The tracheostomy tube may be stitched in or secured around the neck and is either single or double lumen (has an inner tube that can be removed for cleaning). The tubes are either fenestrated or nonfenestrated.

Fenestrated tubes allow the passage of air and secretions into the mouth. These are good for weaning.

Humidification

Heated humidification is used for the short term and is the gold standard. A heat moisture exchanger is used for patients with minimal secretions or who are mobile.

Procedures

Open suction

The aim is to remove secretions and prevent blockages in the tracheostomy tube, bronchial obstruction, and alveolar collapse.

- Use a catheter with diameter no more than one 1/2 the internal tracheotomy diameter. [(Size of outer diameter) − 2 x 2 = x; e.g., 8.0 mm − 2 x2 = 12].
- Negative pressure should be 100–150 mmHg.
- Wear gown, gloves, and protective eyewear.
- Attach a sterile catheter to suction equipment, ensuring a good seal, and leave most of the packaging in place.
- Place under the nondominant arm.
- Put a clean, disposable glove on the dominant hand and do not touch anything other than the catheter tip.
- Pull the packaging away with the nondominant hand.
- Open the suction port.
- Introduce the tip of the catheter into the tracheostomy tube with the dominant hand gently but quickly.
- Depth of insertion should be 0.5–1.0 cm beyond the end of the tracheostomy tube (about 1/3 the length of catheter).

- Insert until the patient coughs.
- Withdraw the tip 0.5 cm and apply suction.
- Continue to withdraw slowly and continuously.
- Close the suction port and discard the glove and catheter.
▶ Suction should last no more than 10 seconds.
▶ Allow sufficient time between passes for recovery.
- Repeat until secretions are cleared.
- After suction, ensure that the patient is reconnected to respiratory support and oxygen and that oxygen levels are returned to normal.

Tube occlusion
- Call for help.
- Reassure the patient.
- Ask the patient to cough, or attempt to clear secretions via suction.
- Remove the inner cannula and replace it with a new one.
- If there is no inner cannula, deflate the cuff and administer oxygen facially, instill 2–5 mL 0.9% saline, and suction to try to clear blockage.
- If you are unable to clear the blockage, a total tube change may be required (try using a smaller size, if necessary).
- If tube insertion fails, then consider mask-to-stoma ventilation (consider suction via stoma).
▶ If respiration stops all together, initiate the proper code, call for anesthesia service, inflate the cuff, and manually ventilate using a catheter mount and rebreather or Ambu-bag.

Swallowing assessment
This should be performed by the appropriate practitioner (e.g., radiologist or speech and language therapist).
- Sit the patient up.
- Suction via tracheotomy prior to cuff deflation.
- *Deflate* cuff fully, if possible, or to maximum degree that the patient can tolerate.
- Ensure that there is an appropriate inner cannula in place.
- Give the patient *sips* of water from a teaspoon and follow the procedure explained on 📖 p. 289.
- Intermittently check for voice quality (ask the patient to say "ah" or count out loud).
- Stop if the patient deteriorates, fatigues, shows signs of persistent coughing or aspiration on suction, or has a persistently "wet" voice.

Hints
- Practice techniques before needing them in an emergency.
- Stridor is a good indication that an airway is partially blocked.
- Always remember to humidify oxygen in tracheotomy patients.

▶▶ Endotracheal (ET) intubation

Theory
There are three main indications for tracheal intubation: relieving airway obstruction, protecting the airway from aspiration, and facilitating artificial ventilation of the lungs.

▶ Remember, if you are inexperienced in this technique, never perform tracheal intubation unsupervized.

▶ In an emergency situation, it is safer to bag and mask the patient or use a laryngeal mask airway if one is available and await assistance.

Equipment
- Laryngoscope (check bulb)—usually size 3 is adequate
- Selection of ET tubes (size 7 in most women and size 8 in most men)
- Sterile lubricant
- 20 mL syringe for cuff inflation
- Tape to tie tube in place
- Rigid stilette or gum-elastic bougie
- Self-inflating bag and oxygen supply
- Stethoscope for confirming correct position of tube
- Suction apparatus with a wide-bore, rigid suction end (Yankauer)

Procedure
- In the awake patient, introduce yourself, confirm the patient's identity, explain the procedure, and obtain verbal consent.
- Wash your hands and put on a pair of gloves.
- Pre-oxygenate the patient with a high concentration of oxygen for a minimum of 15 seconds.

▶ Remember, intubation must take no longer than 30 seconds.

- Position the neck such that it is distally extended and proximally slightly flexed, with a small pillow underneath the head—an exaggeration of the normal cervical lordosis.

▶ If a cervical injury is suspected, the head and neck should be maintained in neutral alignment.

- Stand at the head of the bed and open the mouth.
- Inspect for loose dentures or foreign material—remove any if present.
- Hold the laryngoscope in the left hand and look down its length as you insert.
- Slide the scope into the right side of the mouth until the tonsillar fossa comes into view.
- Now move the blade to the left so that the tongue is pushed into a midline position.
- Advance blade, following the posterior edge of the soft palate until the uvula comes into view.
- Advance blade over the base of the tongue, and the epiglottis should pop into sight.
- With blade positioned between the epiglottis and base of the tongue (vallecula), apply traction in the line of the handle of the laryngoscope.

- This movement should lift the epiglottis and expose the V-shaped glottis behind.
- Once the triangular-shaped laryngeal inlet is in view, position the ET tube between the vocal cords so that the tube is just distal to them.
  - Use mark on the tube above the cuff to indicate correct position.
  - This is around 21 cm in a female and 22 cm in a male.
- If difficulty is experienced passing ET tube into the larynx, pass a gum-elastic bougie first and then try passing a lubricated ET tube over this.
- Once the ET tube is in position, inflate the cuff while ventilating through the ET tube with a self-inflating bag (Fig. 18.27).
- Verify correct positioning of the tube by observing chest movement and auscultate at the sides of the chest in the mid-axillary line (both sides of the chest should move equally, and you should hear breath sounds at both lung bases).
- Secure the ET tube with a tie.
- Obtain a chest X-ray to confirm the tube position. The ET tube has a radio-opaque line within it.
- Document the details of the procedure in the patient notes.

Important note

▶ The insertion of the ET tube should take no more than 30 seconds from start to finish. If 30 seconds pass and the tube is not in the correct position, remove all the equipment and bag/mask ventilate the patient until you are ready to try again.

Some complications of ET intubation

- Trauma to teeth, airway, larynx, or trachea
- Aspiration
- Airway obstruction
- Tube misplacement
- Hypoxia from prolonged attempts
- Tracheal stenosis (late complication)

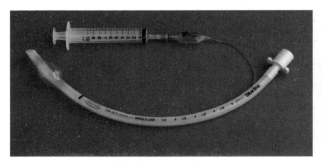

Fig. 18.27 ET tube with attached syringe. The cuff has been inflated to demonstrate.

▶▶ Noninvasive ventilation (NIV)

Theory

NIV is the application of positive pressure ventilatory support via a facial or nasal interface and not via an airway (ET tube, tracheostomy) (see Box 18.6 for setup). NIV should be operated only by trained staff in an appropriate area. It may be used in acute conditions in the hospital or in chronic conditions at home.

Patients need to be spontaneously breathing, maintaining their airway (i.e., conscious), and compliant. It is not a substitute for mechanical ventilation unless this has been decided as the ceiling of treatment.

Pressures are usually documented in cmH_2O (rather than mmHg), and it is good practice that the decision of maximal pressure to be used is documented in the medical notes so that if a patient continues to deteriorate, the intensivist, pulmonologist, or anesthesiologist has an appropriate management strategy in place.

Contraindications

These include undrained pneumothorax and pulmonary hemorrhage. It is good practice to review a recent chest X-ray to rule these out before beginning.

Cautions

These comprise bullae, unstable cardiovascular system, abscess, facial trauma, basal skull fracture, recent bronchial or esophageal surgery, persistent vomiting, and high bronchial tumor.

CPAP

Continuous **P**ositive **A**irways **P**ressure (CPAP) maintains a single pressure continuously throughout both inspiratory and expiratory phases.

It is used in the treatment of type I respiratory failure (obstructive sleep apnea and cardiopulmonary edema, and occasionally in pulmonary embolus, pneumonia, and weaning from ventilation).

BiPAP

Bilevel **P**ositive **A**irways **P**ressure (BiPAP) ventilation uses different pressures on expiration (EPAP) and on inspiration (IPAP). Higher EPAP increases functional residual capacity (FRC), while higher IPAP augments tidal volume. The system is normally pressure driven but can be volume driven.

It is used in the treatment of type II respiratory failure (i.e., hypoventilation, chronic neuromuscular conditions, and exacerbations of COPD).

Box 18.6 Setting up NIV

This is not something that the inexperienced provider will be expected to do. The following is a brief guide that should allow you to understand what is involved.

CPAP

Equipment
- Mask, head strap, positive end-expiratory pressure (PEEP) valves (5–7.5–10 cmH₂O)
- Circuit, safety pop-off/blow-off valve
- High-flow generator for oxygen and air
- Heated humidification

Procedure
- Explain the procedure to the patient and obtain verbal consent.
- Use measuring templates to assess appropriate-size interface and minimize air leaks.
- Set oxygen and flow rate and ensure that the PEEP valve opens a small distance only and never fully closes.
- Start with a low pressure and slowly increase for patient comfort and to gain compliance.
- Aim to reduce the work of breathing.
- Continuously monitor ABG/SaO₂, heart rate, and BP. Watch for abdominal distension.

BiPAP

Equipment
- Mask (facial/nasal), prongs, full face mask, head strap
- Circuit, exhalation port
- Entrained oxygen, if required
- Heated humidification
- Ventilator (NIPPV1/2/3, Breas, BiPAP vision)

Procedure
- Explain the procedure to the patient and obtain verbal consent.
- Use measuring templates to assess appropriate-size interface and minimize air leaks.
- Start with low pressures and slowly increase for patient comfort and to gain compliance. (Trial data in COPD is based on pressures of 20/5.)
- Setting inspiratory and expiratory times will need to be continuously reassessed, as respiratory rate will change over time.
- Initially aim to match the patient's own ventilatory pattern, but eventually aim to ↓ respiratory rate and ↑ tidal volume/flow using the minimal pressures possible.
- Monitor ABG/SaO₂, heart rate, and BP at 1 and 4 hours. Watch for abdominal distension.

▶ Pleural fluid sampling (thoracentesis)

Theory

After identifying a pleural effusion, a small volume of fluid may be aspirated and sent for biochemical, cytological, and microbiological analysis.

A neurovascular bundle runs on the inferior/inner aspect of each rib; to avoid this, needles for aspiration are inserted immediately *above* a rib.

Equipment

- Instrument stand
- Sterile/wound care pack
- Sterile gloves
- Antiseptic solution
- 5 mL syringe
- 20 mL syringe
- 1 vial of local anesthetic (usually 1% lidocaine)
- Selection of needles (2 green, 1 orange/blue)
- 2 sterile sample containers
- 1 pair of culture bottles
- Biochemistry tube for glucose sample

Procedure

- Introduce yourself, check the patient's identity, explain the procedure, obtain verbal consent, and unwrap the equipment.
- Position the patient to sit upright on the edge of the bed, leaning forward with arms raised—use a pillow on a raised bedside. table for the patient to lean on (see Fig. 18.29).
- Percuss upper border of the effusion posteriorly, and choose a site one or two intercostal spaces below that.
- Mark the chosen spot at the upper edge of a rib with a pen.
- Wash your hands and put on sterile gloves.
- Clean the marked area with the antiseptic solution on a cotton ball. Work outward in a spiraling fashion.
- Pause to reconfirm patient identity, the procedure, and site.
- Draw up 5 mL of the lidocaine with the green needle.
- Swap the needle for an orange one and infiltrate the skin, creating a surface bleb.
- Swap for a green (18G) needle and infiltrate anesthetic deeper. Advance needle in a step-wise manner, drawing back the syringe each time it is advanced to ensure vasculature is avoided (Fig. 18.30) and infiltrating anesthetic before advancing again.
- Once you reach the pleural cavity, a flashback of pleural fluid may be obtained.
- Take the 20 mL syringe, attach a green (18G) needle and aspirate 20 mL of pleural fluid, being careful to use the anesthetized tract.
- Withdraw the needle and cover the wound with a suitable dressing (dry gauze and medical sticky tape will suffice).
- Put 4 mL of fluid in each bottle and send to the laboratories for
  - Biochemistry (pH, protein, LDH, amylase, glucose)
  - Cytology
  - Microbiology (MC&S plus TB stain and culture, if indicated)

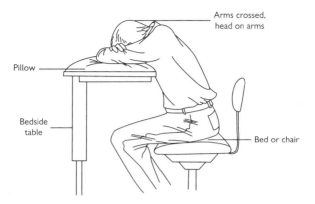

Fig. 18.28 Position patient comfortably leaning forward—use a bedside table and pillow for them to lean on with their arms crossed.

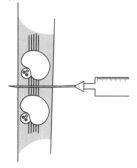

Fig. 18.29 Insert needle just above a rib, at the lower border of the intercostal space, to avoid the neurovascular bundle.

- Request a chest X-ray post-procedure to check for pneumothorax only if the procedure was difficult or high risk.

Hints

▶ If pH needs to be measured, the sample must be sent to the laboratory immediately.

❶ Some laboratories will not measure pH—check before you begin. An alternative is to save a small amount of fluid, draw it up in a primed blood gas syringe, and run it through a blood gas analyzer to gain an instant pH measurement.

- In larger individuals, the pleural cavity may be at some depth from the skin. If this is the case, use a longer needle—needles of IV catheters are often significantly longer despite being the same gauge.

▶▶Chest tube insertion

Theory

Tubes are inserted to drain either fluid (pleural effusion/empyema) or air (pneumothorax) from the pleural cavity. In both cases, the insertion of the tube is almost entirely identical.

The tube is connected to a container with a small amount of water (creating an airtight seal), so there is no direct connection between the pleural cavity and air. On inspiration, the negative intrathoracic pressure draws water up the tube (about 4 cm); on expiration, the water level falls and (if draining a pneumothorax) air bubbles through the water. This one-way valve allows air or fluid to drain from the chest but not re-enter.

The method described below is the *Seldinger technique*. While other techniques exist for wide-bore tubes, these are now only used in the setting of blunt trauma and cardiothoracic surgery, or for other problems such as extensive surgical emphysema overlying a pneumothorax.

Equipment

- Instrument stand
- 10 mL 1% lidocaine
- 10 mL syringe
- 1 orange (14 gauge) needle
- 1 green (18 gauge) needle
- Sterile gloves
- Sterile pack (containing cotton balls, container, drape)
- Barrier pad (Blue pad/Chux)
- Suitable dressing

- Seldinger chest tube kit (containing chest tube, in-troducer, chest drain needle, syringe, scalpel, 3-way tap, guide wire)
- Suture (no. 15)
- Povidone-iodine solution
- Chest drain tubing
- Chest drainage bottle
- 500 mL sterile water

Procedure

- Introduce yourself, confirm the identity of the patient, explain the procedure, and obtain verbal consent.
- Double-check the history and chest X-ray to be *sure* of which side needs the drain.
- Position the patient sitting on a chair or the edge of their bed, arms raised. Instead of asking the patient to hold their arm over their head, it is often easier to ask them to cross their arms and lean on a bedside table with a pillow, raised level with their shoulders (see Fig. 18.28).
- Triple-check the side by briefly examining the patient (tap out dullness of an effusion or listen for the ↓ breath sounds of a pneumothorax).
- The usual site for insertion is in the mid-axillary line, within a triangle formed by the diaphragm, the latissimus dorsi, and the pectoralis major (Fig. 18.30). For apical pneumothoraces, you may wish to choose the second intercostal space in the mid-clavicular line.
- Place the barrier pad on the bed to absorb any spillage.
- Mark your chosen spot (just *above* a rib to avoid hitting the neurovascular bundle; see Fig. 18.29) with a pen.

- Sterilize the area with antiseptic solution or povidone-iodine on cotton balls, working in a spiral pattern outward from the insertion point.
- Pause to reconfirm the patient identity, procedure, and site.
- Using the syringe and the orange needle, anesthetize the skin (see 📖 p. 512), forming a subcutaneous bleb.
- Swap the orange needle for the green (18G) one and anesthetize deeper, remembering to aspirate before injecting, to ensure that you have not hit a vessel. Anesthetize right down to the pleural cavity and only stop when you aspirate air or pleural fluid.
- Use the scalpel to make a small cut in the skin.
- Now use the drain-kit needle with the curved tip and syringe (in some kits, this has a central stylet that needs to be removed first). With the curved tip facing down (up for a pneumothorax), advance through the anesthetized route until you are aspirating either air or fluid again.
- Remove the syringe and hold the needle steady.
- Thread the guide wire through the needle into the pleural cavity (this usually comes precoiled but often needs to be retracted slightly first to straighten the curve on the tip). See Fig. 18.31.
- Once the wire is half-way in the chest, discard the covering.
- Now withdraw the needle from the chest but **be sure to not remove the guide wire**—KEEP HOLD OF iT AT ALL TIMES.
- Thread the needle right off the end of the guide wire. You should now have the wire in the chest, but nothing else.
- Thread the introducer over the guide wire and into the chest, twisting back and forth as you go to open up a tract for the drain's passage. You can then slide the introducer back off the wire—but be careful not to pull the wire out of the chest.
- The chest drain has a central stiffener in place; leave this in situ. Now thread the drain over the wire and into the chest, curving downward. Always HOLD ON TO THE WIRE with one hand—you may need to pull the wire out of the chest slightly so that it protrudes from the end of the drain before you push the drain into the chest. You don't want to push it right into the chest and lose it!
- Once the drain is in place, withdraw the wire and the central stiffener.
- Quickly attach the 3-way tap and make sure all the ports are closed.
- You can now stitch the drain in place (Fig. 18.32). This needn't be complicated—a simple stitch just above the drain will suffice with the ends then wrapped tightly around the drain, knotted several times.
- Fix the drain in place with a suitable dressing.
- Attach the drain to the tubing and the tubing to the drain collection bottle, which you have prefilled with 500 mL of sterile water.
- Open the 3-way tap. You should either see the fluid start to flow or air start to bubble in the collection bottle. Ask the patient to take a few deep breaths and watch the water level in the tubing to ensure it is rising and falling.
- Warn the patient not to knock the bottle over and to keep it below the level of their umbilicus.
- Request a post-insertion chest X-ray.

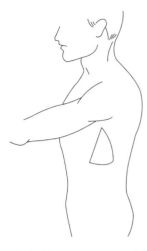

Fig. 18.30 Correct positioning of the patient for chest drain insertion and ideal site of drain insertion.

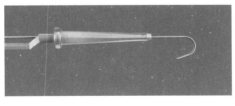

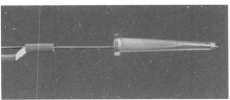

Fig. 18.31 Prepare the guide wire before starting the procedure by retracting slightly so as to straighten the curved tip.

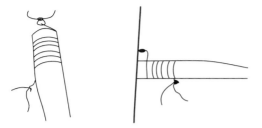

Fig. 18.32 Diagrammatic representation of a suitable stitch to hold the drain in place.

⚠ Nasogastric (NG) tube insertion

Theory

In this procedure, a plastic tube is inserted through the nose, down the back of the throat and esophagus, and into the stomach.

The bore of the tube (large = 16, medium = 12, small = 10) is dictated by the tube's intended purpose. For short- or medium-term nutritional support in patients with a defective swallow, a fine-bore tube is used. Larger bores are used to drain the stomach contents and decompress intestinal obstruction.

- *Contraindications:* severe facial trauma and basal skull fractures
- *Complications:* aspiration, tissue trauma, electrolyte loss, tracheal or duodenal intubation, perforation of esophagus or stomach

Equipment

- Disposable gloves
- Protective gown
- Drape
- Lubricant gel
- NG tube
- Cup of water and straw
- 50 mL syringe
- Drainage bag (if necessary)
- Adhesive tape or steristrips
- Emesis basin
- Paper towel
- Suction pump (if indicated)

Procedure

- Introduce yourself, confirm the patient's identity, explain the procedure, and obtain verbal consent.
- Wash your hands thoroughly, and put on gloves and gown.
- Ideally, the patient should be seated upright (often, the head tilted slightly forward can aid insertion).
- Examine the patient's nose for deformity or obstructions and decide which nostril to use.
- Use the tube to measure the distance xiphoid process → earlobe → tip of nose and note the distance.
- Lubricate the first 4–8 cm of tube. You may also wish to use local anesthetic spray on the patient's throat, if available.
- Pass the tube into the nostril and then posteriorly, a short distance at a time. You will feel it turn the corner at the nasopharynx and another slight obstruction as it passes into the esophagus.
- If the patient is able, ask them to swallow as the tube passes the pharynx—a brief sip of water may help here.
- Advance the tube as far as the premeasured distance.
- To check for correct placement, you may wish to aspirate some stomach contents with the syringe and test the fluid's pH (it should be <6).
- Secure the tube to the patient's nose with some tape. You may also wish to curl it back over their ear and secure it to their cheek.
- Request a chest X-ray and confirm the tube's position (*below* the diaphragm in the region of the gastric bubble) before using for feeding.
- Record the procedure in the patient's notes.

▶ **Hints**
- If resistance is felt, try rotating the tube while advancing it. Never force it.
- Partially cooling the tube can stiffen the tube, making it easier to pass.

▶ No longer considered appropriate, an alternate test for correct placement was to insert a small bolus of air (20–30 mL) via the tube with the syringe while listening to the epigastrium with the stethoscope. One would thus hear the air entering the stomach.

▶▶ Ascitic tap

Theory

In this procedure, a needle is inserted through the abdominal wall, allowing withdrawal of a small amount of fluid for diagnostic purposes.

Equipment

- 1 green (18 gauge) needle
- 1 orange (14 gauge) needle
- 10 mL syringe
- 20 mL syringe
- 5–10 mL 1% lidocaine solution
- Povidone-iodine or antiseptic solution
- Microbiology culture bottles (anaerobic and aerobic)
- Sterile pack (including gloves, cotton balls, and container)
- 2 sterile collection bottles
- Biochemistry tube (glucose)
- Hematology tube

Procedure

- Introduce yourself, confirm the identity of the patient, explain the procedure, and obtain verbal consent.
- Ensure that the patient has emptied their bladder.
- Position the patient lying supine or in the lateral decubitus position, leaving the right side available. Undress this side, exposing abdomen.
- Percuss the extent of the ascitic dullness (📖 p. 239).
- Mark your chosen spot in the region of the right iliac fossa (preferably) within the area of dullness (Fig. 18.33).
- Clean the area thoroughly with antiseptic, and put on sterile gloves.
- Pause to reconfirm patient identity and the procedure and site.
- Infiltrate the skin and subcutaneous tissues with lidocaine via the orange needle and 10 mL syringe and wait a minute for it to take effect.
- Attach the green needle to the 20 mL syringe and insert it into the abdomen, perpendicular to the skin. Advance the needle as you aspirate until fluid is withdrawn.
- Aspirate as much fluid as possible (up to the 20 mL).
- Remove the needle and apply a suitable sterile dressing.
- Put >4 mL of fluid in each bottle and send to the lab for the following:
  - Biochemistry—standard collection bottle (albumin, LDH, amylase)
  - Biochemistry—accurate glucose collection tube (glucose)
  - Cytology
  - Hematology (total and differential white cell count)
  - Microbiology (C&S)

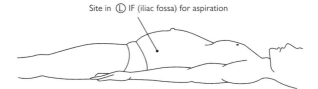

Site in Ⓛ IF (iliac fossa) for aspiration

Fig. 18.33 Performing a diagnostic ascitic tap.

▶▶ Abdominal paracentesis (drainage)

Theory

In this procedure, a drain is inserted into the abdominal cavity, allowing drainage of large amounts of ascitic fluid for therapeutic purposes.

The procedure below relates to a Bonanno drainage kit—the essence is the same as for other catheter kits (Fig. 18.34), although minor details may differ. Refer to the manufacturer's instructions.

Equipment

- 1 orange (14 gauge) needle
- 1 green (18 gauge) needle
- 2 × 10 mL syringes
- 5–10 mL 1% lidocaine solution
- Povidone-iodine or antiseptic solution
- Sterile pack (including gloves, cotton balls, and container)
- Bonanno abdominal catheter pack (catheter, sleeve, puncture needle, and adaptor clamp)
- Catheter bag
- Catheter bag stand
- Scalpel

Procedure

- Introduce yourself, confirm the identity of the patient, explain the procedure, and obtain verbal consent.
- Ensure that the patient has emptied their bladder.
- Position the patient lying supine or in the lateral decubitus position, leaving the right side available. Undress this side, exposing abdomen.
- Percuss the extent of the ascitic dullness (📖 p. 239).
- Mark your chosen spot in the region of the right iliac fossa (preferably) within the area of dullness.
- Clean the area thoroughly with antiseptic and put on sterile gloves.
- Pause to reconfirm patient identity and the procedure and site.
- Infiltrate the skin and subcutaneous tissues with lidocaine via the orange needle and 10 mL syringe and wait a minute for it to take effect.
- Attach the green needle to the other 10 mL syringe and insert into the abdomen, perpendicular to the skin. Advance the needle as you aspirate until fluid is withdrawn.
- Prepare the catheter kit—straighten the catheter (which is curled in the pack) using the plastic covering sheath provided.
- Take the needle provided in the pack and pass through the sheath such that the needle bevel is directed along inside the curve of the catheter (Fig. 18.35). Continue until the needle protrudes from the catheter tip.
- Close off the rubber at the end of the catheter.
- Make a small incision in the skin with the scalpel.
- Grasp catheter needle ~10 cm above the distal end and, with a firm thrust, push needle through the abdominal wall to ~3 cm deep.
- Disengage needle from the catheter hub and advance catheter until the suture disc is flat against the skin.
- Withdraw needle.
- Connect adaptor-clamp to the catheter hub and securely attach the rubber portion of the clamp into a standard drainage catheter bag.

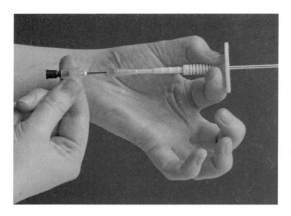

Fig. 18.34 The assembled catheter components.

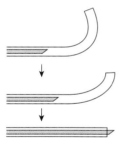

Fig. 18.35 Inserting the needle into the curved catheter.

- Carefully suture the catheter into the abdominal wall—you may also need to apply further tape to ensure the catheter won't fall out.
- Ensure that the clamp is open to allow fluid to drain.

Hints

- In cirrhotic patients, protein loss should be replaced (and hemodynamic stability maintained) by infusing human albumin solution (HAS) IV at a rate of 100 mL of 20% HAS for every 3 L of ascitic fluid drained—check local protocols with the gastroenterology department.
- Usually catheters are not left in place for >24 hours.
- During drainage, the flow may stop, which suggests that the drain is blocked. This may be positional, and simply moving the patient may solve the problem.

⚠ Male urethral catheterization

Theory
A urinary catheter has a balloon near the tip that is inflated via a side-arm near the other end. Once inside the bladder, the inflated balloon prevents it from falling, or being pulled, out.

Equipment
- Catheter pack (containing a basin, a small bowl with cotton balls, a sterile towel, sterile gauze, and sterile gloves)
- Antiseptic solution or vial of saline
- Appropriate urological anesthetic gel
- 10 mL water-filled syringe
- Catheter bag (leg bag if situation is not acute)
- Male catheter (12F or 14F)

Procedure
- Wash your hands thoroughly. Confirm the patient's identity, explain the procedure, and obtain verbal consent.
- Unwrap all the equipment onto an instrument stand in an aseptic fashion and pour saline solution over the cotton balls.
- Position the patient supine with genitalia exposed. Raise the bed to a comfortable height.
- Wash your hands again and put on gloves. Create a hole in the center of the towel, or use a fenestrated drape, and drape over the patient so the penis can be reached through the hole.
- From here on, use your nondominant hand to hold the penis with some gauze.
- Clean the penis with the wet cotton balls, working away from the meatus. Remember to retract the foreskin and clean beneath.
- Lift penis to a vertical position, carefully position the nozzle of the lubricant gel inside the meatus, and instill the full 10 mL slowly. (If proving problematic, this can be aided by gentle milking action.)
- Position kidney bowl between patient's thighs to catch spillages later.
- The catheter will be in a plastic wrapper with a tear-away portion near the tip. Remove this portion, being careful not to touch the catheter.
- Insert the tip of the catheter into the urethral meatus and advance slowly but firmly by feeding it out of the remaining wrapper.
- On passing through the prostate, some resistance may be felt, which, if excessive, may be countered by adjusting the angle of the penis by pulling it to a horizontal position between the patient's legs.
- On entering the bladder, urine should start to drain. Advance the catheter far enough to ensure the balloon is beyond the urethra.
- Inflate the balloon with the 10 mL of water via the secondary catheter lumen.
- ⓘ Warn the patient to alert you to any pain, and watch his face.
- Remove the syringe and withdraw the catheter until resistance is felt.
- Attach draining tube and catheter bag.
- Replace the foreskin, and clean and re-dress the patient as necessary.

Hints
- You may wish to verify the presence of a full bladder with a bladder ultrasound before starting.
- Lack of urine drainage may be caused by blockage by anesthetic gel, an empty bladder, or catheter misplacement.
- Attempt to aspirate urine with a catheter-tipped syringe. Feel for a full bladder. If there is any doubt about position of the catheter, remove it immediately (deflating balloon first) and seek appropriate consultation.
- Always record the residual volume—this is essential in cases of urinary retention.
- Consider the use of prophylactic antibiotics before the procedure.
- Complications include pain, infection, misplacement, and trauma.
- Patients with prostate disease can often experience some mild hematuria following catheterization. Don't worry about this, but watch carefully and be sure the bleeding doesn't continue or form into clots.
▶ Be aware of latex allergy!

⚠ Female urethral catheterization

Theory

A urinary catheter has a balloon near the tip that is inflated via a side-arm near the other end. Once inside the bladder, the inflated balloon prevents it from falling, or being pulled, out.

Female staff will usually catheterize females.

❶ Consider antibiotic prophylaxis.

Equipment

- Catheter pack (containing a basin, a small vessel with cotton balls, a sterile towel, and sterile gauze)
- Sterile gloves
- Saline solution
- 5 mL 1% lidocaine/lubricant gel in prefilled syringe
- 10 mL water-filled syringe
- Catheter bag
- Female catheter (12F or 14F)

Procedure

- Wash your hands thoroughly. Confirm the patient's identity, explain the procedure, and obtain verbal consent.
- Unwrap all the equipment onto a cleaned (antiseptic) instrument stand in an aseptic fashion and pour saline over the cotton balls.
- Position the patient supine with knees flexed and hips abducted with the heels together. Raise the bed to a comfortable height.
- Wash your hands again and put on gloves. Lay the towel and drape it over the patient so the genitalia are exposed.
- From here on, use your nondominant hand to hold the labia apart, approaching the patient from the right-hand side, leaning over her ankles in order to reach the genitalia from below.
- Clean genitalia with the wet cotton balls (using each once only), working in a pubis–anus direction (see Fig. 18.36).
- Carefully position the nozzle of the lubricant gel inside the meatus and instill most of the 5 mL.
- Position the bowl between the patient's thighs to catch spillages.
- The catheter will be in a plastic wrapper with a tear-away portion near the tip. Remove this portion, being careful not to touch the catheter, and apply a little lidocaine gel to the catheter tip.
- Insert the tip of the catheter into the urethral meatus and advance slowly but firmly by feeding it out of the remaining wrapper.
- On entering the bladder, urine should start to drain. Advance the catheter fully to ensure the balloon is beyond the urethra.
- Inflate the balloon with 10 mL of water via the catheter side-arm.
- ❶ Warn the patient to alert you to any pain and watch her face.
- Remove the syringe and withdraw the catheter until resistance is felt.
- Attach draining tube and catheter bag.
- Clean and re-dress the patient as necessary.
- Record the residual urinary volume.

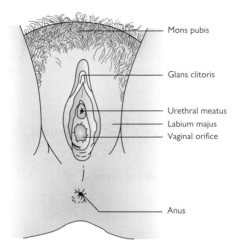

Fig. 18.36 Diagrammatic representation of the female external genitalia showing position of the urethral meatus.

Hints
- Some female patients are easier to catheterize in a different position— lying on their side with knees raised.
- Lack of urine drainage may be caused by blockage by lubricant gel, an empty bladder, or catheter misplacement.
- Attempt to aspirate urine with a catheter-tipped syringe. Feel for a full bladder. If there is any doubt about the position of the catheter, remove it immediately (deflating balloon first) and seek advice.
- Complications
  - Pain
  - Infection
  - Misplacement and trauma
- ▶ Be aware of latex allergy!

▶▶ Suprapubic catheterization

Theory

Suprapubic catheterization is sometimes seen as a safer and more efficient means of controlling bladder drainage than urethral catheterization, particularly if the patient has had treatment or surgery involving the vagina, urethra, ureter, or prostate. Patients may in fact find this more acceptable than urethral catheterization. Also, it allows assessment of when the patient is able to void spontaneously, without having to remove (and possibly replace) a urethral catheter.

The catheter is inserted directly into the bladder, through the abdominal wall just superior to the pubic symphysis. Safe placement under local anesthesia requires a very full bladder.

The procedure below relates to the Bonanno Suprapubic tray. The essentials of the technique remain the same for other catheterization systems, although small details may differ—refer to the pack instructions.

Many urologists currently favor the Bard Addacath system.

Equipment

- Instrument (Mayo) stand
- 1 Bonanno Suprapubic catheter tray (contains puncture needle, catheter with sleeve, and adaptor clamp)
- 1 drainage bag
- Povidone-iodine or antiseptic solution
- 2 x 10 mL syringes
- 5–10 mL 1% lidocaine
- 1 green needle
- 1 orange needle
- Sterile pack (containing gloves, swab, and container)
- Fine, nonabsorbable suture

Procedure

- Introduce yourself, confirm identity of the patient, explain the procedure, and obtain verbal consent.
- Position the patient supine with genitalia exposed. Raise the bed to a comfortable height.
- Unwrap all the equipment onto an instrument stand in an aseptic fashion and pour antiseptic solution over the cotton balls.
- Before commencing, make sure that the patient has a palpable bladder. If not, distend the bladder with 500–700 mL of saline solution instilled via a urethral catheter (if urethral route is available and feasible).
- ▶ If the bladder is not full, **proceed no further**.
- Put on sterile gloves, and prep the suprapubic area with antiseptic solution.
- Pause to reconfirm patient identity and the procedure and site.
- The point of insertion is in the midline, two finger-breadths above the pubic symphysis and well below the upper edge of palpable bladder.
- Assemble the Bonanno catheter components (see Fig. 18.34).
- Advance the catheter sleeve along the course of the radio-opaque catheter from a proximal position adjacent to the suture disc to the distal end of the catheter to allow straightening of the coiled catheter.
- Infiltrate the insertion area with the lidocaine.

- Carefully insert the 18-gauge puncture needle into the catheter so that the heel of the needle bevel is directed along inside the curve of the catheter and move in a clockwise direction, until the bevel extends beyond the catheter tip (Fig. 18.35).
- Slide the straightener sleeve off the distal end of the catheter.
- Grasp the catheter needle ~9 cm above the distal end and, with a firm thrust, push the needle through the abdominal wall, heading in a slightly caudal direction, until you feel resistance disappear.
- Check position of the catheter in the bladder by removing the black vent plug, and aspirate urine with a 10 mL syringe.
- Disengage needle from the catheter hub and advance catheter until the suture disc is flat against the skin.
- Withdraw needle.
- Connect adaptor-clamp to the catheter hub and securely attach the rubber portion of the clamp into a standard drainage catheter bag.
- Carefully suture the catheter into the abdominal wall—you may also need to apply further tape to ensure the catheter won't fall out.
- Ensure that the clamp is open to allow urine to drain.

Hints
- It may be easier to use a scalpel to make a small stab incision before inserting the needle.

⚠ Basic suturing

Theory

Basic suturing, or stitching, has many practical applications outside the field of surgery.

Whether you are called upon to suture a central line in place or are stitching up a laceration, it's a skill you should practice before you need to use it. There are many useful texts and articles that describe in more detail the fine art of suturing, and we refer you to these. Undoubtedly, the best way to learn is by watching a surgeon and then doing it yourself. In most clinical skills labs you should find the necessary equipment to practice these skills.

Equipment

- Instrument (Mayo) stand
- Dressing pack
- 21-gauge green needle
- 25-gauge orange needle
- 10 mL and 20 mL syringes
- Gauze
- Antiseptic solution
- Sutures
- Tape
- Sterile gloves
- Sharps bin
- Toothed forceps
- Needle holder
- Scissors
- Scalpel

(selection depending on site and nature of wound)

Procedure

- Introduce yourself, confirm identity of the patient, explain the procedure, and obtain verbal consent.
- First assess the wound and decide on the size of the suture material.
  - Remember that there are alternative ways to achieve wound closure, such as glue, staples, and steri-strips. Always consider the most appropriate means of closing a wound.
- Before suturing, irrigate the wound and remove any foreign bodies and any nonviable or infected tissue.
- Use a needle holder such as toothed forceps, where possible, to minimize the risk of needle-stick injury.
- Hold the needle 2/3 of the way from the needle tip.
- Lift the skin edge farthest away without pinching or damaging it.
- Pierce the skin with the needle at 90°.
- Rotate your wrist to pass the needle into the middle of the wound.
- Release the forceps and clasp the needle again as it protrudes into the wound, rotating it out of the wound.
- Next press the near side with the closed forceps to evert the skin edge, and pass the needle through, taking a smooth semicircular course to exit at 90° to the wound edge. See Fig. 18.37.
- This method ensures a square bite and good eversion of the wound.
- Now perform a surgeon's knot.
  - Wrap the long end of the thread around the forceps, which is used to transfer the coil around the short end (grab the short tail and pull in toward you, pulling the long end away).
  - Repeat the cycle.

- Remember to cut the ends of the thread off, leaving a few mm so that they can be easily removed later.

▶ When removing sutures, clean the wound with antiseptic solution, use forceps or a blade, and pull the suture out across rather than away from the wound.

The time taken to remove nonabsorbable sutures depends on location:

- Face: 5–7 days or less
- Scalp: 7–10 days
- Limbs and trunk: 12–14 days

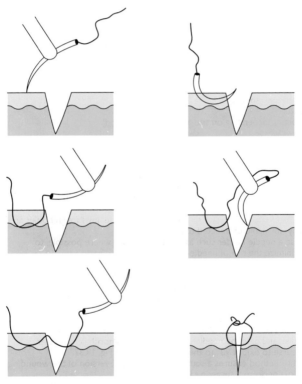

Fig. 18.37 Diagrammatic representation of the stages involved in a basic suture.

► Lumbar puncture

Theory

A needle is introduced between the lumbar vertebrae at a level below termination of the spinal cord. It then passes through the dura into the subarachnoid space and a sample of cerebrospinal fluid (CSF) is obtained.

Lumbar puncture (LP) is used for diagnostic and therapeutic purposes, which are too numerous to list.

Equipment

- Sterile gloves
- Sterile pack (containing drape, cotton balls, and container)
- Antiseptic solution
- Sterile gauze dressing
- 5–10 mL 1% lidocaine
- 2 ×10 mL syringe
- Biochemistry tube for glucose
- Orange needle (14 gauge)
- Green needle (18 gauge)
- LP needle
- LP manometer
- 3-way tap (may be included in LP kit)
- Sterile collection tubes

Procedure

- Introduce yourself, confirm identity of the patient, explain the procedure, and obtain verbal consent.
- Position patient lying on their left-hand side with the neck, knees, and hips flexed as much as possible (ask the patient to clasp their hands around their knees, if they are able). Put a pillow between the patient's knees to prevent the pelvis from tilting (see Fig. 18.38).
- Ensure that the patient can hold this position comfortably.
- Identify the iliac crest—the disc space vertically below this (as you are looking) will be ~L3–L4.
- Mark the space between the vertebral spines with a pen.
- Wash your hands and put on sterile gloves.

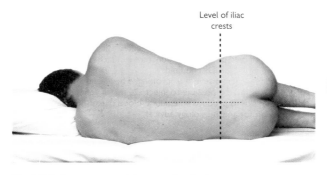

Level of iliac crests

Fig. 18.38 Correct position of the patient for a lumbar puncture.

- Unwrap all equipment and ensure that it fits together correctly.
- Apply the drapes around the area and sterilize with the antiseptic solution and cotton balls in outward-spiral motions.
- Pause to reconfirm patient identity and the procedure and site.
- Inject the lidocaine (using a 10 mL syringe and the orange needle) at the marked site to raise a small wheal.
- Swap out the orange needle for the green one and infiltrate the lidocaine deeper. Take care to aspirate before injecting to ensure that blood vessels are avoided.
- Wait for ~1 minute for the anesthetic to take effect.
- Introduce the spinal needle (22G usually) through the marked site at about 90° to the skin, heading slightly toward the umbilicus. Keep the bevel facing up the patient's spine.
- Gently advance the needle through the ligaments (to ~5 cm depth).
- At this point, a further push of the needle should produce a give as the needle enters the subarachnoid space (this takes a little practice to feel with confidence).
- If at any point the needle strikes bone and cannot be advanced, withdraw slightly, re-aim it, and advance in a stepwise fashion until the gap is found.
- Withdraw the stylet from the needle. CSF should begin to drip out.
- Measure the CSF pressure—connect the manometer to the end of the needle via the 3-way tap (the CSF will rise up the manometer, allowing you to read off the number).
- Open the tap and allow the CSF to drip into the three collection tubes, about 5 or 6 drips per tube. The tubes should be labeled "1," "2," and "3," in order of collection. Collect a few more drips into the biochemistry tube for glucose measurement.
- Replace the stylet and remove the needle. Apply a sterile dressing.
- Send the fluid for analysis.
  - Cell count (bottles 1 and 3)
  - Microscopy, culture, and sensitivities (M,C&S) (bottles 1 and 3)
  - Biochemistry: glucose, protein (bottle 2)
- Advise the patient to lie flat for 1 hour, and ask nursing staff to check CNS observations regularly during that time.

Hints

- Always use the smallest-gauge spinal needle available.
- Treatment of mild post–lumbar puncture headache (PLPH) is supportive with NSAIDs and fluids.
- If the patient suffers a severe or prolonged headache after the procedure, it may be possible to inject ~20 mL of venous blood into the LP site to produce an epidural blood patch (EBP), a "blood patch"—ask for anesthesiology advice!

▶▶ Pericardial aspiration

Theory

Emergency pericardial aspiration (drainage of fluid from the pericardial cavity) may be performed in cardiac tamponade or large pericardial effusions where there is hemodynamic compromise. This procedure can also be used to obtain diagnostic pericardial fluid.

Equipment

- Sterile gown and gloves
- Antiseptic solution
- Sterile towels
- 10 mL syringe
- 50 mL syringe
- Three-way tap
- ECG monitoring, defibrillator and resuscitation equipment
- Local anesthetic
- Needles
- 18-gauge catheter

Procedure

- If the patient is conscious, introduce yourself, confirm the identity of the patient, explain the procedure, and obtain verbal consent.
- Establish IV access and connect the ECG monitor with full resuscitation equipment at hand.
- Provide adequate sedation, if necessary.
- Put on sterile gloves and gown.
- Pause to reconfirm patient identity and the procedure and site.
- If time permits, use local anesthesia to infiltrate the insertion site.
- Attach the 18-gauge catheter to the 50 mL syringe.
- Introduce needle at 45^0 to the skin immediately below and to the left of the xiphoid process to a depth of 6–8 cm, in a direction aiming for the tip of the scapula.
- Aspirate continuously and watch the ECG.
  - If the needle touches the ventricle, an injury pattern (depressed ST segment) or arrhythmia may be seen—withdraw the needle slightly.
- Aspirate pericardial fluid through the syringe and 3-way tap.
- Aspiration should produce immediate hemodynamic improvement.
- You can check if the fluid you are aspirating is pure blood if it clots quickly. Heavily bloodstained pericardial fluid does not clot.
- Perform a chest X-ray and echocardiogram after the procedure.
- You may wish to insert a pericardial drain (seek consultation).
- Document the details of the procedure in the notes.

Possible complications

- Pneumothorax
- Arrhythmia
- Myocardial puncture
- Damage to the coronary arteries

⚠ **Defibrillation**

Theory

Electrical defibrillation is the only effective therapy for cardiac arrest caused by ventricular fibrillation (VF) or pulseless ventricular tachycardia (VT). The American Heart Association (AHA) has long supported early attempted defibrillation, because the chances of successful defibrillation decline at a rate of 7–10% with each minute of delay.

In the hospital setting, two types of defibrillator may be encountered: the traditional manual defibrillator and the newer automated external defibrillators (AED).

There are two types of AED: most are semiautomatic and advise the need for a shock, but this has to be delivered by the operator, when prompted. Some also have the facility to enable the operator to override the device and deliver a shock manually, without any prompts. A few fully automatic AEDs are also available.

In recognition of changing guidelines, the reader is directed to the AHA Web site: www.americanheart.org for the most current resuscitation guidelines.

Equipment

- Defibrillator
- Gel pads

Procedure for manual defibrillation

- Switch on the defibrillator and ensure that the skin is dry and free of excess hair.
- Attach the ECG electrodes accordingly:
  - Red under right clavicle
  - Yellow under left clavicle
  - Green at the umbilicus
- Ascertain that the ECG rhythm is shockable (VF/pulseless VT).
- Place the defibrillation gel pads on the patient's chest (Fig. 18.39):
  - One just to the right of the sternum, below the clavicle
  - The other just lateral to the cardiac apex
- Shave chest hair only if it is excessive and will interfere with electrical contact.
- Select 360J on the defibrillator.
- Place the paddles firmly on the gel pads.
- Press the charge button on the paddles to charge the defibrillator and shout, "**stand clear—charging.**"
- Check that all staff have stepped back *(including yourself)* and that no one is touching the patient or their bed.
- ▶ Ensure that high-flow oxygen has also been removed.
- ▶ Check the monitor again to ensure a shockable rhythm.
- Shout **"stand clear—shocking"** and press both discharge buttons simultaneously to discharge the shock.
- Follow protocol overleaf (Fig. 18.40). Return paddles to defibrillator before continuing with cardiopulmonary resuscitation (CPR).

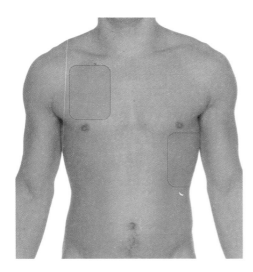

Fig. 18.39 Correct position of gel pads or AED electrodes on patient. Ensure that they are not touching or overlying any wires, oxygen tubing, or any other conducting material. Ensure that the patient's chest is dry and shaved if particularly hairy.

Procedure for AEDs (Fig. 18.41)

- Switch on the defibrillator, ensure the skin is dry and free of excess hair, and attach the electrode pads (same position as the gel pads in manual defibrillation; see Fig. 18.39).
- Continue CPR while this is done if more than one assistant is present.
- Make sure no one is touching the patient during ECG analysis by AED.
- Follow the voice prompts.
  - These are usually programmable, and the American Heart Association recommends that they be set as follows:
    - A single shock only when a shockable rhythm is detected
    - No rhythm, breathing, or pulse check after the shock
    - A voice prompt for immediate resumption of CPR after the shock.
    - Two minutes allowed for CPR using a ratio of 30 compressions to 2 rescue breaths before a voice prompt to assess the rhythm, breathing, or a pulse is given.
- ▶ If a shock is indicated, shout "**stand clear**" and perform visual checks to ensure no personnel are in contact with the patient or their bed and that any oxygen has been removed.
- Push the shock button and continue as directed.

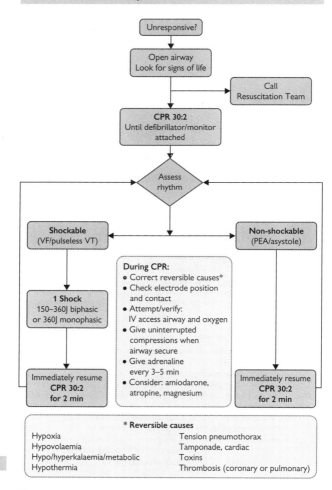

Fig. 18.40 Algorithm for advanced life support using a manual defibrillator. Reproduced with permission from the Resuscitation Council (UK) guidelines. It is recommended to consult the latest AHA guidelines when available.

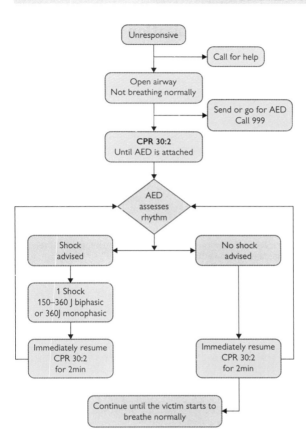

Fig. 18.41 AED algorithm. Reproduced with permission from the Resuscitation Council (UK) guidelines..

▶▶ Knee joint aspiration

Theory
In the context of a swollen joint, a joint aspiration is performed for both diagnostic (to identify infectious and crystal arthropathies) and therapeutic (to relieve tense effusions and hemarthroses) purposes.

A sample of fluid may be removed and sent for microscopy, culture and sensitivity and to be examined for crystals under polarized light.

This same procedural approach may be used for joint injections (e.g., steroids and local anesthetic to suppress inflammation).

Equipment
- 5–10 mL 1% lidocaine
- 1 x 20 mL syringe
- 1 x 5 mL syringe
- 1 x 21-gauge (green) needle
- 1 x 25-gauge (orange) needle
- Sterile gloves
- Antiseptic solution
- Sterile bottles
- Dressing pack with cotton balls

Procedure
- Introduce yourself, confirm the identity of the patient, explain the procedure, and obtain verbal consent.
- Ensure that the patient is relaxed and lying comfortably on the couch or bed with the knee exposed and slightly flexed.
- Palpate the outline of the patella and the medial joint line (aspiration is easier on the medial side).
- Wash your hands and put on a pair of sterile gloves.
- Clean the site with the cotton balls and antiseptic solution.
- Pause to reconfirm patient identity and the procedure and site.
- Infiltrate the insertion site with local anesthetic. Use 1–2 mL of 1% lidocaine using the 25-gauge orange needle and a 5 mL syringe. Remember to aspirate before injecting.
- Take a 20 mL syringe and attach a 21-gauge green needle.
- Insert the needle at an angle of about 45^0 in the gap between the lower border of the patella and the medial joint line (Fig. 18.42).
- If the needle is in the joint space (about 2 cm in), you should be able to freely aspirate synovial fluid. Aspiration can be aided by pressing on the opposite side of the joint with your free hand.
- Once the syringe is full, remove it from the joint and transfer the fluid into sterile specimen bottles.
- Send to microbiology for microscopy, culture, and sensitivity and a further sample to the biochemistry department to look for crystals.
- Following aspiration, ask the patient to rest the knee for 24–48 hours.
- Record in the notes the procedural details, including the color of the synovial fluid and the investigations requested.

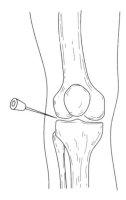

Fig. 18.42 Aspiration of the knee joint—insert the needle at about 45° heading distally below the patella.

Data interpretation

ECG: an introduction

The first step in making sense of an electrocardiogram (ECG) printout is to understand the electrical conduction process in the normal heart.

Electrophysiology of the heart

Cardiac myocytes

In their resting state, the surface of cardiac myocytes (muscle cells) is polarized with a potential difference of 790 mV across the cell membrane (negatively charged intracellularly and positively charged extracellularly).

Depolarization (reversal of this charge) results in movement of calcium ions across the cell membranes and subsequent cardiac muscle contraction. It is this change in potential difference that can be detected by the ECG electrodes and represented as deflections on a tracing.

Basics of the tracing

It is easiest to imagine an electrode 'looking' at the heart from where it is attached to the body.

Depolarization of the myocytes that spreads toward the electrode is seen as an upward deflection, electrical activity moving away from the electrode is seen as downward deflection, and activity moving to one side but neither toward nor away from the electrode is not seen at all (Fig. 19.1).

Electrical conduction pathway

In the normal heart, pacemaker cells in the sinoatrial (SA) node initiate depolarization. The depolarization first spreads through the atria, and this is seen as a small upward deflection (the P wave) on the ECG.

The atria and the ventricles are electrically isolated from each other. The only way in which the impulse can progress from the atria to the ventricles normally is through the atrioventricular (AV) node. Passage

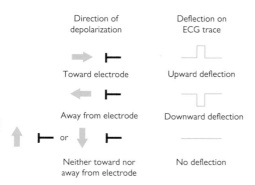

Fig. 19.1 Diagrammatic representation of how the electrodes monitor waves of depolarization.

through the AV node slows its progress slightly. This can be seen on an ECG as the isoelectric interval between the P wave and QRS complex, the PR interval.

Depolarization then continues rapidly down the rapidly conducting Purkinje fibers—bundle of His, then down left and right bundle branches—to depolarize both ventricles (Fig. 19.2). The left bundle has two divisions (fascicles). The narrow QRS complex on ECG shows this rapid ventricular depolarization.

Repolarization of the ventricles is seen as the T wave. Atrial repolarization causes only a very slight deflection, which is hidden in the QRS complex and not seen.

▶ The P wave and QRS complex show the electrical depolarization of atrial and ventricular myocardium, respectively, but the resultant mechanical muscle contraction, which usually follows, cannot be inferred from the ECG trace (e.g., in pulseless electrical activity [PEA]).

12-lead ECG
Leads
Electrodes are placed on the limbs and chest for a 12-lead recording. The term *12-lead* refers to the number of directions that the electrical activity is recorded from, not number of electrical wires attached to the patient.

The six chest leads ($V_{1–6}$) and six limb leads (I, II, III, aVR, aVL, aVF) comprise the 12-lead ECG. These reflect the electrical activity of the heart from various directions. The chest leads correspond directly to the six electrodes placed at various points on the anterior and lateral chest wall (see Fig. 19.3). The six limb leads represent the electrical activity through a combination of the four electrodes placed on the patient's limbs, e.g., lead I is generated from the right and left arm electrodes.

▶ Remember there are 12 ECG leads—12 different views of the electrical activity of the heart—but only 10 actual electrodes placed on the patient's body.

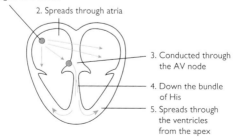

1. Impulse begins at SA node

2. Spreads through atria

3. Conducted through the AV node

4. Down the bundle of His

5. Spreads through the ventricles from the apex

Fig. 19.2 Electrical conduction pathway in the normal heart.

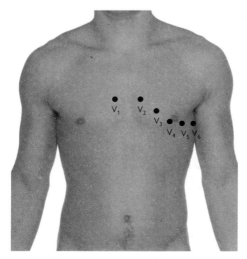

Fig. 19.3 V_{1-6} electrode placement on the chest wall.

⚠ Additional leads can be used (e.g., V7–9 extending laterally around the chest wall) to look at the heart from further angles, such as in suspected posterior myocardial infarction (MI).

ECG orientation
When a wave of myocardial depolarization flows toward a particular lead, the ECG tracing shows an upward deflection. A downward deflection represents depolarization moving away from that lead. The key to interpreting the 12-lead ECG is thus to remember the directions at which the different leads view the heart.

The six limb leads look at the heart in the coronal plane (see Fig. 19.4).
• aVR views the right atrium.*
• aVF, II, and III view the inferior or diaphragmatic surface of the heart.
• I and aVL examine the left lateral aspect.
The six chest leads examine the heart in a transverse plane.
• V_1 and V_2 look at the right ventricle.
• V_3 and V_4 look at the septum and anterior aspect of the left ventricle.
• V_5 and V_6 look at the anterior and lateral aspects of the left ventricle.
Although each of the 12 leads gives a different view of electrical activity of the heart, for simplicity's sake when considering the standard ECG trace we can describe the basic shape common to all leads (Fig. 19.5).

*All the vectors in lead aVR will be negative in the normal ECG.

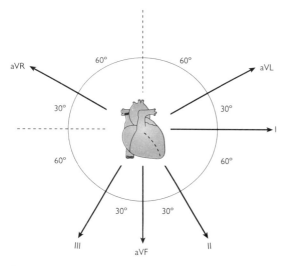

Fig. 19.4 The respective views of the heart of the six limb leads. Note the angles between the directions of the limb leads—these become important when calculating the cardiac axis.

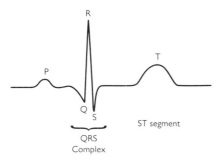

Fig. 19.5 Basic shape of the ECG tracing.

ECG tracing

Waves
- *P wave* represents atrial depolarization and is a positive (upward) deflection, except in aVR.
- *QRS complex* represents ventricular depolarization and comprises
  - *Q wave*—so called if the first QRS deflection is negative (downward). Pathological Q waves are seen in infarction (📖 p. 612).
  - *R wave*—the first positive (upward) deflection. It may or may not follow a Q wave.
  - *S wave*—a negative (downward) deflection following the R wave
- *T wave* represents ventricular repolarization and is normally a positive (upward) deflection, concordant with the QRS complex.

> 🛈 Remember, Q waves appear following an MI, so they should be absent from the normal ECG trace.

Rate
The heart rate can be calculated by dividing 300 by the number of large squares between each R wave (with machine trace running at the standard speed of 25 mm/sec and deflection of 1 cm/10 mV).
- 3 large squares between R waves = rate 100
- 5 large squares = rate 60
Normal rate is 60–100 beats per minute (bpm).
- Rate <60 = bradycardia
- Rate >100 = tachycardia

Intervals and timing
- *PR interval:* from start of the P wave to start of the QRS complex. This represents the built-in delay in electrical conduction at the AV node. Normally <0.20 seconds (5 small squares at standard recording speed)
- *QRS complex:* width of the QRS complex. Normally <0.12 seconds (3 small squares at standard rate)
- *R–R interval:* from the peak of one R wave to the next. This is used in calculation of the heart rate (see above).
- *QT interval:* from start of the QRS complex to end of the T wave. It varies with heart rate. Corrected QT = QT/square root of the R–R interval. Corrected QT interval should be 0.38–0.42 seconds.

Rhythm
- Is rhythm (and time between successive R waves) regular or irregular?
  - If irregular but in a clear pattern, then it is 'regularly irregular' (e.g., types of heart block—see 📖 p. 599).
  - If irregular but with no pattern, then it is 'irregularly irregular' (e.g., atrial fibrillation).

ECG axis

Cardiac axis
The cardiac axis, or *QRS axis*, refers to the overall direction of depolarization through the ventricular myocardium in the coronal plane.

Zero degrees is taken as the horizontal line to the left of the heart (the right of your diagram).

The normal cardiac axis lies between −30° and +90° (Fig. 19.6). An axis outside of this range may suggest pathology, either congenital or acquired.

Cardiac axis deviation may be seen in healthy individuals with distinctive body shapes—right-axis deviation if tall and thin, left-axis deviation if short and stocky.

Calculating the axis

Look at Fig. 19.4. Leads I, II, and III all lie in the coronal plane (along with aVR, aVL, and aVF). By calculating the relative depolarization in each of these directions, one can calculate the cardiac axis. To accurately determine the cardiac axis, use leads I, II, and III, as described below.

- Draw a diagram like the one in Fig. 19.7 showing the three leads—be careful to use the correct angles.
- Look at ECG lead I. Count the number of millimeters (mm) above the baseline that the QRS complex reaches.
- Subtract from this the number of mm below the baseline that the QRS complex reaches.
- Now measure this number of centimeters along line I on your diagram and make a mark (measure backward for negative numbers).
- Repeat this for leads II and III.
- Extend lines from your marks, perpendicular to the leads (Fig. 19.6).
- The direction from the center of the diagram to the point at which all these lines meet is the cardiac axis.

Calculating the axis—short cuts

There are many shorter ways of roughly calculating the cardiac axis. These are less accurate, however.

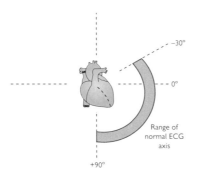

Fig. 19.6 The normal ECG axis.

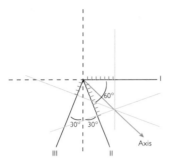

Fig. 19.7 Calculating the ECG axis using leads I, II, and III. See text on previous page.

Box 19.1 Causes of axis deviation

Left axis deviation (<–30°)
• Left ventricular hypertrophy
• Left bundle branch block (LBBB)
• Left anterior hemiblock (anterior fascicle of the left bundle)
• Inferior MI
• Cardiomyopathies
• Tricuspid atresia

Right axis deviation (>+90°)
• Right ventricular hypertrophy
• Right bundle branch block (RBBB)
• Anterolateral MI
• Right ventricular strain (e.g., pulmonary embolism)
• Cor pulmonale
• Fallot's tetralogy (pulmonary stenosis)

An easy method is to look at only leads I and aVF. These are perpendicular to each other and make a simpler diagram than the one described above.

(AV) conduction abnormalities
In the normal ECG, each P wave is followed by a QRS complex. The isoelectric gap between is the PR interval and represents slowing of the impulse at the AV junction. Disturbance of the normal conduction here, leads to heart block.

Causes of heart block include ischemic heart disease, idiopathic fibrosis of conduction system, cardiomyopathies, inferior and anterior MI, drugs, such as digoxin, B-blockers, and verapamil, and physiological factors (first degree) in athletes.

First-degree heart block
The PR interval is fixed but prolonged at >0.20 seconds (5 small squares at standard rate). See rhythm strip 1 (Fig. 19.8).

Second-degree heart block
Not every P wave is followed by a QRS complex.
- *Möbitz type I:* PR interval becomes progressively longer after each P wave until an impulse fails to be conducted at all. The interval then returns to the normal length and the cycle is repeated (rhythm strip 2; Fig. 19.8). This is also known as the *Wenckebach phenomenon.*
- *Möbitz type II:* PR interval is fixed but not every P wave is followed by a QRS complex. The relationship between P waves and QRS complex

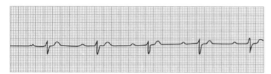

Rhythm strip 1—first-degree heart block.

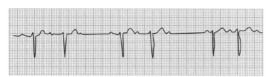

Rhythm strip 2—second-degree heart block Möbitz type I.

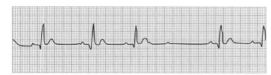

Rhythm strip 3—second-degree heart block Möbitz type II.

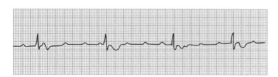

Rhythm strip 4—third-degree (complete) heart block.

Fig. 19.8 Rhythm strips showing AV conduction abnormalities.

may be 2:1 (two P waves for every QRS), 3:1 (three P waves per QRS), or random. See rhythm strip 3 (Fig. 19.8).

Third-degree heart block

This is also called *complete heart block*; see rhythm strip 4 (Fig. 19.8). There is no conduction of impulse through the AV junction. Atrial and ventricular depolarization occur independent of one another. Each has a separate pacemaker triggering electrical activity at different rates (rhythm strip 4).

The QRS complex is an abnormal shape, as the electrical impulse does not travel through ventricles via normal routes (see Ventricular Escape Rhythm, ☐ p. 609).

⊕ In third-degree heart block, P waves may be seen merging with QRS complexes if they coincide.

⊕ If in doubt about the pattern of P waves and QRS complexes, mark out the P-wave intervals and the R–R intervals separately, then compare.

▶ P waves are best seen in leads II and V_1.

Ventricular conduction abnormalities

Depolarization of both ventricles usually occurs rapidly through left and right bundle branches of the His–Purkinje system (see Fig. 19.9). If this process is disrupted as a result of damage to the conducting system, depolarization will occur more slowly through nonspecialized ventricular myocardium. The QRS complex, usually <0.12 seconds' duration, will become prolonged and is described as a *broad*.

Right bundle branch block (RBBB)

Conduction through the AV node, bundle of His, and left bundle branch will be normal but depolarization of the right ventricle occurs by the slow spread of electrical current through myocardial cells (Fig. 19.10). The result is delayed right ventricular depolarization, giving a second R wave known as R' (R prime).

RBBB suggests pathology in the right side of the heart but can be a normal variant.

ECG changes
- RSR pattern seen in V_1
- Cardiac axis usually remains normal unless left anterior fascicle is also blocked (bifascicular block), which results in left axis deviation.
- T wave ↓ in anterior chest leads (V_1–V_3)

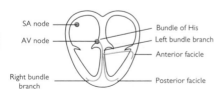

Fig. 19.9 Diagrammatic representation of the conducting system of the heart.

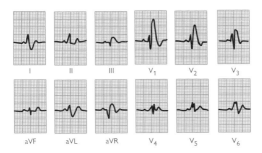

Fig. 19.10 Typical 12-lead ECG showing RBBB.

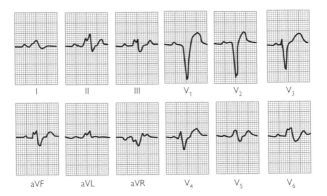

Fig. 19.11 Typical 12-lead ECG showing LBBB.

Some causes of RBBB
- Hyperkalemia
- Congenital heart disease (e.g., Fallot's tetralogy)
- Pulmonary embolus
- Cor pulmonale
- Fibrosis of conduction system

Left bundle branch block (LBBB)

Conduction through the AV node, bundle of His, and right bundle branch will be normal but depolarization of the left ventricle occurs by the slow spread of electrical current through myocardial cells (Fig. 19.11). The result is delayed left ventricular depolarization.

LBBB should always be considered pathological.

ECG changes
- M pattern seen in V_6
- T wave ↓ in lateral chest leads (V_5–V_6)

Some causes of LBBB
- Hypertension
- Ischemic heart disease
- Acute MI
- Aortic stenosis
- Cardiomyopathies
- Fibrosis of conduction system

ⓘ LBBB on the ECG causes abnormalities of the ST segment and T wave. You should not comment any further on these parts of the tracing.

> **Box 19.2 Bundle branch block mnemonic**
>
> - In LBBB, the QRS complex in V_1 looks like a *W* and like an *M* in V_6. This can be remembered as **WiLLiaM**. There is a *W* at the start, an *M* at the end, and an *L* in the middle, for 'left.'
> - Conversely, in RBBB, the QRS complex in V_1 looks like an *M* and in V_6, like a *W*. Combined with an *R*, for 'right,' you have **MaRRoW**.

Sinus rhythms

Supraventricular rhythms arise in the atria. They may be physiological in some causes of sinus brady and tachycardia or be caused by pathology within the SA node, the atria, or the first parts of the conducting system.

Normal conduction through the bundle of His into the ventricles will usually give narrow QRS complexes.

Sinus bradycardia

This is a bradycardia (rate <60 bpm) at the level of the SA node. The heart beats slowly, but conduction of the impulse is normal (rhythm strip 1, Fig. 19.12).

Some causes of sinus bradycardia
- Drugs (B-blockers, verapamil, amiodarone, digoxin)
- Sick sinus syndrome
- Hypothyroidism
- Inferior MI
- Hypothermia
- ↑ Intracranial pressure (ICP)
- Physiological (athletes)

Sinus tachycardia

This is a tachycardia at the level of the SA node—the heart is beating too quickly but conduction of impulse is normal (rhythm strip 2, Fig 19.12).

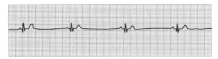

Rhythm strip 1—sinus bradycardia.

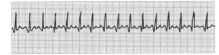

Rhythm strip 2—sinus tachycardia.

Fig. 19.12 Rhythm strips from lead II showing a sinus bradycardia (rhythm strip 1) and sinus tachycardia (rhythm strip 2).

ECG features
- Ventricular rate >100 (usually 100–150 bpm)
- Normal P wave before each QRS

Some causes of sinus tachycardia
- Drugs (epinephrine/adrenaline, caffeine, nicotine)
- Pain
- Exertion
- Anxiety
- Anemia
- Thyrotoxicosis
- Pulmonary embolus
- Hepatic failure
- Cardiac failure
- Hypercapnia
- Pregnancy
- Constrictive pericarditis

Supraventricular tachycardias

These are tachycardias (rate >100 bpm) arising in the atria or the AV node. As conduction through the bundle of His and ventricles will be normal (unless there is other pathology in the heart), the QRS complexes appear normal.

There are four main causes of a supraventricular tachycardia that you should be aware of: atrial fibrillation, atrial flutter, junctional tachycardia, and re-entry tachycardia.

Atrial fibrillation (AF)

This is disorganized contraction of the atria in the form of rapid, irregular twitching. There will thus be no P waves on the ECG.

Electrical impulses from the twitches of the atria arrive at the AV node randomly. They are then conducted via the normal pathways to cause ventricular contraction. The result is a characteristic ventricular rhythm that is *irregularly irregular* with no discernable pattern (Fig. 19.13, rhythm strip 1).

ECG features
- No P waves. Rhythm is described as irregularly irregular.
- Irregular QRS complexes
- Normal appearance of QRS
- Ventricular rate may be ↑ (fast AF)—typically 120–160 per minute.

Some causes of atrial fibrillation
- Idiopathic
- Ischemic heart disease
- Thyroid disease
- Hypertension
- MI
- Pulmonary embolus
- Rheumatic mitral or tricuspid valve disease

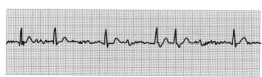

Rhythm strip 1—atrial fibrillation.

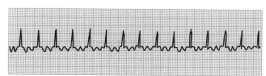

Rhythm strip 2—atrial flutter with 2:1 block.

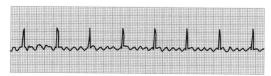

Rhythm strip 3—atrial flutter with 4:1 block.

Fig. 19.13 Rhythm strips from lead II showing some supraventricular tachycardias.

Atrial flutter

This is abnormally rapid contraction of the atria. The contractions are not disorganized or random, as in AF, but are fast and inadequate for the normal movement of blood. Instead of P waves, the baseline will have a typical saw-tooth appearance (sometimes known as *F waves*).

The AV node is unable to conduct impulses faster than ~200/min. Atrial contraction faster than that leads to impulses failing to be conducted. For example, an atrial rate of ~300/min will lead to every other impulse being conducted, giving a ventricular rate (and pulse) of ~150/min. In this case, it is called *2:1 block* (Fig. 19.13, rhythm strip 2). Other ratios of atrial to ventricular contractions may occur.

A variable block at the AV node may lead to an irregularly irregular pulse indistinguishable from that of AF on clinical examination.

ECG features
- Saw-tooth appearance of baseline
- Normal appearance of QRS complexes

Causes of atrial flutter
Similar to those of AF (see previous page)

Junctional (nodal) tachycardia

Here the area in or around the AV node depolarizes spontaneously; the impulse will be immediately conducted to the ventricles. The QRS complex will be of a normal shape but no P waves will be seen.

ECG features
- No P waves
- QRS complexes are regular and normal shape
- Rate may be fast or may be of a normal rate

Some causes of junctional tachycardia
- Sick sinus syndrome (including drug-induced)
- Digoxin toxicity
- Ischemia of the AV node, especially with acute inferior MI
- Acutely after cardiac surgery
- Acute inflammatory processes (e.g., acute rheumatic fever) that may involve the conduction system
- Diphtheria
- Other drugs (e.g., most antiarrhythmic agents)

Wolff–Parkinson–White syndrome

In Wolff–Parkinson–White (WPW) syndrome, there is an extra conducting pathway between the atria and the ventricles (the bundle of Kent)—a break in the normal electrical insulation. This accessory pathway is not specialized for conducting electrical impulses so does not delay the impulse as the AV node does. However, it is not linked to the normal conduction pathways of the bundle of His.

Depolarization of the ventricles will occur partly via the AV node and partly by the bundle of Kent. During normal atrial contraction, electrical activity reaches the AV node and the accessory pathway at roughly the same time. While it is held up temporarily at the AV node, the impulse passes through the accessory pathway and starts to depolarize the ventricles via nonspecialized cells (pre-excitation), distorting the first part of the R wave and giving a short PR interval. Normal conduction via the bundle of His then supervenes. The result is a slurred upstroke of the QRS complex called a *delta wave* (see Fig. 19.14).

This is an example of a *fusion beat*, in which normal and abnormal ventricular depolarization combine to give a distortion of the QRS complex.

▶ *Re-entry tachycardia*

The accessory pathway may allow electrical activity to be conducted from the ventricles back up to the atria.

For example, in a re-entry tachycardia, electrical activity may be conducted down the bundle of His, across the ventricles, and *up the accessory pathway* into the atria (Fig. 19.15), causing them to contract again, and the cycle is repeated (Fig. 19.16). This is called a *re-entry circuit*.

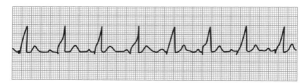

Fig. 19.14 Rhythm strip showing WPW syndrome.

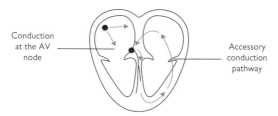

Conduction at the AV node

Accessory conduction pathway

Fig. 19.15 Diagrammatic representation of re-entry tachycardia.

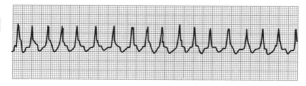

Fig. 19.16 Rhythm strip showing a re-entry tachycardia.

Box 19.3 Classification of Wolff–Parkinson–White syndrome

The bundle of Kent may connect the atria with either the right or the left ventricle. Thus, WPW is classically divided into two groups according to the resulting appearance of the QRS complex in the anterior chest leads. In practice, this classification is simplistic, as 11% of patients may have more than one accessory pathway.

- *Type A:* upright delta wave and QRS in V_1
  - May be mistaken for RBBB or posterior MI
- *Type B:* downward delta wave and QRS in V_1, positive elsewhere
  - May be mistaken for LBBB or anterior MI

Ventricular rhythms

Most ventricular rhythms originate outside the usual conduction pathways, meaning that excitation spreads by an abnormal path through the ventricular muscle to give broad or unusually shaped QRS complexes.

Ventricular tachycardia (VT)

There is a focus of ventricular tissue depolarizing rapidly within the ventricular myocardium. VT is defined as three or more successive ventricular extrasystoles at a rate of >120/min. Sustained VTs last >30 seconds.

VT may be *stable*, showing a repetitive QRS shape (monomorphic; Fig.19.17, rhythm strip 1) or *unstable*, with varying patterns of the QRS complex (polymorphic).

It may be impossible to distinguish VT from an SVT with bundle branch block on a 12-lead ECG.

ECG features

- Wide QRS complexes that are irregular in rhythm and shape
- AV dissociation—independent atrial and ventricular contraction
- May see fusion and capture beats on ECG as signs of atrial activity independent of ventricular activity. This is said to be pathognomonic.
  - **Fusion beats:** depolarization from AV node meets depolarization from ventricular focus, causing hybrid QRS complex
  - **Capture beats:** atrial beat conducted to ventricles causing a normal QRS complex in among the VT tracing
- Rate can be up to 130–300/min.
- QRS concordance: all QRS complexes in chest leads are either mainly positive or mainly negative—suggests ventricular origin of tachycardia.
- Extreme axis deviation (far negative or far positive)

Some causes of ventricular tachycardia

- Ischemia (acute including MI or chronic)
- Electrolyte abnormalities (↓ K, ↓ Mg)
- Aggressive adrenergic stimulation (e.g., cocaine use)
- Drugs, especially antiarrhythmics

Ventricular fibrillation (VF)

This is disorganized, uncoordinated depolarization from multiple foci in the ventricular myocardium (Fig. 19.17, rhythm strip 2).

ECG features

- No discernible QRS complexes
- A completely disorganized ECG

Some causes of ventricular fibrillation

- Coronary heart disease
- Cardiac inflammatory diseases
- Abnormal metabolic states
- Proarrhythmic toxic exposures
- Electrocution
- Tension pneumothorax, trauma, and drowning
- Large pulmonary embolism
- Hypoxia or acidosis

Box 19.4 Fine VF

This is VF with a small-amplitude waveform (Fig. 19.17, rhythm strip 3). It may resemble asystole on the ECG monitor (see Fig. 19.18, rhythm strip 5, 📖 p. 609), particularly in an emergency situation.

In a clinical situation, you should remember to increase the gain on the monitor to ensure that what you think is asystole is not really fine VF, as the management for each is very different.

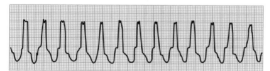

Rhythm strip 1—monomorphic ventricular tachycardia (VT).

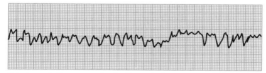

Rhythm strip 2—ventricular fibrillation (VF).

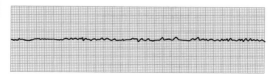

Rhythm strip 3—"fine" ventricular fibrillation.

Fig. 19.17 Rhythm strips showing ventricular rhythms.

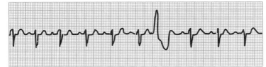

Rhythm strip 1—a single ventricular extrasystole.

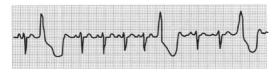

Rhythm strip 2—multiple, unifocal, ventricular extrasystole.

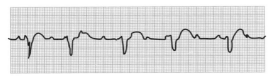

Rhythm strip 3—ventricular escape in the case of complete heart block.

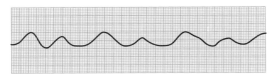

Rhythm strip 4—agonal rhythm.

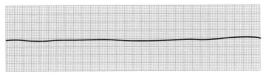

Rhythm strip 5—asystole.

Fig. 19.18 Rhythm strips showing some ventricular rhythms.

Other ventricular rhythms

Ventricular extrasystoles (ectopics)
These are ventricular contractions originating from a focus of depolarization within the ventricle. As conduction is via abnormal pathways, the QRS complex will be unusually shaped (Fig. 19.18, rhythm strips 1 and 2).

Ventricular extrasystoles are common and harmless if there is no structural heart disease. If they occur at the same time as a T wave, the *R-on-T phenomenon*, they can lead to VF.

Ventricular escape rhythm
This occurs as a backup when conduction between the atria and the ventricles is interrupted (as in complete heart block).

The intrinsic pacemaker in ventricular myocardium depolarizes at a slow rate (30–40/min) (see Fig. 19.18, rhythm strip 3).

The ventricular beats will be abnormal and wide with abnormal T waves following them. This rhythm can be stable but may suddenly fail.

Asystole
This is a complete absence of electrical activity and is not compatible with life (see Fig. 19.18, rhythm strip 5).

There may be a slight wavering of the baseline, which can be easily confused with fine VF in emergency situations (see Box 19.5).

Agonal rhythm
This is a slow, irregular rhythm with wide ventricular complexes that vary in shape (Fig. 19.18, rhythm strip 4). This is often seen in later stages of unsuccessful resuscitation attempts as the heart dies. Complexes become progressively broader before all recognizable activity is lost (asystole).

Box 19.5 Torsades de pointes

Torsades de pointes, literally meaning 'twisting of points,' is a form of polymorphic VT characterized by a gradual change in the amplitude and twisting of the QRS axis (Fig. 19.19). In the United States, it is known as *cardiac ballet*.

Torsades usually terminates spontaneously but frequently recurs and may degenerate into sustained VT and VF.

Torsades results from a prolonged QT interval. Causes include congenital long-QT syndromes and drugs (e.g., antiarrhythmics). Patients may also have ↓ K and ↓ Mg.

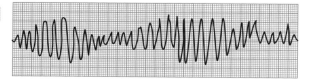

Fig. 19.19 Torsades de pointes. The axis of the QRS complex rotates—seen from a fixed position, there is a repeated change of amplitude.

P- and T- wave abnormalities

P wave

This represents depolarization of the small muscle mass of the atria. The P wave is thus much smaller in amplitude than the QRS complex.

Normal
- In sinus rhythm, each P wave is closely associated with a QRS complex.
- P waves are usually upright in most leads, except aVR.
- P waves are <3 small squares wide and <3 small squares high.

Abnormal
- Right atrial hypertrophy will cause tall, peaked P waves (Fig. 19.20, rhythm strip 1). Causes include pulmonary hypertension (in which case the wave is known as *P pulmonale* and *tricuspid valve stenosis*).
- Left atrial hypertrophy will cause the P wave to become wider and twin-peaked, or *bifid* (Fig. 19.20, rhythm strip 2). This is usually caused by mitral valve disease, in which case the wave is known as *P mitrale*.

T wave

This represents repolarization of the ventricles. The T wave is most commonly affected by ischemic changes. The most common abnormality is inversion, which has a number of causes.

Normal
- Commonly inverted in V_1 and aVR
- May be inverted in V_1–V_3 as normal variant

Abnormal
- Myocardial ischemia or MI (e.g., non-Q-wave MI) can cause T-wave inversion (Fig. 19.20, rhythm strip 3). Changes need to be interpreted in light of clinical picture.
- Ventricular hypertrophy causes T inversion in those leads focused on the ventricle in question. For example, left ventricular hypertrophy will give T changes in leads V_5, V_6, II, and aVL.
- Bundle branch block causes abnormal QRS complexes due to abnormal pathways of ventricular depolarization. The corresponding abnormal repolarization gives unusually shaped T waves, which have no significance in themselves.
- Digoxin causes a characteristic T-wave inversion with a down-sloping of the ST segment known as the *reverse tick* sign. This occurs at therapeutic doses and is not a sign of digoxin toxicity (see Fig. 19.20, rhythm strip 4).
- Electrolyte imbalances cause a number of T-wave changes.
  - ↑ K can cause tall tented T waves.
  - ↓ K can cause small T waves and U waves (broad, flat waves occurring after the T waves; Fig. 19.20, rhythm strip 5).
  - ↑ Ca can cause small T waves with a prolongation of the QT interval (↓ Ca has the reverse effect).
  - Other causes of T-wave inversion include subarachnoid hemorrhage and lithium use.

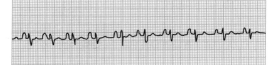

Rhythm strip 1—peaked P waves.

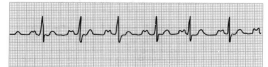

Rhythm strip 2—bifid P waves.

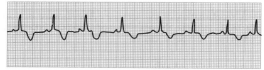

Rhythm strip 3—T wave inversion after myocardial infarction.

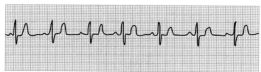

Rhythm strip 4—Hyperkalemia with peaked T waves.

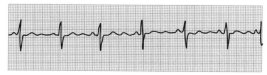

Rhythm strip 5—Hyperkalemia with small T waves and U waves.

Fig. 19.20 Rhythm strips showing some P-and T-wave abnormalities.

ST segment

This is the portion of the ECG from the end of the QRS complex to the start of the T wave and is an isoelectric line in the normal ECG (see Fig. 19.5, 📖 p. 595.). Changes in the ST segment can represent myocardial ischemia and, most importantly, acute MI (Fig. 19.21, rhythm strip 1).

ST elevation

The degree and extent of ST elevation is of crucial importance in ECG interpretation, as it determines whether reperfusion therapy (thrombolysis or primary PCI) is considered in an acute MI.

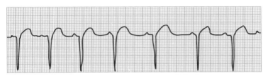

Rhythm strip—Lead V₂ showing acute myocardial infarction.

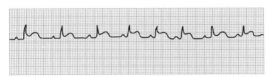

Rhythm strip—Pericarditis. The ST elevation is usually described as 'saddle-shaped'.

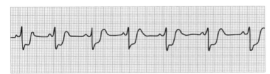

Rhythm strip—Ischemia.

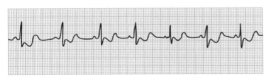

Rhythm strip—Digoxin use showing the 'reverse-tick'.

Fig. 19.21 Rhythm strips showing some ST segment abnormalities.

Causes of ST elevation
- Acute MI—convex ST elevation in affected leads (the tombstone appearance), often with reciprocal ST depression in opposite leads
- Pericarditis—widespread concave ST elevation (saddle-shaped; Fig. 19.21, rhythm strip 2)
- Left ventricular aneurysm—ST elevation may persist over time.

ST depression
ST depression can be horizontal, upward sloping, or downward sloping.

Causes of ST depression
- Myocardial ischemia—horizontal ST depression and an upright T wave (Fig. 19.21, rhythm strip 3). May be the result of coronary artery disease or other causes (e.g., anemia, aortic stenosis)
- Digoxin toxicity—downward sloping (reverse tick; Fig. 19.21, rhythm strip 4)
- Nonspecific changes—ST segment depression that is often upward sloping may be a normal variant and is not thought to be associated with any underlying significant pathology.

▶ In exercise ECG testing, which looks to induce ischemic changes, the extent, timing, and nature of ST changes can help quantify the probability of ischemic heart disease.

Myocardial infarction
In the first hour following an MI, the ECG can remain normal. However, when changes occur, they usually develop in the following order:
- ST segment becomes elevated and T waves become peaked.
- Pathological Q waves develop.
- ST segment returns to baseline and T waves invert.

The leads in which these changes take place can help you identify which part of the heart has been affected and, therefore, which coronary artery is likely to be occluded.
- *Anterior:* V_2–V_5
- *Anterolateral:* I, aVL, V_5, V_6
- *Inferior:* III, aVF (sometimes II also)
- *Posterior:* The usual depolarization of the posterior of the left ventricle is lost, giving a dominant R wave in V_1. Imagine it as a mirror image of the Q wave you would expect with an anterior infarction.
- *Right ventricular:* often no changes on the 12-lead ECG. If suspected clinically, leads are placed on the right of the chest, mirroring the normal pattern and are labeled V_1R, V_2R, V_3R, and so on.

Hypertrophy
If the heart is faced with having to overcome pressure overload (e.g., left ventricular hypertrophy in hypertension or aortic stenosis) or higher systemic pressures (e.g., essential hypertension), it will ↑ its muscle mass in response. This muscle mass can result in changes in the ECG.

Atrial hypertrophy
This can lead to changes in the P wave.

Ventricular hypertrophy

This can lead to changes in the cardiac axis, QRS complex height and depth, and the T wave.

Left ventricular hypertrophy (LVH)
- Tall R wave in V_6 and deep S wave in V_1
- May also see left axis deviation
- T-wave inversion in V_5, V_6, I, aVL
- Voltage criteria for LVH includes the following:
  - R wave >25 mm (5 large squares) in V_6
  - R wave in V_6 + S wave in V_1 >35 mm (7 large squares)

Right ventricular hypertrophy
- Dominant R wave in V_1 (i.e., R wave bigger than S wave)
- Deep S wave in V_6
- May also see right axis deviation
- T-wave inversion in V_1–V_3

Paced rhythms

Temporary or permanent cardiac pacing may be indicated for a number of conditions, such as complete heart block or symptomatic bradycardia. These devices deliver a tiny electrical pulse to an area of the heart, initiating contraction. This can be seen on the ECG as a sharp spike.

Many different types of pacemakers exist, and can be categorized according to the following:
- The chamber paced (atria or ventricles or both)
- The chamber used to detect the heart's electrical activity (atria or ventricles or both)
- How the pacemaker responds—most are inhibited by the normal electrical activity of the heart

On the ECG, look for the pacing spikes (see Fig. 19.22), which may appear before P waves if the atria are paced, before the QRS complexes if the ventricles are paced, or both.

ⓘ Be careful not to mistake the vertical lines that separate the different leads on some ECG printouts as pacing spikes!

▶ Paced complexes do not show the expected changes described elsewhere in this section. Thus you are unable to diagnose ischemia in the presence of pacing.

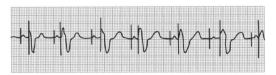

Fig. 19.22 Rhythm strip showing dual-chamber pacing.

Chest X-rays: introduction

Experienced clinicians and radiologists who look at a chest film and immediately give a diagnosis are able to do so through years of practice and the development of pattern recognition. For the nonspecialist, careful review of chest radiographs requires systematic examination of the film, including all systems and body parts in it.

While there is no 'correct' method, you should ensure that all is examined. You can do this by region; we do it by organ system. See Box 19.6 for a framework for reporting chest X-ray (CXR) results.

> **Box 19.6 Framework for reporting a chest film**
>
> - Name
> - DOB
> - Exam date
> - Technical considerations
>   - Stationary vs. portable
>   - Type of film
>   - Position of patient
>   - Projection
>   - Orientation
>   - Rotation
>   - Exposure
>   - Inspiration
>   - Inclusion
> - Clinical review

Technical considerations

▶ It should be remembered that the CXR is not a slice of the chest. It is a two-dimensional *representation* of all the internal structures, created by X-rays passing through them. Features can overlie each other, hiding abnormalities or creating unusual features with compound images. As such, the image can be influenced by a whole host of external factors.

Projection

This refers to the direction at which the X-ray beam passes.

- *PA (posterior–anterior):* The cassette is placed in front of the patient and X-rays pass from the back. This is a standard CXR.
- *AP (anterior–posterior):* The cassette is placed at the back of the patient and X-rays are fired from in front. An AP film may be taken in the ill or injured patient who is unable to stand in front of the X-ray machine.
- *Lateral:* These views are from either the left or the right of the patient. The direction of the beam has consequences for the appearance of the intrathoracic structures. As the X-rays leave the machine, they diverge. Thus objects near the cassette will appear their true size, but objects further from the cassette (i.e., nearer the source of radiation) will appear enlarged (see Fig. 19.23).

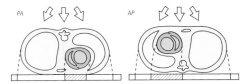

Fig. 19.23 An exaggeration of X-ray beam divergence. Note that when the heart is closer to the origin of the beam, it appears larger on the resultant image.

This is particularly important for viewing the heart—it is not possible to accurately judge heart size on an AP film, as the heart lies much further from the cassette.

Position

Standard X-rays are taken with the patient standing. Any deviation from this will usually be marked on the film, allowing you to learn more about the patient and adjust your assessment of the image.

- *Sitting:* suggests a severe illness as the patient is unable to stand
  - The diaphragm will be artificially raised, inflation of the lungs will be reduced, soft tissues at the front of the patient may be folded.
- *Supine or prone:* suggests a very severe illness (patient is unable to sit).
  - Structures will be displaced within the chest, with abnormal distribution of blood supply to the lungs; fluid levels will not be seen.

Orientation

- Films should have position markers. Often only one side is labeled (e.g., *R*, for the right of the patient).
- The image should be presented as if you are looking at the patient—that is, the patient's right on your left, and vice versa.
- Ensure that the marker is on the correct side—watch for the relatively rare cases of dextrocardia.

Rotation

Films should be taken with the patient facing directly away from the source (for PA films).

You should ensure that this is the case, as rotation can cause abnormal appearances of the mediastinum and other structures.

- Look at the spinous processes of the thoracic vertebrae—these should appear at the center of each bone.
- Look also at the distance between the medial ends of the clavicles and the spinous process of the nearest vertebra—these should be equal.

Exposure

The appropriate exposure depends largely on patient size. Too little will cause the lungs to appear too white, too much will make structures appear too dark (Fig. 19.24) and subtle signs may be lost.

- As a rule of thumb, you should *just* be able to make out the thoracic vertebral bodies through the image of the heart.

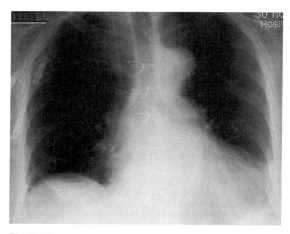

Fig. 19.24 Radiograph showing an inadequate image quality. The lung fields appear too black and the apices of the lungs are not included in the image.

Inflation

A chest X-ray should be taken with fully inflated lungs. A poor inspiration can make the lungs appear denser, draw the trachea to the right, and make the heart appear abnormally large.

- There should be ≥ 9 ribs visible posteriorly.
  - Count from the top down, but be careful, as it is often easy to confuse the first couple of ribs and the clavicles.
  - To be sure, find the anterior end of the first rib and trace it posteriorly; the second rib often appears quite close below.
▶ See Fig. 19.25 for a comparison of adequate and inadequate lung inspiration.

Inclusion

Does the film show all the structures that you wish it to? You should be able to see the apices of both lungs and both costophrenic angles.

Box 19.7 Densities

▶ Be aware that there are five basic densities on X-rays:
- *Black:* gas
- *Dark gray:* fat
- *Light gray:* soft tissues and fluid
- *White:* bone and calcification
- *Intense white:* metal

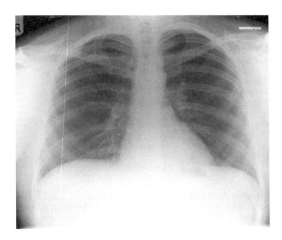

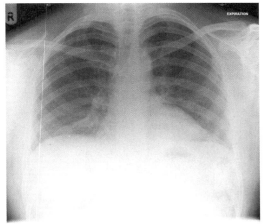

Fig. 19.25 Radiographs of the same patient showing the effect of inspiration. The upper image has a good inspiration, the lower is inadequate. Note how the lungs appear denser in the lower image and the heart is enlarged.

Clinical interpretation

Heart and mediastinum

The key to understanding the mediastinum is knowledge of the normal anatomy. All the structures, apart from the trachea, appear as fluid or soft-tissue density and are hard to distinguish separately. Much can be learned by looking at the shape of the mediastinum (Fig. 19.26).

Examine the following:

- Mediastinal border, looking for abnormality
- Trachea and bronchi
- Heart, looking for visible valves (metal heart valves will appear opaque on the CXR—see Fig. 19.52, 📖 p. 638)
- Cardiac size: should be <1/2 of the thoracic width on a PA film. Measure carefully (with a ruler).
- Look for masses, calcification, or free air (pneumomediastinum).

Abnormalities

- Venous engorgement: look at the lung fields.
- Hiatal hernia: may be seen as a rounded object sitting behind the heart or causing distortion of the normal mediastinal outline. There may be a visible fluid level within it (Fig. 19.27).
- Enlarged heart: enlargement of one or more chamber may be seen on the mediastinal outline or simply by enlargement of the heart size (Fig.19.28).
- Pericardial effusion: massive enlargement of the heart with a classical boot shape (Fig. 19.29)
- LV aneurysm: seen as an enlarged left side of the heart—look for calcification, which will appear white.
- Pericardial calcification: seen as a patchy white outline of the heart

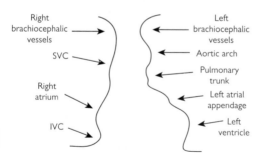

Fig. 19.26 Diagram illustrating the normal outline of the mediastinum and the structures giving rise to the shape.

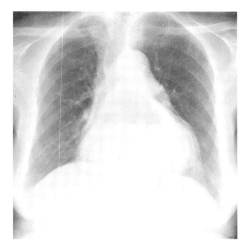

Fig. 19.27 Radiograph showing a large hiatal hernia. A fluid level can be seen within the herniated stomach behind the heart.

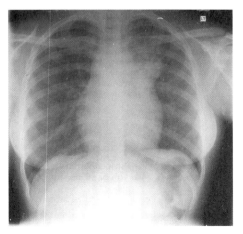

Fig. 19.28 Radiograph showing a mass in the upper portion of the mediastinum on the left.

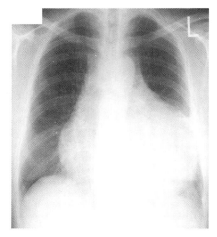

Fig. 19.29 Radiograph showing a large pericardial effusion. The heart appears grossly enlarged with a typical boot shape.

Hila

The *hila* are the regions at which the lungs connect to the central circulation. They appear as opaque regions on the right and the left side of the mediastinum. Most of the image is created by the pulmonary arteries and veins coming to and from the heart.

The hila should be rounded and symmetrical. As the left pulmonary artery is slightly superior to the right, the left hilum appears ~1 cm higher than the right. On each side, the bronchi appear as lucent structures.

Look for the following:
- Difference in density
- Asymmetry
- Loss of the normal concavity
- ▶ Check for rotation of the film.

Causes of hilar enlargement

- *Vascular:* smoothly enlarged and irregularly shaped. Arterial enlargement is due to congestion or aneurysm or pulmonary hypertension (usually bilateral).
  🔵 Pulmonary hypertension will also cause ↓ peripheral vasculature in the lung field (Fig. 19.30).
- *Lymph nodes:* smoothly enlarged, regular masses within the hila. Causes include neoplastic (bronchial carcinoma, lymphoma, metastatic), infective (especially TB—look also for peripheral abscesses or miliary shadowing), and infiltrative (sarcoid—look also for pulmonary nodules) (Fig. 19.31).
- *Other masses:* irregular masses, sometimes with poorly defined edges

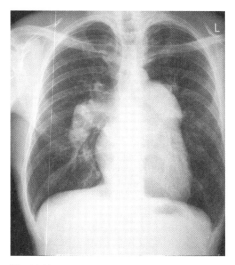

Fig. 19.30 Radiograph showing pulmonary hypertension. The engorged pulmonary arteries are clearly visible at both hila.

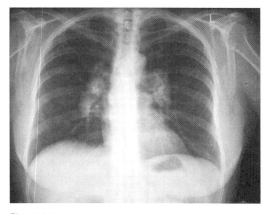

Fig. 19.31 Radiograph showing bilateral hilar lymphadenopathy, in this case, due to sarcoidosis.

Look at each bone in detail, including the shoulder girdles, ribs, clavicles, and thoracic vertebrae. Look at the density and trabecular pattern. Look for the following:
- Lytic lesions
- Sclerosis
- Erosions
- Fractures
- Dislocation

Vertebrae
Ensure that the size and density are uniform and the spaces equal. Remember to look for paraspinous soft tissue masses.

Ribs
- Trace each from the back to the front, note width of space between.
- New fractures appear as sharp lines—look for associated complications, such as surgical emphysema and pneumothorax.
- Old fractures appear as widened areas of rib, often with a slight distortion of the line of the bone.

Lytic lesions
Bone looks as if it is smudged. This may be the only sign of metastatic disease.

Soft tissues
Remember that chest cavities are surrounded on all sides by soft tissue, including the front and the back. Look at all the regions visible. Look for calcification and free air.

Surgical emphysema
Air pockets exist in the soft tissues (Fig. 19.32). Anterior or posteriorly, this can be difficult to see, and may only be seen indirectly by distortion of the image of the other structures. Laterally, side-on views of the pockets of air can be seen as radiolucent, lozenge-shaped or tapering structures.

Breasts
Female and male breast tissue overlying the inferior part of the lung may give the appearance of an increase in lung density. Look for missing breasts as a clue to underlying disease (Fig. 19.33).

Nipples
Nipples often appear as rounded opacities that could be mistaken for lesions within the lung.

Abdomen
One should be able to see air in the stomach as a bubble below the left hemidiaphragm. Often, there is an air-fluid level within it creating a shape with a rounded top and a horizontal lower edge.

A gastric bubble on the right may indicate either situs inversus or mis-labeling of the film.

Look below the diaphragm for free air (pneumoperitoneum), often seen as a wisp of radiolucency between the liver and the right hemidiaphragm or above the gastric bubble (Fig. 19.34).

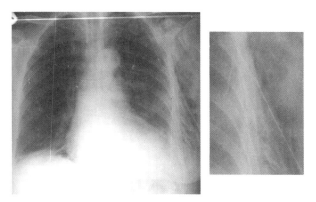

Fig. 19.32 Radiograph showing extensive surgical emphysema on the left of the chest. Insert shows a close-up. Also visible is the chest tube causing the problem.

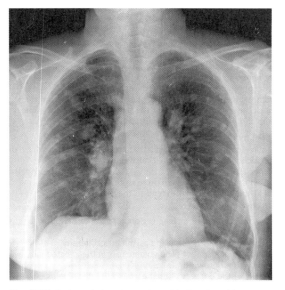

Fig. 19.33 Radiograph showing a patient with disseminated breast cancer. Aside from the multiple pulmonary lesions, there is a lack of breast shadow on the left, indicating that this patient has had a left mastectomy.

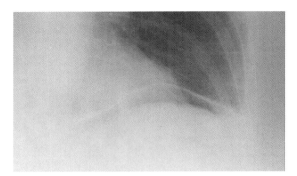

Fig. 19.34 Close-up showing free air below the left hemidiaphragm.

Lungs

Readers should review normal lung anatomy. The points pertinent to the physical examination are also relevant to the radiographic examination.

Normal

Seen head on, the oblique fissures are not visible. As the upper lobes lie anterior to the lower lobes, the lung field on the CXR is both the upper and lower lobes (on the left). Normal features include the following:

- Lung fields are of equal density.
- The right hemidiaphragm is slightly higher than the left.
- Sharp costophrenic angles and cardiophrenic angles
- The horizontal fissure in the right lung passes horizontally from the midpoint of the right hilum to about the sixth rib in the axillary line.
- The pleura should be thin and symmetrical.

Examining the film

Scan the entire lung, looking for areas that are too black, too white, or abnormally placed. Look for abnormal calcification.

▶ Look especially at the first ribs, behind the heart, and behind the diaphragms, where lesions can often be missed.

▶ Ensure that the lung markings extend to the periphery.

Collapse

On film, loss of air in a lobe or lung region appears dense. Look for the following:

- Changes to the normal anatomy and asymmetrical density
- Mediastinal and tracheal shift (The volume loss in the affected lung will pull the mediastinum toward the lesion.)
- Loss of clarity of the borders of the heart and the diaphragms (Collapse nearby will cause a blurred outline.)

Right upper lobe

Collapses are upward and to the midline (Fig. 19.35). The horizontal fissure may be elevated and mediastinum shifted to the right. There is a white mass to the right of the upper part of the mediastinum.

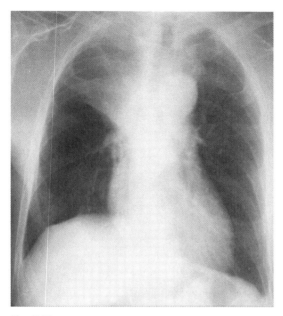

Fig. 19.35 Radiograph showing right upper lobe collapse.

Right middle lobe
This is difficult to see on PA film. It may be seen as a slight blurring of the right heart border and elevation of the right hemidiaphragm (Fig. 19.36).

On lateral film, collapse here is seen as a triangle of white with its apex at the hilum and base anteriorly.

Right lower lobe
A triangular area of white is between the right heart border and diaphragm, causing both to be indistinct.

Left upper lobe
Collapse is hard to see; the left hemithorax is hazy with loss of clarity at the left heart border (Fig. 19.37). Collapse is easier to see on lateral film.

Left lower lobe
There is a sail-like shape of white (Fig. 19.38), but hidden behind the heart border so it is difficult to spot. Look for a double edge to the heart.

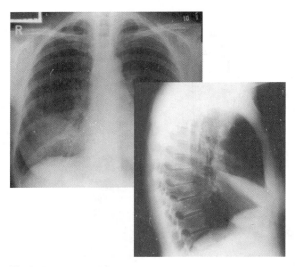

Fig. 19.36 Radiographs showing right middle lobe collapse. This is seen only as a slight increase in density to the right of the heart on the PA film. The collapse is much easier to see here than on the lateral film.

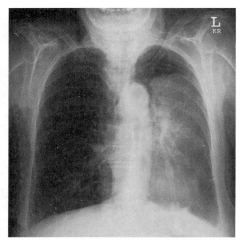

Fig. 19.37 PA radiograph showing left upper lobe collapse.

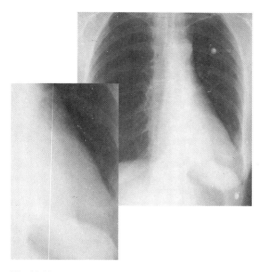

Fig. 19.38 Radiograph showing left lower lobe collapse—note the sail-like shape of white behind the heart.

Consolidation

Consolidation is usually a sign of infection—fluid within the alveolar spaces, making an area of the lung appear denser (Fig. 19.39). Look for the following:

- Focal area of ↑ density with indistinct margins
- Heterogeneous alveolar shadowing
- Not present on previous X-rays (Focal fibrosis may appear similar but is usually long-standing with a chronic course.)
- There may be a sharp demarcation at lobar margins (right upper lobe consolidation may be seen with a sharp horizontal lower border where it meets the right middle lobe) (see Box 19.8).
- *Air bronchograms:* as the airways remain patent, an air-filled bronchus passing through an area of consolidation may be seen as a radiolucent (black) tube.

Fibrosis

Increased density of the lung tissue in fibrosis causes a reticulonodular (net-like with nodules) pattern of opacity. As it progresses, it may cause a honeycomb appearance of the lung. Be careful to differentiate fibrosis from edema or consolidation.

Features of fibrosis (Figs. 19.40 and 19.41) are as follows:

- Often bilateral, although not necessarily symmetrical
- Causes ↓ lung volumes

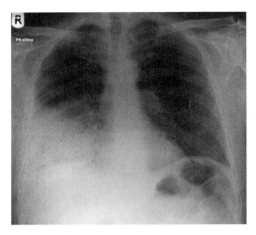

Fig. 19.39 Radiograph showing right lower lobe consolidation.

Box 19.8 Differentiating right lower zone consolidation
Consolidation at the base of the right lung may either be in the right middle lobe and/or right lower lobe. Look for blurring of the structures nearby.
- **The right middle lobe** does not touch the diaphragm—consolidation here will cause blurring of the right heart border, whereas the diaphragm remains distinct.
- **The right lower lobe** lies against the diaphragm but very little of it touches the heart—consolidation here will cause blurring of the right hemidiaphragm but leave the right heart border relatively distinct.

- If focal, draws the mediastinum toward the affected side
- Causes blurring of the heart and diaphragm borders
- Has a distinctive reticulonodular pattern

Pulmonary edema
This causes an alveolar pattern of shadowing. If due to congestive cardiac failure, there will also be changes in the appearance of the heart.
   Features of pulmonary edema secondary to heart failure (Fig. 19.42):
- Enlarged heart
- Bilateral, although not necessarily symmetrical, lung shadowing
- Classically, in middle and upper zones, causing a bat's wing appearance

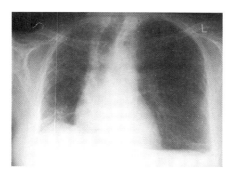

Fig. 19.40 Radiograph showing a patient post–lung transplant. The right lung is the patient's native lung and is severely fibrosed—note the reticular shadowing and the ↓ volume. The left lung is the healthy donated lung.

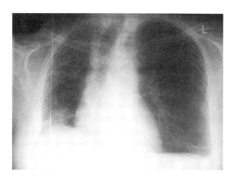

Fig. 19.41 Close-up of a radiograph showing pulmonary fibrosis.

- Pulmonary venous engorgement
  - The vessels appear to extend further than normal into the lung field.
  - Vessels in the upper zone appear larger than normal (often >5 mm diameter)—upper lobe blood diversion.
- *Kerley's B lines:* short, horizontal white lines close to the lung periphery, usually extending horizontally into the lung field. They are found particularly at the bases and caused by edema of the interlobular septa.

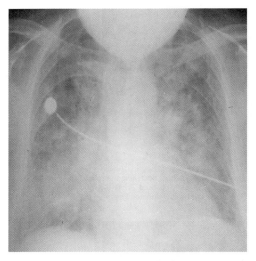

Fig. 19.42 Radiograph showing severe pulmonary edema. There is extensive alveolar shadowing in both lung fields, and the heart is enlarged. Note also the ECG lead attached to the patient's chest—a sign of the clinical severity.

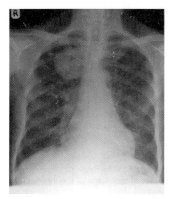

Fig. 19.43 Radiograph showing a right upper zone mass.

Coin lesions

The lung masses often have well-demarcated borders. They could also represent a focal area of consolidation or a pleural lesion (Fig. 19.43). Look for the following:

- Calcification within the lesion (rare if malignant)
- Air bronchogram within lesion (indicating consolidation, not a mass)
- Cavitation
- Changes in the bones and soft tissues nearby
- Lymph node enlargement in the hila
- Other lesions

Cavitating lesions

These lung lesions have a central cavity, creating a circular radiographic appearance. If there is fluid within the lesion, an air-fluid level may be seen (Fig. 19.44). Look at the rest of the film for clues to the nature of the lesion (i.e., lymphadenopathy, other lesions, signs of infection). Possible causes include lung abscess, neoplasm, or focal area of infarction.

Bronchiectasis

This can be difficult to diagnose on a plain X-ray. The combination of airway enlargement, airway wall thickening, and alveolar shadowing can, however, give a distinct appearance.

- *Ring shadows:* affected bronchi are seen head on. They appear as small rings—several together give a bunch-of-grapes appearance.
- *Tramline shadows:* affected bronchi are seen side on. They appear as short parallel lines.

Pneumonectomy

This is rare. The side from which the lung was removed will appear densely white (a whiteout) (Fig. 19.45). As such, it should be carefully differentiated from a large pleural effusion or dense consolidation. There may also be the following:

- Mediastinal shift toward the affected side (An effusion would push the mediastinum the other way.)
- Total absence of lung markings on the affected side

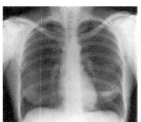

Fig. 19.44 Radiograph showing an abscess in the left lung—note the distinct air-fluid level within the rounded lesion (insert).

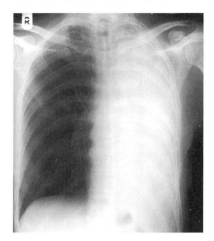

Fig. 19.45 Radiograph showing a previous left pneumonectomy. The mediastinum has shifted so far to the left that it is almost impossible to distinguish amid the density of the left side of the chest.

- ↓ Density of the remaining lung as it expands to fill the space available
- Signs of previous surgery (e.g., rib resections, sutures)

Pleural lesions

Lesions in the pleura may be seen to overlie the lung field, or may be seen laterally at the lung edge. Pleural plaques caused by asbestos exposure are often seen as a heterogeneous lesion with irregular and spiculated edges (holly-leaf appearance) (Fig. 19.46).

Remember that the pleura also covers the diaphragm—look for the linear appearance of plaques seen side-on. Be careful not to mistake pleural lesions for lung lesions.

Pleural effusion

An effusion will appear as a white area at the base of the lung (if the patient is standing or sitting up). It often has a well-demarcated upper border with a meniscal edge as the fluid tracks up lateral to the lung (Fig. 19.47). As the overlying lung is unable to inflate fully, there may be the appearance of increased lung density with a blurred upper border of the effusion. Look for mediastinal shift (it will move away from the effusion, if large) (Fig. 19.48).

⊙ Small effusions may only be seen as a blunting of the costophrenic angle on the affected side. Remember that ~500 mL of fluid can hide behind the hemidiaphragm before it becomes visible on a PA chest film.

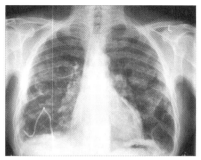

Fig. 19.46 Radiograph showing extensive pleural plaque disease. Close-up shows one of the lesions—note the characteristic holly-leaf appearance.

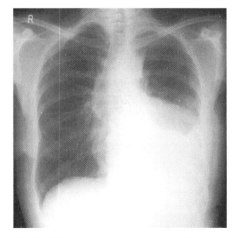

Fig. 19.47 Radiograph showing large pleural effusion on the left. Note the meniscus as the fluid tracks laterally beside the lung.

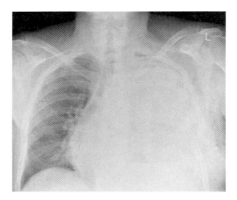

Fig. 19.48 Radiograph showing a massive pleural effusion causing almost a complete whiteout of the left lung field. Note how the mediastinum is shifted away from the affected side.

Air outside the lung will appear as a black area, often as a sliver between the lung and the thoracic wall. Look for the following:
- A darker area peripherally, often superior in an erect film
- The lung markings do not reach the edge of the lung field—look carefully, do not mistake a bulla for a pneumothorax. Examine the rest of the lung for similar areas.
- A visible, albeit thin, demarcation between the lung and the free air (Fig. 19.49)

Small pneumothoraces can be hard to spot, try
- Turning the film on its side (one can often see horizontal lines easier than vertical ones).
- Asking for an expiratory film (the lungs will appear more dense and the pneumothorax will take up relatively more of the lung field).

Tension pneumothorax
❶ This is a medical emergency, as ↑ pressure in the chest reduces venous return to the heart.
- The lung may appear small and shriveled within the lung field.
- The mediastinum is shifted away from the affected side (Fig. 19.50).
- A lowered hemidiaphragm is on the affected side.

COPD
This is difficult to spot on a chest X-ray. The lung fields may appear less dense than normal with reduced lung markings. The chest may be hyperinflated, often with an elongated appearance to the mediastinum. Look for bullae and be careful to differentiate from a pneumothorax.
▶ The key sign is flattening of the diaphragms (Fig. 19.51).

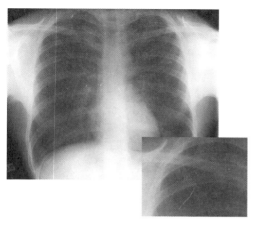

Fig. 19.49 Radiograph showing a right-sided pneumothorax. It is difficult to spot. Close-up shows the pleural edge as a tiny but distinct demarcation between the lung tissue and the free air.

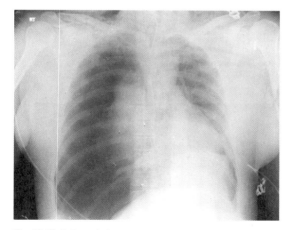

Fig. 19.50 Radiograph showing a right-sided tension pneumothorax. There are no lung markings on the right of the chest. The mediastinum is shifted to the left and the right hemithorax is overinflated.

Iatrogenic features and foreign bodies
Clothes, buttons, zippers, or even a cigarette packet in a shirt pocket can give misleading and often amusing appearances on the chest film.

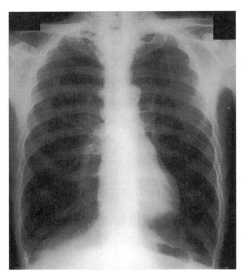

Fig. 19.51 Radiograph showing COPD. Note the ↓ density of the lung fields.

(a)   (b)

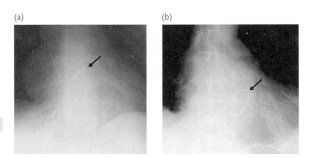

Fig. 19.52 Close-ups of radiographs showing (a) aortic valve replacement and (b) mitral valve replacement.

NG tubes

A correctly placed NG tube (Fig. 19.53) will appear as a thin radio-opaque line descending through the mediastinum, below the diaphragm, and ending somewhere in the region of the gastric bubble. If the tube does not reach the stomach but is seen to pass inferior to the carina, it is almost certainly in the esophagus and will need to be inserted further rather than reinserted. Tubes seen entering either major bronchus (Figs. 19.54 and 19.55) should be removed immediately.

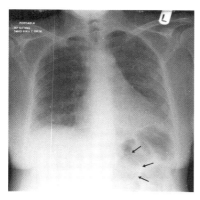

Fig. 19.53 Radiograph showing a correctly placed NG tube.

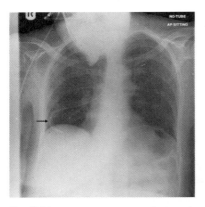

Fig. 19.54 Radiograph showing an NG tube in the right bronchus.

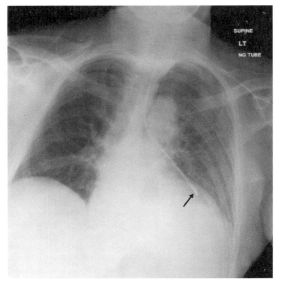

Fig. 19.55 Radiograph showing an NG tube in the left bronchus.

Abdominal X-rays: introduction

A systematic viewing strategy will aid you in the interpretation of abdominal films. Certain key points to inspect on every abdominal X-ray include technical quality, gas pattern, calcification, bones, and soft tissue.

Technical assessment

Always begin your inspection by checking the following:
- Name of patient
- DOB
- Age of patient
- Sex of patient
- Date when film was taken
- Left and right markers
- Note the projection of the film.
  - Almost all abdominal X-rays are AP; other views include upright, supine, or decubitus—these are usually marked on the film.

Views

- *Standard abdominal X-ray:* also known as an *AXR*, 'flat plate,' or KUB (kidneys, ureters, bladder); it is a supine view (Fig. 19.56).
- *Upright film* is useful in identifying the presence of free intraperitoneal air and intestinal air-fluid levels.
- The *left/right lateral decubitus** is especially useful in severely ill patients who are suspected of having free intraperitoneal air and are unable to stand or sit.
  - Decubitus films can be identified by fluid levels lying parallel to the long axis of the body, instead of at right angles to it as on conventional erect films.

Penetration

- A film that is too light (underpenetrated) or too dark (overpenetrated) is of little diagnostic value (see Box 19.9).
- As a general rule, if you can see the bones in the spine, the technical quality should suffice.
- With overexposed or overpenetrated films, it is recommended that you inspect these areas with a bright light behind them (present on most viewing boxes).

Gas pattern

The large bowel lies around the periphery of the abdomen and normally shows haustral indentations. It should contain feces and gas.
- In the large bowel, loops are considered dilated if diameter is >5 cm.

The small bowel is more central, shows mucosal folds across its width (valvulae conniventes), and contains fluid and gas.
- The diameter of the normal small bowel should not exceed 2.5–3 cm.
  ▶ Become familiar with the normal gas pattern on an abdominal X-ray. Abnormal positioning of bowel loops may indicate the presence of an abdominal mass.

**From the Latin *decumbere:* 'to lie down' on the left or right side.

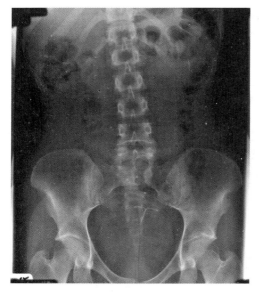

Fig. 19.56 A standard abdominal X-ray showing a normal abdomen. Incidentally, this patient has a T-shaped copper contraceptive device in her uterus, which is visible on the film.

Box 19.9   Densities

▶ Be aware that there are five basic densities on X-rays:
- *Black:* gas
- *Dark gray:* fat
- *Light gray:* soft tissues and fluid
- *White:* bone and calcification
- *Intense white:* metal

Fluid levels

Air-fluid levels are seen as a clear horizontal demarcation between an area of light gray fluid and darker gray or black gas. Small fluid levels in the small and large bowel are a normal finding.

However, distended loops of bowel with air-fluid levels in a diffuse pattern are highly suggestive of a mechanical obstruction. The bowel loops frequently have a hairpin (180° turn) appearance.

To demonstrate fluid levels, you need an erect or decubitus film.

Extraluminal gas

Carefully inspect for signs of extraluminal gas (outside the bowel lumen). This may be either free (pneumoperitoneum) or contained within an abscess cavity, the retroperitoneum, the bowel wall, or the biliary or portal venous systems of the liver.

Free intraperitoneal air suggests a ruptured viscus in the absence of immediate previous surgery.

A subtle sign to look for free gas is the *double wall* sign. Here, both sides of the wall of loops of bowel become visible because of air on the inside and outside of the bowel.

Pneumoperitoneum

Request an erect chest film in suspected cases of pneumoperitoneum and look for bilateral dark crescents of free gas under the hemidiaphragms (Fig. 19.57).

Calcification

There are several structures that may become calcified, particularly with ↑ age of the patient. These may sometimes cause confusion if mistaken for intestinal structures:

- Costal cartilages
- Aorta
- Iliac and splenic arteries

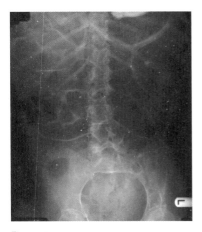

Fig. 19.57 An AXR showing a severe pneumoperitoneum. Note how the bowel wall can be clearly seen; it has air both on the outside and the inside.

- Pelvic phleboliths (small round opacities sometimes containing lucent centers in the pelvic venous plexus)
- Mesenteric lymph nodes

▶ Make careful note of abnormal calcifications (Fig. 19.58), such as biliary and urinary calculi, calcified aneurysms, tumors, pancreatic calcification in chronic pancreatitis, and calcified kidneys in nephrocalcinosis.

Bones

Examine the bones, looking for secondary malignant disease (possibly seen as rounded lucent lesions), degenerative changes, and osteoporosis (cortical thinning).

Remember to look at all the bones and joints within the field:

- Pelvis
- Vertebrae
- Lowermost ribs
- Sacroiliac joints
- Femoral heads

Soft tissues

Scan the film and identify the following:

- Lower borders of the liver and spleen
- Renal outlines
- Psoas muscles

Masses

Abdominal masses are frequently revealed by displacements or distortions of normal viscera.

Distended bladder is the most common mass encountered in the pelvis; alternatively, a mass here may be ovarian or uterine pathology.

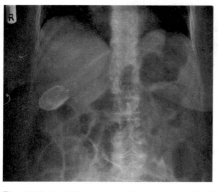

Fig. 19.58 An AXR showing calcification in the gall bladder.

Gross liver enlargement may be indicated by a large mass in the right side of the abdomen, which may extend to the iliac crest. Look for an absence of gut shadows and increased density here.

Gross splenic enlargement is seen as a mass extending inferomedially from the left upper quadrant. There may be elevation of the left hemidiaphragm and downward displacement of the left kidney and stomach. There may also be associated liver and lymph node enlargement.

Normal *renal* length is ~3–3.5 lumbar vertebrae plus their discs. The left kidney is usually higher and slightly larger than the right one. A discrepancy of more than 1.5 cm between the two sides should be viewed with suspicion.

▶ The loss of the psoas margin or renal outline generally indicates an inflammatory condition in the retroperitoneum.

Radiology: pelvis

Normal
The symphysis pubis joint space should be no wider than 5 mm and there should be alignment of the pubic rami. Look closely at the main pelvic ring and the two obturator rings to exclude any abnormality in the bony cortex. Examine the sacroiliac joints to ensure consistent width on either side. The sacral foramina should appear symmetrical and undisrupted.

Pelvic fractures
Stable
- Avulsion fractures—e.g., ischial tuberosity (hamstring avulsion)
- Iliac wing fracture: Duverney's
- Sacral fractures: Denis classification
- Ischiopubic rami fractures
- Acetabular fractures
- Coccygeal fractures: X-rays are *not* indicated here, as they will not change management.
- ① Avulsion fractures are often due to forceful muscle contraction.

Unstable
The pelvic ring is disrupted in two or more places (Fig. 19.59).

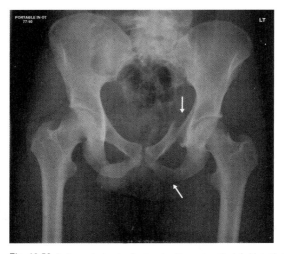

Fig. 19.59 Radiograph showing fractured pubic rami on the left. Note that both the superior and inferior pubic rami are broken—it is not usually possible to break only one.

- *Straddle fracture:* both obturator rings
- *Bucket-handle fracture:* sacroiliac and contralateral ischiopubic rami (not to be confused with the bucket-handle fracture indicative of child abuse)
- *Malgaigne fracture:* sacroiliac and ipsilateral ischiopubic rami
- *Open-book fracture:* both sacroiliacs and both ischiopubic rami

Hints

▶ If you detect a fracture of the main pelvic ring, look hard to exclude a second disruption to the ring—either a fracture or joint widening at the symphysis pubis/sacroiliacs.

   ▶ Pelvic fractures can result in severe damage to internal organs.

Pediatrics

- *Normal development:* be careful not to misinterpret the normal cartilaginous junction (synchondrosis) between pubic and ischial bones as a fracture.

Radiology: hips and femurs

Normal
The joint space between the femoral head and acetabulum should not appear narrowed at any point. Examine the femoral neck for a normal trabecular (bony mesh) pattern and absence of sclerotic areas. Look for a smooth, undamaged cortex as you trace the outline of the proximal femur and femoral shaft.

Fractures
Fractures of the proximal femur are common in the elderly and carry significant mortality risk. Avascular necrosis is a potential complication if the fracture involves the femoral neck and results from disruption of the blood supply to the femoral head (retinacular vessels).

Fractures about the hip are typically characterized by location as femoral neck, intertrochanteric (between the greater and lesser trochanters), and subtrochanteric (Fig. 19.60).

Femoral neck fractures can be further graded on their radiological appearance using the *Garden classification*, presented in Box 19.10.

Hints
▶ Ask for lateral as well as AP views when requesting hip X-rays.
❶ *Hip fracture* is used loosely, but incorrectly, to describe all proximal femoral fractures. Strictly speaking it only relates to intracapsular fractures (those within the joint capsule).
❶ Fractures described as *subcapital* (just below the femoral head) and *transcervical* (across the femoral neck) are both intracapsular fractures.

Degenerative changes
Classical X-ray changes in osteoarthritic degenerative disease at the hip (Fig. 19.61), as with other joints, include the following:

(a)   (b)

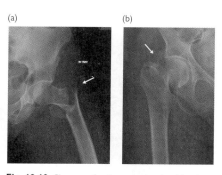

Fig. 19.60 Close-up of radiographs showing (a) an intertrochanteric fracture on the left and (b) fractured neck of the femur.

Box 19.10 Garden classification*

- I—fracture line across the neck stops short of inferior cortex. No displacement. Trabecular angulation across fracture
- II—fracture extends right across the neck. No displacement. No trabecular angulation (no deviation of bony mesh lines)
- III—fracture extends right across the neck. Some displacement and/or rotation of femoral head
- IV—femoral head severely (often completely) displaced

* The value of this classification is disputed.

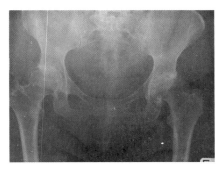

Fig. 19.61 Radiograph showing severe degenerative changes at both hips.

- ↓ Joint space
- Osteophyte formation (bony spurs)
- Bone cysts
- Subarticular sclerosis

Dislocation of hip joint

Of all such cases, 90% are posterior dislocations, with the femoral head seen superior and lateral to the acetabulum. Check for sciatic nerve injury (10%).

🛈 Posterior dislocation strongly suggests that major force was applied; consider trauma elsewhere.

Pediatrics

- *Slipped femoral epiphysis:* Look for misalignment on lateral X-ray of the shaft and neck of the femur with the epiphysis (teenagers).
- *Legg-Calve-Perthes disease* (aseptic necrosis of femoral epiphysis): Look for sclerosis and flattening of the epiphysis and cysts in metaphysic (preteens).
- *Developmental dysplasia of the hip* (congenital dislocation): The femoral head fails to lie within the acetabulum. If missed, osteoarthritis and gait defects ensue. This is diagnosed neonatally with ultrasound.

Radiology: knees

Normal

AP and lateral views are provided as standard. The joint space should be maintained across the joint. On AP film, the lateral tibial condyle margin should be no more than 5 mm outside the femoral condyle margin. On lateral film the distance from the tibial tuberosity to the inferior aspect of the patella should be similar to the length of the patella.

Abnormal

Distal femur fractures

All of the following fractures are readily identifiable on plain X-ray:
- Supracondylar
- Condylar (medial or lateral)
- Intercondylar

Proximal tibial fractures

These are often a result of being hit by car. Lateral (80%) tibial plateau fractures are more common (think impact site).

On X-rays, look for an impacted sclerotic area and lateral displacement of tibial condyle, in addition to fracture itself. A lateral view of the knee can show a fat-fluid (marrow-blood) level in the suprapatellar bursa, which may be the only sign of intra-articular fracture.

- Depressed plateau fracture—lateral or medial
- Split fracture—proximal fibula and lateral tibial condyle both affected
- Combined split depressed fracture—combination of depressed plateau and split fracture
- Medial condyle fracture—less common
- Comminuted fracture of lateral and medial tibial condyles
- Segond fracture—avulsion fracture superolateral aspect proximal tibia. Associated with ligamentous and meniscal injury
- Intercondylar eminence fracture (tibial spine)—associated with anterior cruciate ligament injury

Patella

Transverse, vertical, comminuted, or avulsion fractures can occur. Oblique or skyline views may be required to identify some vertical fractures. Patella dislocation is usually lateral. Rupture of patellar ligament leads to superior displacement of the patella.

Neck of fibula fractures

Think about accompanying ligamentous (collateral and cruciate) injury.

Proximal third of fibula fractures

Look for associated ankle fracture.

Degenerative changes

Knee joint changes are similar to those at the hip.

Knee dislocation

In knee dislocation, 75% of cases are posterior. There is potential for significant injury to the popliteal and peroneal blood vessels.

Hints

ⓘ Most meniscal or ligamentous injuries have no X-ray changes.
▶ Examine the hip when patients complain of a painful knee—it could be referred pain.

Pediatrics

- *Bipartite patella:* normal variant. Secondary ossification center, usually in superiolateral region. May stay unfused throughout adulthood. Do not confuse this with fracture.
- *Osgood–Schlatter disease:* recurrent minor trauma leads to swelling and pain at quadriceps tendon insertion. Avulsion of tibial tubercle may be seen on X-ray. Boys are affected more than girls.
- *Osteochondritis dissecans:* chronic trauma causes articular cartilage and subchondral bone disruption. Most commonly seen at lateral side of medial femoral epicondyle. Remember the mnemonic *LAME:* Lateral Aspect Medial Epicondyle.

Radiology: shoulder

AP and either axial (armpit view), lateral scapular (Y view), or apical oblique views are usually provided.

Abnormal

Glenohumeral dislocation
- *Anterior dislocations:* (95%) humeral head lies anterior and inferior to glenoid
- *Posterior dislocation:* often missed. Look for a rounded symmetrical humeral head (due to internal rotation).
- *Inferior dislocation (luxatio erecta):* rare (neurovascular damage more likely)

Fractures
- *Clavicle fracture:* readily identified on AP film. 80% lateral 1/3
- *Fracture-dislocations:* humeral greater tuberosity often involved
- *Humeral head or neck fracture:* oblique or impacted fractures seen on X-ray (Fig. 19.62)
- *Humeral shaft fracture:* transverse, spiral, or comminuted
- *Scapula fracture:* uncommon. May require trans-scapular view.
- *Supraspinatus rupture:* may see bony avulsion on X-ray

Acromioclavicular (AC) injury
On the AP view, the inferior cortex of the clavicle and that of the acromion process should be aligned. Normal AC distance should be ≤8 mm. Look for widening of the AC joint and any associated fractures.

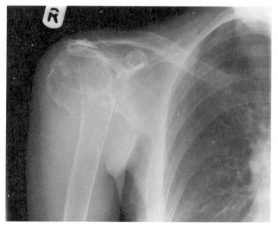

Fig. 19.62 Radiograph showing fractured neck of humerus on the right.

AC injury is graded according to degree of separation:
- *Grade I:* ligamentous involvement only. Slight separation
- *Grade II:* subluxation but with some bony overlap
- *Grade III:* AC joint fully dislocated. Coracoclavicular ligament ruptured

Adhesive capsulitis (frozen shoulder)
On X-ray, joint space narrowing and osteoporotic changes due to disuse are apparent.

Sternoclavicular dislocation
Anterior dislocations are more common (Fig. 19.63). There is risk of injury to large vessels and the trachea with posterior dislocation.

Calcific tendonitis
This is exquisitely painful; rapid relief is with local steroidal injections. Look for abnormal calcium in soft tissues around the joint on X-ray.

Hints
▶ AP views of posterior dislocation may appear normal. The axillary view may be helpful.
- Fracture of the glenoid can be a complication of anterior dislocation.
🔵 Look for any fracture fragments with anterior dislocation.
   Stress views (giving the patient weight to hold on the affected side) can make AC injury more obvious on X-ray.

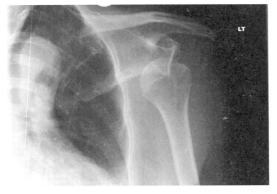

Fig. 19.63 Radiograph showing anterior dislocation of the humerus on the left.

Radiology: cervical spine

Examining C-spine films

Three views are advisable—lateral, AP, and open mouth (the latter to get a clear view of the odontoid peg). Remember, the peg is the upward extension of the body of C2—the axis.

Lateral view

- Can you see all seven cervical vertebrae, including the top of T1?
- Trace three superimposed parallel curved lines running down the neck to look for steps or misalignments (see Fig. 19.64).
- Check the gap between the anterior aspect of the peg and anterior arch of C1—it should be ≤3 mm in adults, ≤5 mm in children.
- Look for prevertebral soft-tissue swelling. This may be only sign of a C-spine fracture (lack of soft tissue swelling does not exclude fracture).
- Inspect for narrowing of disc spaces.

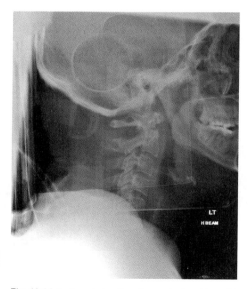

Fig. 19.64 Radiograph showing a fractured odontoid peg. Note that the first cervical vertebra is displaced posteriorly. Several additional lines appear on the film, caused by the head and neck brace that the patient is wearing.

AP view
- Ensure that the spinous processes are aligned (some may be bifid).
- Measure the gaps between spinous processes. These should be approximately equal (but are allowed to be up to 50% wider than the gaps directly above or below).

Open-mouth (odontoid peg) view
- Check that the peg is intact.
- Are the lateral aspects of C1 and C2 aligned?
- Look for equal gaps on both sides of the peg.

C-spine injuries

Stable
- *Unilateral facet dislocation:* spinous processes misaligned on AP
- Posterior arch of C1 fracture
- *Wedge fracture:* ↓ height of anterior vertebral body. Delayed instability is possible.
- *Extension teardrop fracture:* avulsion fracture, anteroinferior aspect C2
- *Burst fracture:* compression fracture between C3 and C7
- *Anterior subluxation:* fanning (widening) seen between adjacent spinous processes on lateral view. Delayed instability is possible.
- *Clay-shoveler's fracture:* oblique avulsion fracture of lower spinous process

Unstable
- Bilateral facet dislocation
- Odontoid fracture (Fig. 19.64)
- *Hangman's fracture:* fracture of C2 pedicles
- *Jefferson's fracture:* fracture to anterior and posterior arches of C1
- *Flexion teardrop fracture:* fracture-dislocation of the vertebral body
- *Hyperextension fracture-dislocation:* anterior displacement of vertebra is common
- Atlanto-occipital disassociation (remember, *atlanto* refers to C1)

Pediatrics
- *Normal variant:* Particularly in children, the base of C2 spinous process may lie 2 mm posterior to the curved line linking the other bases.
- *Pseudosubluxation:* Normal ligamentous laxity causes anterior displacement of C2 or C3.

Hints
🛈 If you see one fracture, look for another—20% of cases are multiple.
🛈 Most C-spine fractures occur near the top (C1–C2) and bottom (C5–C7) of the neck.

Radiology: thoracic and lumbar spine

Examining spinal films

Lateral and AP views are provided as standard.

- Examine the height of each vertebra—they should be approximately equal and the same front and back.
- Look for the normal concave shape of the back of each vertebral body. The gaps between vertebrae (the disc spaces) should be equal.
- Trace the lines of the anterior and posterior vertebral bodies. Look for any steps, ridges, or misalignments.
- On the AP view, the lumbar pedicles should become slightly further apart going down the spine.

Abnormalities

Thoracic (T) and lumbar (L) spine fractures

- Wedge (compression) fracture (Fig. 19.65)
  - ↓ Height of vertebral body with wedge shape
  - Loss of concave shape to posterior vertebral body

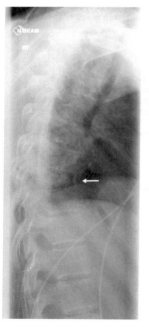

Fig. 19.65 Radiograph showing a wedge fracture of a thoracic vertebra.

- Burst fracture: vertebral body crushed into >2 pieces (comminuted)
- Fracture-dislocations: high suspicion of spinal cord injury
- Chance fracture: horizontal splitting of vertebra
- Transverse process fracture
- Spinous process fracture

Spondylolysis
- Degeneration of intervertebral discs leads to narrowing of disc space and osteophyte formation.

Spondylolisthesis
- Anterior subluxation of vertebral body (congenital or after injury)

Hint
- 90% fractures are at T11–L4.

Lung function tests

Simple lung function tests can help with the diagnosis and monitoring of common respiratory diseases, such as asthma and chronic obstructive pulmonary disease (COPD). Recognizing patterns of abnormality of these tests is an essential skill in data interpretation.

Peak expiratory flow rate

Peak expiratory flow rate (PEFR) is the maximum flow rate recorded during a forced expiration. Predicted readings vary according to age, sex, height, and ethnicity (see Fig. 19.66).

Interpreting PEFR

PEFR readings less than the patient's predicted, or usual best reading, demonstrate airflow obstruction in the large airways.

PEFR readings are useful in determining the severity and thus most appropriate treatment algorithm for asthma exacerbations:
- PEFR 80–100% best or predicted—mild asthma attack
- PEFR 50–80% best or predicted—moderate asthma attack
- PEFR <50% best or predicted—severe asthma attack
- PEFR <33% best or predicted—life-threatening asthma attack
- ❶ PEFR readings are subject to considerable personal variation.
- ❶ Note the diurnal variations in PEFR with asthma.
- ▶ Don't confuse PEFR with forced expiratory volume in 1 second (FEV_1).

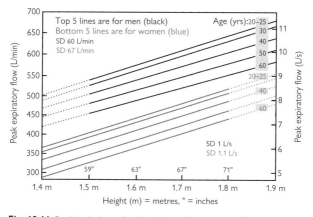

Fig. 19.66 Predicted values of peak expiratory flow rate according to age, sex, and height. Reproduced with permission from Longmore M, et al. (2004). *Oxford Handbook of Clinical Medicine*, 6th ed. Oxford: Oxford University Press.

Reversibility testing

Improvement in PEFR or FEV₁% 15% following bronchodilator therapy (e.g., salbutamol) shows reversibility of airflow obstruction and can help to distinguish asthma from poorly reversible conditions, such as COPD.

Spirometry

Spirometry is the measurement of airflow and functional lung volumes. Fig. 19.67 shows the pattern of lung volumes in a healthy individual during normal breathing, and maximum inspiration and expiration with a single breath.

Patients are asked to blow, as fast as possible, into a mouthpiece attached to a spirometer. This records the rate and volume of airflow. Unlike measuring PEFR, patients must continue blowing out for as long as possible. The test is repeated until two similar readings are achieved.

Two key values are

- *FEV₁:* forced expiratory volume in the first second.
- *FVC:* forced vital capacity—the total lung volume from maximum inspiration to maximum expiration, in forced exhalation.

Modern machines will often calculate the patient's predicted values for FEV₁ and FVC, which, like PEFR, are dependent on age, sex, height, and ethnicity. Usually 70–85% of the FVC is expired in the first second, giving the volume–time graph shown in Fig. 19.68.

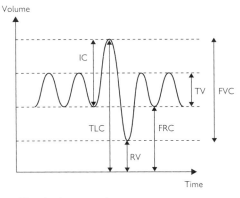

IC   = Inspiratory capacity
TLC = Total lung capacity
RV   = Residual volume
FRC = Functional residual capacity
TV   = Tidal volume
FVC = Forced vital capacity

Fig. 19.67 Normal pattern of lung volumes.

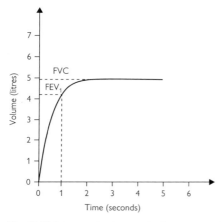

Fig. 19.68 Spirogram showing normal volume–time graph.

Flow volume loops can also be generated from spirometry data and show the flow at different lung volumes. These are useful in distinguishing intra- and extrathoracic causes of obstruction as well as in assessing for small airways obstruction.

▶ Spirometry is valuable in assessing anesthetic risk prior to elective surgery and vital for the diagnosis of COPD.

❶ Don't confuse PEFR with FEV_1. While these may correlate well in asthma, a normal PEFR does not exclude a reduced FEV_1 in COPD.

Gas transfer

Measuring the capacity of a gas to diffuse across the alveolar–capillary membrane can provide important information. DLCO (carbon monoxide diffusion capacity) measures the uptake from a single breath of 0.3% CO. It is reduced in interstitial lung disease and emphysema.

Other tests

Pulmonology practices calculate static lung volumes with a body plethys-mograph or through helium rebreath and dilutional techniques:

• TLC—total lung capacity
• RV— residual volume

Both of these can help in identifying patterns of lung disease and assessing patients prior to lung surgery.

Common patterns of abnormality

Abnormal patterns of lung function fall broadly into two types, obstructive and restrictive (see Table 19.1).

Table 19.1 Obstructive v. restrictive spirometry results

Pattern	FEV1	FVC	FEV₁/FVC ratio	TLC	RV
Obstructive	↓	↔/↓	<75%	↑ (or ↔)	↑
Restrictive	↓	↓	>75%	↓	↓

See Fig. 19.69 for spirograms showing obstructive and restrictive volume–time graphs.

Obstructive
When airflow is obstructed, although FVC may be reduced, FEV_1 is much more reduced, hence the FEV_1/FVC ratio falls. It can also take much longer to fully exhale.
▶ FVC can be normal in mild to moderate obstructive conditions.
  Conditions causing an obstructive defect include the following:
• COPD
• Asthma
• Bronchiectasis
• Cystic fibrosis
• Foreign bodies, tumors, and stenosis following tracheotomy (all localized airflow obstruction)

Restrictive
The airway patency is not affected in restrictive lung conditions, so the PEFR can be normal. But the FEV_1 and FVC are reduced because of the restrictive picture.
  Conditions causing a restrictive defect include the following:
• Fibrosing alveolitis of any cause
• Skeletal abnormalities (e.g., kyphoscoliosis)
• Neuromuscular diseases (e.g., motor neuron disease)
• Connective tissue diseases
• Late-stage sarcoidosis
• Pleural effusion
• Pleural thickening
▶ Mixed obstructive and restrictive defects can also be found.

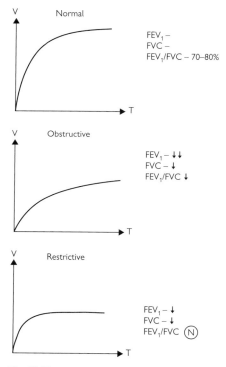

Fig. 19.69 Spirograms showing obstructive and restrictive volume–time graphs.

Arterial blood gas analysis

While clinical examination skills will enable you to detect many important conditions, at times we all need help from the analysis of blood and other fluids. Even the most experienced provider can't determine the $PaCO_2$ just by the laying on of hands (although they might tell you otherwise).

A systematic approach

The printout from the ABG machine can have a bewildering number of results. Initially, just focus on the pH, $PaCO_2$, and HCO_3^-, in that order (see Box 19.11).

pH
Is it low (acidosis) or high (alkalosis)?

$PaCO_2$
Remember, CO_2 is acidic.

- If $PaCO_2$ is raised and there is acidosis (pH <7.35), you can deduce a *respiratory acidosis*.
- If $PaCO_2$ is low and there is alkalosis (pH >7.45), then the lack of acid gas has led to a *respiratory alkalosis*.
- Conversely, if $PaCO_2$ is low and there is acidosis, the respiratory system is not to blame and there must instead be a *metabolic acidosis*.
  - Confirm this by looking at the ***HCO_3^-***; it should be low—remember it is alkaline and acts as a buffer.
- If $PaCO_2$ is high or normal and there is alkalosis, then again the respiratory system will not be to blame and there must instead be a *metabolic alkalosis*.
  - Confirm this by looking at the ***HCO_3^-***; it should be raised.

PaO_2
❶ Note what FiO_2 (fraction of inspired oxygen) the patient was breathing when the sample was taken.

Hypoxia is PaO_2 of <60 mmHg (8.0 kPa) and can result from ventilation–perfusion (V/Q) mismatch—e.g., pulmonary embolism—or from alveolar hypoventilation—e.g., COPD, pneumonia.

- *Type I respiratory failure:* hypoxia and $PaCO_2$ ≤45 mmHg
- *Type II respiratory failure:* hypoxia and $PaCO_2$ ≥50 mmHg
- ▶ If the PaO_2 is very low, consider venous blood contamination.

Box 19.11 Reference ranges

- *pH:* 7.35–7.45
- *$PaCO_2$:* 35–45 mm Hg
- *PaO_2:* 80–100 mm Hg
- *HCO_3^-:* 21–28 mEq/L
- *Base excess:* ±2 mEq/L

Compensatory mechanisms

Mechanisms controlling pH are activated when acid–base imbalances threaten. Thus, renal control of H^+ and HCO_3^- ion excretion can result in compensatory metabolic changes. Similarly, blowing off or retaining CO_2 via control of respiratory rate can lead to compensatory respiratory changes. This can complicate interpretation of ABG results.

▶ A normal pH does not exclude acid–base disturbance (Table 19.2)—there may be adequate compensation or a mixed picture.

▶ A compensated picture suggests chronic disease.

Base excess and (standard) HCO_3^- effectively measure the same thing. Small variations of above-normal values exist between facilities.

Table 19.2 Some acid–base disturbances

Disturbance	pH	PaCO$_2$	HCO$_3^-$
Respiratory acidosis	↓	↑	↔ (↑ if compensated)
Metabolic acidosis	↓	↔ (↓ if compensated)	↓
Respiratory alkalosis	↑	↓	↔ (↓ if compensated)
Metabolic alkalosis	↑	↔ (↑ if compensated)	↑

Acidosis

A relative excess of cations (e.g., H^+), unless adequately compensated, will result in acidosis (more correctly, acidemia).

Respiratory acidosis

In this condition, pH is ↓, PaCO$_2$ ↑ is (HCO_3^- may ↑ be if compensated) (Box 19.12). Conditions that can lead to respiratory acidosis are as follows:

• COPD, asthma, pneumonia, pneumothorax, pulmonary fibrosis
• Obstructive sleep apnea
• Opiate overdose (causing respiratory depression)
• Neuromuscular disorders (e.g., Guillain–Barré, motor neuron disease)
• Skeletal abnormalities (e.g., kyphoscoliosis)
• Congestive cardiac failure
⬤ In COPD, find patient's normal PaCO$_2$—it may be abnormally high.

Box 19.12 Example of respiratory acidosis (on room air)

pH 7.29, PaCO$_2$ 56, PaO$_2$ 70, HCO$_3^-$ 25
The *cause* in this case is acute exacerbation of COPD.

Metabolic acidosis

This involves pH, ↓ HCO$_3^-$ ↓ (PaCO$_2$ may be ↓ if compensated) (see Box 19.13).

Anion gap (Na$^+$ + K$^+$) − (HCO$_3^-$ + Cl$^-$): Normal range is 8–16 mEq/L (Note: Reference values vary and an alternative formula is available.)

It is useful to calculate the anion gap to help distinguish causes of metabolic acidosis. An ↑ anion gap points to ↑ production of unmeasurable anions. Conditions that can lead to metabolic acidosis involve either an increased or normal anion.

↑ Anion gap
- Diabetic ketoacidosis
- Renal failure (urate)
- Lactic acidosis (tissue hypoxia or excessive exercise)
- Salicylates, ethylene glycol, biguanides

Normal anion gap
- Chronic diarrhea, ileostomy (loss of HCO$_3^-$)
- Addison's disease
- Pancreatic fistula
- Renal tubular acidosis
- Acetazolamide treatment (loss of HCO$_3^-$)

Box 19.13 Example of metabolic acidosis (on room air)

pH 7.25, PaCO$_2$ 40, PaO$_2$ 96, HCO$_3^-$ 12
The *cause* in this case is diabetic ketoacidosis

Alkalosis

A relative excess of anions (e.g., HCO$_3^-$), unless adequately compensated, will result in alkalosis (more correctly, alkalemia)

Respiratory alkalosis

This involves ↑ pH, ↓ PaCO$_2$ (HCO$_3^-$ may be ↓ if compensated) (Box 19.14). Conditions that can lead to respiratory alkalosis are as follows:
- Hyperventilation, secondary to
  - Panic attack (anxiety)
  - Pain
- Meningitis
- Stroke, subarachnoid hemorrhage
- High altitude

Box 19.14 Example of respiratory alkalosis (on room air)

pH 7.53, PaCO$_2$ 28, PaO$_2$ 85, HCO$_3^-$ 22
The *cause* in this example is anxiety.

▶ Sensory changes (tingling in hands, face, lips) with hyperventilation are due to ↓ ionized calcium.

Metabolic alkalosis

This involves ↑ pH, ↑ HCO_3^- ($PaCO_2$ may be ↑ if compensated) (Box 19.15). Conditions that can lead to metabolic alkalosis are as follows:

- Diuretic drugs (via loss of K^+)
- Prolonged vomiting (via acid replacement and release of HCO_3^-)
- Burns
- Base ingestion

Mixed metabolic and respiratory disturbance

In clinical practice, patients can develop a mixed picture in which acid–base imbalance is the result of both respiratory and metabolic factors (Box 19.16). For example, in critically ill patients, hypoventilation leads to ↓ PaO_2, and O_2-depleted cells then produce lactic acid.

Box 19.15 Example of metabolic alkalosis (on room air)

pH 7.50, $PaCO_2$ 36, PaO_2 92, HCO_3^- 27
The *cause* in this example is vomiting

Box 19.16 Example of mixed respiratory and metabolic acidosis (on room air)

pH 7.0, $PaCO_2$ 59, PaO_2 86, HCO_3^- 14
The *cause* in this example is septic shock.

Cerebrospinal fluid (CSF)

CSF is produced by the choroid plexus lining the cerebral ventricles and helps cushion and support the brain. Samples are usually obtained by means of lumbar puncture.

Normal adult CSF

Normal values will vary by laboratory.
- Opening pressure   50–200 mm H_2O
- Red cells   0
- WBC   0–5
- Lymphocytes   40–80%
- Neutrophils   0–6%
- Protein   15–45 mg/dL
- Glucose   60–80% of blood glucose)
- IgG   0–4.5 mg/dL

▶ CSF glucose is abnormal if it is < 50% of blood glucose level
ℹ Premature babies, newborns, children, and adolescents have different normal ranges

Interpreting CSF

Table 19.3 is only a general guide. Be guided by CSF results (see Box 19.17) together with the clinical picture.

Table 19.3 Characteristics of CSF according to underlying pathology

Pathology	Appearance	Protein	Glucose CSF–blood ratio)	Cells
Bacterial meningitis	Turbid	↑	↓	Neutrophils
Viral meningitis	Clear	↔/↑	↑/↔	Lymphocytes
Viral encephalitis	Clear	↔/↑	↓	Lymphocytes
TB meningitis	Fibrin webs	↑	↓↓	Lymphocytes Neutrophils
Fungal meningitis	Clear/turbid	↑	↓	Lymphocytes
Subarachnoid hemorrhage	Xanthochromia	↔/↑	↑	Red cells
Multiple sclerosis	Clear	↔/↑	↔/↑	Lymphocytes
Guillain–Barré syndrome	Clear	↑	↔/↑	
Cord compression	Clear	↑	↔	
Malignancy	Clear	↑	↓	Malignant

Box 19.17 Further CSF tests

- Culture
- Gram stain
- Ziehl–Neelsen stain (TB)
- India ink (cryptococcus)
- Electrophoresis (oligoclonal bands in multiple sclerosis)
- Cytology (malignant cells)
- Serological tests (syphilis)
- Viral polymerase chain reaction (PCR)

Urinalysis

Dipstick urinalysis offers speedy and noninvasive testing that can help with the diagnosis of common conditions such as urinary tract infections (UTIs) and diabetes mellitus (DM). Samples can be sent to the laboratory for further analysis, including microscopic analysis and culture/sensitivity.

Box 19.18 Methods of collecting urine for analysis

- Random sample (contamination likely)
- Mid-stream sample (less contamination)
- First-void urine (for intracellular organisms—e.g., *Chlamydia*)
- Early-morning sample (to look for acid-alcohol fast bacilli—TB)
- Suprapubic aspiration
- Via catheter bag
- Via urine bag (pediatrics)
- 24-hour collection

Dipstick

Dipstick testing gives semiquantitative analysis of the following:
- Protein (normally negative)
- Glucose (normally negative)
- Ketones (normally negative)
- Nitrites (normally negative)
- Blood (normally negative)
- Leucocytes (normally negative)
- Bilirubin (normally negative)
- pH (normally acidic with range 4.5–8.0)
- Specific gravity (normal range 1.000–1.030)
▶ Test the urine within 15 minutes of obtaining the sample.
❶ Color vision must be intact to interpret the dipstick chart.
▶ Urine pregnancy-testing is equally convenient and is indicated in females of childbearing age who present with abdominal symptoms.
▶ Various foods (e.g., beets, asparagus, blackberries) and drugs (e.g., rifampicin, tetracyclines, levodopa, phenytoin, chloroquine, vitamins, iron supplements) can change the color of urine.

Microscopy, culture, and sensitivity (M,C&S)

Microscopy enables identification of bacteria and other microorganisms, urinary casts (formed in the tubules or collecting ducts from proteins or cells), crystals, and cells (including renal tubular and transitional epithelial cells, leukocytes, and red blood cells). Organism growth and antibiotic sensitivities and can also be determined.
▶ Microscopy and culture/sensitivity may not be indicated for patients with uncomplicated UTI diagnosed on clinical history and dipstick and started on antibiotics.
▶ Asymptomatic bacteriuria is more common in pregnancy (up to 7%) and can lead to pyelonephritis and potential fetal complications.

Characteristic urinalysis findings

- *UTIs:* nitrites, leukocytes
- *Diabetes mellitus:* glucose
- *Diabetic ketoacidosis:* ketones
- *Cholestasis (obstructive jaundice):* bilirubin
- *Prehepatic jaundice:* urobilinogen
- *Glomerulonephritis:* protein, blood
- *Renal stones:* blood
- *Renal carcinoma:* blood
- *Nephrotic syndrome:* protein ++
- *Renal TB:* leukocytes, no organisms grown (sterile pyuria)
- *Sexually transmitted infections* (chlamydia, gonorrhea): sterile pyuria

▶ Suspected UTIs in children must be investigated with the consideration that they may be indicators of anatomical abnormalities or possible sexual abuse.

Pleural and ascitic fluid

Pleural effusion

Fluid in the pleural space can be classified as *exudate* (protein content >30 g/L) or *transudate* (protein content <30 g/L). At borderline levels, if the pleural protein is >50% serum protein, then the effusion is an exudate. Blood, pus, and chyle (lymph with fat) can also form an effusion. See 📖 p. 561 for pleural tap guidance.

Box 19.19 Tests for pleural fluids

- Microscopy, culture (conventional ± TB culture), and sensitivity (Gram stain, Ziehl–Neelsen stain)
- Cytology (malignant cells)
- Biochemistry
  - Protein
  - Glucose (↓ if rheumatoid or pneumonia related)
  - Amylase (↑ in pancreatitis)
  - LDH (↑ in empyema, malignancy, rheumatoid)

▶ A large effusion needs a chest drain.
▶ If you suspect malignant pleural disease, consider pleural biopsy.
ⓘ Unilateral effusion suggests localized disease (malignancy, pneumonia).
ⓘ Pleural fluid may be purulent (e.g., empyema) and therefore difficult to aspirate.

Transudate causes

These involve ↑ venous or ↓ oncotic pressure.

- Heart failure
- Hypoproteinemia (liver failure, malabsorption, nephrotic syndrome)
- Hypothyroidism
- Constrictive pericarditis
- Meig's syndrome (ovarian fibroma + pleural effusion)

Exudate causes

These involve ↑ capillary permeability.

- Pneumonia
- Empyema
- Malignancy (lung, pleura, lymph)
- Pulmonary infarction
- TB
- Systemic lupus erythematosus (SLE)
- Rheumatoid arthritis
- Dressler's syndrome (post-MI)

Ascites

Fluid in the peritoneal cavity can result in abdominal distension and short-ness of breath. As with pleural fluid, analysis of an aspirated sample can aid diagnosis. See 📖 p. 569 for ascitic tap guidance.

> **Box 19.20 Tests for ascites**
>
> • MCS (bacterial peritonitis, TB)
> • Cytology (malignant cells, macrophages in inflammatory diseases)
> • Biochemistry (amylase, protein)

▶ Spontaneous bacterial peritonitis = neutrophils >250/mm³
▶ Further tests you may consider for a patient with ascites include liver function tests (LFTs), hepatitis serology, antimitochondrial antibodies (pri-mary biliary cirrhosis), ultrasound of liver or pelvis, and esophagogastrodu-odenoscopy (EGD) (varices).
❶ It is useful to check platelets and clotting profile before inserting drain.
❶ Chylous ascites can result from obstruction of lymph drainage.

Causes
• Decompensated liver disease
• Infection (bacterial peritonitis, TB)
• Malignancy (liver, ovary)
• Right-sided heart failure
• Pancreatitis
• Portal vein occlusion
• Nephrotic syndrome

Serum/ascites albumin gradient (SAAG)
• Used to classify ascites as exudate or transudate
• SAAG = serum albumin concentration/ascitic fluid albumin concentration

SAAG >1.1 g/dL (transudate)
• Cirrhosis with portal hypertension
• Cardiac failure
• Nephrotic syndrome

SAAG <1.1 g/dL (exudate)
• Malignancy
• Pancreatitis
• TB

Index